Stroke Medicine

Sumanjit K. Gill • Martin Brown
Fergus Robertson • Nicholas Losseff
Editors

Stroke Medicine

Case Studies from Queen Square

Second Edition

Springer

Editors
Sumanjit K. Gill
Institute of Neurology, UCL
National Hospital for Neurology and Neurosurgery
London, UK

Martin Brown
UCL Stroke Research Centre, UCL Queen Square Institute of Neurology
University College London
London, UK

Fergus Robertson
National Hospital for Neurology and Neurosurgery
London, UK

Nicholas Losseff
National Hospital for Neurology and Neurosurgery
London, UK

ISBN 978-3-031-58187-8 ISBN 978-3-031-58188-5 (eBook)
https://doi.org/10.1007/978-3-031-58188-5

This Springer imprint is published by the registered company Springer Nature Switzerland AG
The registered company address is: Gewerbestrasse 11, 6330 Cham, Switzerland

• *for our patients*

Editorial team

Preface

The details of the case are important: their analysis distinguishes the expert from the journeyman. CM Fisher [1]

This update of the first edition includes both new and revised chapters to reflect the immense changes within stroke medicine which have happened over the last ten years. This edition includes cases where clinicians have used advanced imaging techniques to both aid diagnosis and select patients for acute intervention. The advantages of mechanical thrombectomy, the difficulties of patient selection, and the complications of this intervention are also discussed. We have designed the publication with the aim of assisting the reader in developing a thorough understanding of neurovascular anatomy, stroke localization, and therapeutic interventions.

As in the first edition, the histories describe real clinical cases and the clinical reasoning behind the diagnosis and treatment is presented with the actual patient outcomes—which are not always perfect. The discussion that follows each case describes the evidence basis of the management and provides a critical reflection on the case management. These cases demonstrate that collaborative working with other specialists increases the odds of good decision-making and that this is a vital skill to foster, in addition to being one of the most enjoyable aspects of clinical practice.

The structure of each chapter means that the reader is "talked through" the case presentation and investigations. This is then followed by a thorough analysis with key learning points to highlight underlying principles. Imaging is included to illustrate the cases with radiological learning points. This book is a suitable companion for anyone interested in developing their knowledge and understanding of neurovascular medicine, including medical students through to experienced physicians.

Reference

1. Caplan L. Fishers rules. Arch Neurol. 1982;39:389–90.

London, UK Sumanjit K. Gill
London, UK Martin Brown
London, UK Fergus Robertson
London, UK Nicholas Losseff

Contents

Chapter 1
Transient Functional Neurological Episodes Associated with Cerebral Amyloid Angiopathy

Benjamin Sacks and David J. Werring

Case Presentation

Clinical History

A 76-year-old right-handed man presented to the Emergency Stroke Unit with a three-day history of stereotyped, self-resolving episodes of left sided weakness and paraesthesia. The patient reported a spreading sensation of tingling, affecting the left side of his face and then progressing down his left arm and into his hand. This was followed 5 min later by numbness in the left arm and face. The whole episode lasted for 20 min before self-resolving. A second, identical episode recurred 48 h later. A third episode of hemisensory disturbance was reported 24 h after the second, this time associated with incoordination of his left hand and a spreading weakness up his left arm which persisted for 15 min. The patient reported no abnormal movements, loss of consciousness, visual loss or speech disturbance. His past medical history included hypothyroidism, hypertension, chronic kidney disease stage 3 (CKD3) and cerebral amyloid angiopathy (CAA). He was an ex-smoker and did not drink alcohol to excess.

B. Sacks (✉) · D. J. Werring
Department of Stroke Medicine, National Hospital for Neurology & Neurosurgery, London, UK
e-mail: benjamin.sacks@ucl.ac.uk; d.werring@ucl.ac.uk

S. K. Gill et al. (eds.), *Stroke Medicine*,
https://doi.org/10.1007/978-3-031-58188-5_1

Examination

He was alert and conversant throughout. Visual fields, limb power, speech, attention and coordination were all normal. There was no evidence of limb jerking, tongue biting or urinary incontinence. Sensation was intact across all modalities. Respiratory, cardiovascular and gastrointestinal systems examinations were unremarkable.

Investigations

At the time of admission, blood tests including a full blood count, clotting screen, lipid profile, glucose level, C-reactive protein, liver and thyroid function tests were all within normal range. His creatinine was 100 μmol/L and his eGFR was 65. The patient was in sinus rhythm with a heart rate of 70 beats per minute. His blood pressure was 138/67 mmHg. A plain computed tomography (CT) scan showed a subtle hyperdensity in the right central sulcus. CT angiography identified mild mixed atheroma with no intracranial or extracranial steno-occlusive disease. Magnetic resonance imaging (MRI) identified a tiny focus of low apparent diffusion coefficient (ADC) projected over the left internal capsule, consistent with an incidental subacute infarction. Susceptibility weighted imaging showed multiple peripheral microbleeds and superficial siderosis, in keeping with a diagnosis of CAA. Of note, the right central sulcus contained a new area of superficial haemosiderosis with an associated microbleed just lateral to this, adjacent to the hand motor area. There was a right marginal sulcus hyperdensity, in keeping with an acute convexity subarachnoid haemorrhage. The patient was discharged with a diagnosis of transient functional neurological episode (TFNE) secondary to CAA.

Discussion

Epidemiology & Pathophysiology

CAA is increasingly recognized as an important cause of intracerebral haemorrhage (ICH), accounting for between 20–30% of all ICH presentations in the elderly [1]. Moderate—severe CAA pathology is present in 8% of people over the age of 75, rising to 12% in those over 85 [2]. The condition is characterized by amyloid-beta peptides (principally Aβ40) accumulating in the basement membranes of small to medium sized cerebral and leptomeningeal arteries [3]. Aβ deposition results in thickening of the tunica adventitia, followed by the tunica media. This results in loss of vascular reactivity and dysregulation of cerebral blood flow. Eventually, the toxic effects of Aβ cause vascular smooth muscle loss and vessel wall thinning. The resultant thin, friable vessels rupture easily. ICH is the most widely recognized complication; however, CAA is better understood as a multifaceted condition which can also present with cognitive impairment or, as in the present case, transient focal neurological symptoms.

Although the precise mechanisms of Aβ accumulation are not understood, it is thought that reduced clearance of Aβ may result from a failure of perivascular drainage pathways, resulting in toxic accumulation and local astrocyte driven cytokine release. This results in a local inflammatory process, causing apoptosis, vascular dysfunction and compromised integrity of the blood brain barrier [4]. There are several known autosomal dominant missense mutations in the amyloid precursor protein (*APP*) gene that can result in early onset Alzheimers and CAA with varying phenotypes. The mutations most uniquely associated with vascular pathology are E693Q (Dutch), E693K (Italian) and L705V (Piedmont) [5].

Phenotypes

CAA can be divided up into three presenting phenotypes, often with significant overlap.

Transient Functional Neurological Episodes

TFNE, sometimes termed "amyloid spells," are self-resolving stereotyped, neurological symptoms that occur in patients with CAA. They typically present with positive symptoms such as spreading paraesthesia, rhythmic limb jerking and visual disturbances (photopsia and visual blurring). More recently, negative symptoms have been recognized as a feature of TFNE and include aphasia, monocular visual loss, sensory loss and limb weakness [6]. These are especially relevant in stroke medicine as they present similarly to transient ischaemic attacks (TIAs). It is important for the clinician to be aware of TFNE as the differential diagnoses, namely TIA and seizure, have drastically different and potentially harmful treatments.

TFNEs are increasingly recognized in association with convexity sub-arachnoid haemorrhages (cSAH), a common finding in CAA. cSAH evolves over weeks to months and is visible as focal collections of cortical superficial siderosis (cSS) on blood sensitive MRI sequences (see Fig. 1.1) [7]. TFNE and cSAH have a positive correlation with the overall burden of leptomeningeal CAA and are both independently associated with an increased risk of ICH [8]. It is therefore crucial that patients presenting with classical TFNE are recognized as such. The core features distinguishing TFNE from TIA are migratory symptoms, sensory disturbance and the presence of recurrent stereotyped events. Of note, both migratory symptoms and sensory disturbances are independently associated with the presence of cSAH [9].

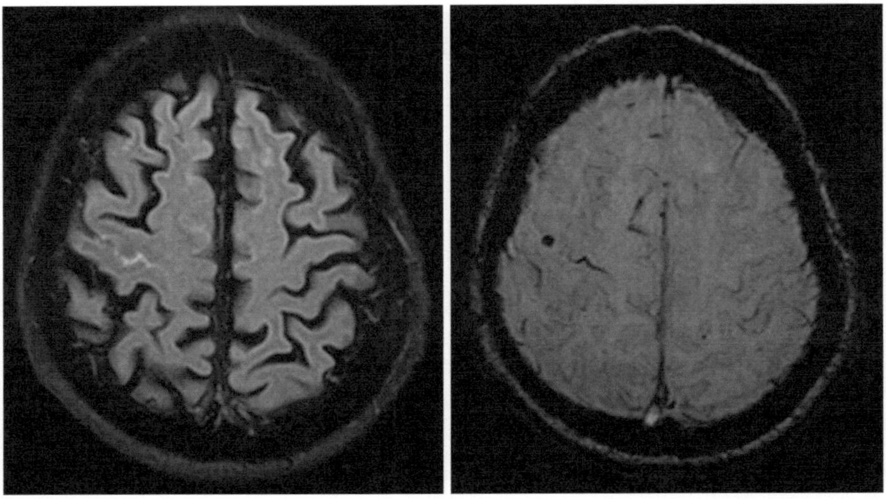

Fig. 1.1 Right marginal sulcus shows hyperintensity on FLAIR imaging (left) with new superficial siderosis and associated microbleed on susceptibility weighted imaging (right). Consistent with cSAH

Intracerebral Haemorrhage

The annual risk of ICH in CAA is between 5–10% [10]. CAA accounts for 75% of all spontaneous ICH in the normotensive elderly population [11]. ICH in CAA is usually peripherally located, with a characteristic 'lobar' distribution and a particular predilection for posterior regions. This is compared to ICH of hypertensive aetiology, which affects deeper structures in the brainstem and basal ganglia. The clinical presentation of ICH is classically headache, nausea, vomiting, focal neurological deficit, depressed consciousness and seizures. The imaging modality of choice is a plain CT scan of the head. An acute ICH will appear as a hyperdense locus of blood with surrounding hypodense perihaematomal cerebral oedema and mass effect. The ICH may have 'finger like projections', a classical feature of CAA related ICH. MRI may show peripherally located microbleeds, cortical superficial siderosis, enlarged perivascular spaces, white matter hyperintensities and evidence or historic 'silent' ICH (see Fig. 1.2).

Cognitive Impairment

The relationship between CAA and dementia is well established. There is a higher prevalence of CAA in elderly patients with dementia than those without. There is also a significant overlap of AD and CAA, and AD patients with CAA have worse cognitive performance than patients with AD alone [12]. CAA patients tend to exhibit poor executive dysfunction, slower processing speed and worse episodic memory as compared to non-CAA subjects. Language skills are also preferentially

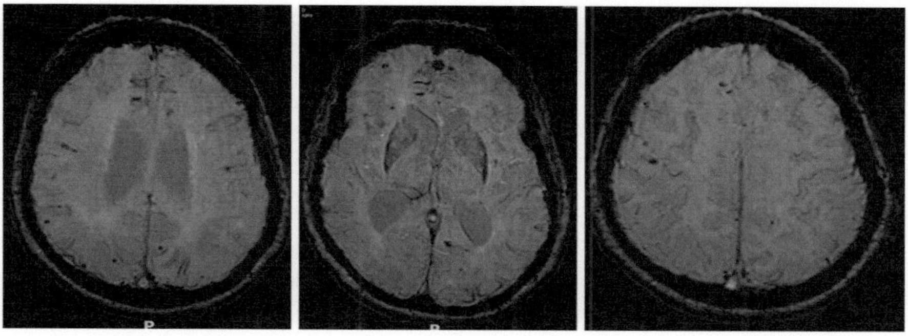

Fig. 1.2 Susceptibility weighted imaging shows multiple peripheral cortical microbleeds

impaired [13]. Cognitive impairment in CAA may manifest as a stepwise decline in function, associated with identifiable vascular events, however it can also progress sub-clinically, in the absence of any ICH or TFNE.

Management

The age demographic most susceptible to CAA is also the age demographic most likely to require antithrombotic or antiplatelet treatment for unrelated comorbidities. Around 30% of patients with TFNE and cSAH are taking antithrombotic medications [14]. One study of patients with lobar ICH showed that 20% left hospital with an anticoagulant medication prescribed [15]. The data on recurrent ICH risk with anticoagulant therapy is inconclusive and there have not been any adequate studies looking at CAA specifically. The current consensus is to hold antithrombotic medications in the acute setting and for up to 8 weeks following a presentation with TFNE [16]. In patients at high risk of thrombosis, direct oral anticoagulants are preferable to vitamin K antagonists as they carry a 50% lower risk of ICH [8]. Left atrial appendage occlusion devices can be considered in patients with atrial fibrillation, however they may still require post procedure antithrombosis.

TFNE heralds a 24.5% risk of ICH within 8 weeks of the event, and a 50% risk within 14 months. This is higher than the risk of recurrent ICH after a first-time ICH presentation in patients with CAA [8]. Most cases of TFNE present once the symptoms have abated. However, if a patient does present acutely, anti-convulsive medications such as leveteracetam and topiramate may be of symptomatic benefit [17]. Due to the potential of cSAH to extend into the parenchyma and manifest an ICH, clinicians are advised to control blood pressure (aim <140/80 mmHg) in patients presenting within 24 h of a TFNE [16]. Patients should be reassured that each TFNE does not necessarily represent new bleeding and usually self resolves.

Statins are generally avoided in CAA due to concerns that they may increase the risk of haemorrhagic events. There is particular concern that statin therapy increases the risk of lobar ICH [18]. In addition to managing blood pressure lifestyle factors such as reducing alcohol intake are also recommended.

Conclusion

CAA is associated with ICH, TFNE and cognitive impairment. TFNE is an increasingly recognized mimic of stroke syndromes. In any patient with episodes of self-resolving, stereotyped focal neurology, TFNE and an underlying diagnosis of CAA should be considered. In patients presenting to stroke departments with characteristic MRI findings of CAA, specialist opinion should be sought.

Key Clinical Learning Points

- Transient functional neurological episodes are common presentations of CAA and may mimic stroke syndromes or seizures.
- CAA is a risk factor for cognitive impairment independent of Alzheimer's dementia.
- Decisions regarding antithrombotic medications require careful consideration by specialist clinicians.
- Adequate blood pressure control is preventative in CAA patients at risk of intracerebral haemorrhage.

Key Radiological Learning Points

- CAA is associated with recurrent lobar haemorrhages which can appear as ICH with 'finger like projections' on CT scanning
- Susceptability weight imaging can show convexity subarachnoid haemorrhage, microbleeds and superficial siderosis
- Other MRI features can include enlarged perivascular spaces, white matter hyperintensities or previous bleeds
- Microbleeds associated with amyloid angiopathy tend to be more peripherally located

References

1. Biffi A, Greenberg SM. Cerebral amyloid angiopathy: a systematic review. J Clin Neurol. 2011;7(1):1–9. https://doi.org/10.3988/jcn.2011.7.1.1.
2. Neuropathology Group; Medical Research Council Cognitive Function and Aging Study. Pathological correlates of late-onset dementia in a multicentre, community-based population

in England and Wales. Neuropathology Group of the Medical Research Council Cognitive Function and Ageing Study (MRC CFAS). Lancet. 2001;357:169–75.
3. https://onlinelibrary.wiley.com/action/showCitFormats?doi=10.1111%2F1754-9485.12726
4. Gatti L, Tinelli F, Scelzo E, Arioli F, Di Fede G, Obici L, Pantoni L, Giaccone G, Caroppo P, Parati EA, Bersano A. Understanding the pathophysiology of cerebral amyloid angiopathy. Int J Mol Sci. 2020;21(10):3435. https://doi.org/10.3390/ijms21103435.
5. Bugiani O, Giaccone G, Rossi G, Mangieri M, Capobianco R, Morbin M, Mazzoleni G, Cupidi C, Marcon G, Giovagnoli A, et al. Hereditary cerebral hemorrhage with amyloidosis associated with the E693K mutation of APP. Arch Neurol. 2010;67:987–95. https://doi.org/10.1001/archneurol.2010.178.
6. Banerjee G, Carare R, Cordonnier C, Greenberg SM, Schneider JA, Smith EE, Buchem MV, Grond JV, Verbeek MM, Werring DJ. The increasing impact of cerebral amyloid angiopathy: essential new insights for clinical practice. J Neurol Neurosurg Psychiatry. 2017;88(11):982–94. https://doi.org/10.1136/jnnp-2016-314697.
7. Charidimou A, Linn J, Vernooij MW, et al. Cortical superficial siderosis: detection and clinical significance in cerebral amyloid angiopathy and related conditions. Brain. 2015;138(Pt 8):2126–39. https://doi.org/10.1093/brain/awv162.
8. Connolly SJ, Eikelboom J, Joyner C, et al. Apixaban in patients with atrial fibrillation. N Engl J Med. 2011;364:806–17. https://doi.org/10.1056/NEJMoa1007432.
9. Stanton JED, Chandratheva A, Wilson D, et al. Clinical features distinguish cerebral amyloid angiopathy-associated convexity subarachnoid haemorrhage from suspected TIA. J Neurol. 2020;267:133–7. https://doi.org/10.1007/s00415-019-09558-9.
10. Charidimou A, Imaizumi T, Moulin S, Biffi A, Samarasekera N, Yakushiji Y, Peeters A, Vandermeeren Y, Laloux P, Baron JC, Hernandez-Guillamon M, Montaner J, Casolla B, Gregoire SM, Kang DW, Kim JS, Naka H, Smith EE, Viswanathan A, Jäger HR, Al-Shahi Salman R, Greenberg SM, Cordonnier C, Werring DJ. Brain hemorrhage recurrence, small vessel disease type, and cerebral microbleeds: a meta-analysis. Neurology. 2017;89(8):820–9. https://doi.org/10.1212/WNL.0000000000004259. Epub 2017 Jul 26. PMID: 28747441; PMCID: PMC5580863
11. Knudsen KA, Rosand J, Karluk D, Greenberg SM. Clinical diagnosis of cerebral amyloid angiopathy: validation of the Boston criteria. Neurology. 2001;56:537–9.
12. Pfeifer LA, White LR, Ross GW, Petrovitch H, Launer LJ. Cerebralamyloid angiopathy and cognitive function: the HAAS autopsy study. Neurology. 2002;58:1629–34.
13. Boyle PA, Yu L, Nag S, et al. Cerebral amyloid angiopathy and cognitive outcomes in community-based older persons. Neurology. 2015;85:1930–6. https://doi.org/10.1212/WNL.0000000000002175.
14. Ni J, Auriel E, Jindal J, et al. The characteristics of superficial siderosis and convexity subarachnoid hemorrhage and clinical relevance in suspected cerebral amyloid angiopathy. Cerebrovasc Dis. 2015;39(5-6):278–86.
15. Iswanathan A, Rakich SM, Engel C, et al. Antiplatelet use after intracerebral hemorrhage. Neurology. 2006;66:206–9. https://doi.org/10.1212/01.wnl.0000194267.09060.77.
16. Smith EE, Charidimou A, Ayata C, Werring DJ, Greenberg SM. Cerebral amyloid angiopathy-related transient focal neurologic episodes. Neurology. 2021;97(5):231–8. https://doi.org/10.1212/WNL.0000000000012234.
17. Roch JA, Nighoghossian N, Hermier M, et al. Transient neurologic symptoms related to cerebral amyloid angiopathy: usefulness of T2*-weighted imaging. Cerebrovasc Dis. 2005;20(5):412–4.
18. Pezzini A, Grassi M, Iacoviello L, et al. Multicenter Study on Cerebral Haemorrhage in Italy (MUCH-Italy) Investigators. Serum cholesterol levels, HMG-CoA reductase inhibitors and the risk of intracerebral haemorrhage. The Multicenter Study on cerebral haemorrhage in Italy (MUCH-Italy). J Neurol Neurosurg Psychiatry. 2016;87:924–9. https://doi.org/10.1136/jnnp-2015-312736.

Chapter 2
Cerebral Amyloid Angiopathy Related Inflammation

P. Obrocki, Sumanjit K. Gill, Richard Perry, and D. J. Werring

Clinical History

A 75-year-old right-handed female presented to with a three-day history of worsening confusion. On further questioning, she reported a 6-month history of new and continuous bitemporal headaches as well as intermittent unsteadiness of gait. Her family also noted two self-limiting episodes of confusion in the last 3 months, both of which completely resolved within 48 h. On this occasion, the patient was found collapsed in the bathroom, with progressively worsening confusion over a course of 3 days.

Her past medical history was notable for hypertension and hypercholesterolaemia with no previous hospital admissions. Patient's regular prescription included amlodipine, however she was poorly compliant with treatment due to side effect of ankle oedema. There was a family history of stroke over 60 years old in both her parents as well as her brother. She denied regular alcohol use and never smoked.

P. Obrocki
Royal Free Hospital NHS Trust, London, London, UK
e-mail: p.obrocki@nhs.net

S. K. Gill (✉)
Institute of Neurology, UCL, National Hospital for Neurology and Neurosurgery, London, UK
e-mail: Sumanjit.Gill@uclh.nhs.uk

R. Perry
National Hospital for Neurology and Neurosurgery, London, UK

University College London, London, UK
e-mail: richard.perry2@nhs.net

D. J. Werring
UCL Queen Square Institute of Neurology, London, UK
e-mail: d.werring@ucl.ac.uk

S. K. Gill et al. (eds.), *Stroke Medicine*,
https://doi.org/10.1007/978-3-031-58188-5_2

Examination

Cranial nerve examination revealed a left homonymous hemianopia and marked left visual neglect (Fig. 2.1) with normal visual acuity and optic disc appearance on fundoscopy. There was a normal range of eye movements with frequent saccadic intrusions. There was no dysarthria, however there was marked poverty of speech. In the upper limbs, there was a left pronator drift with mild pyramidal pattern of weakness and hyperreflexia on the same side with left sensory neglect. There was no evidence of tremor, dysmetria or dysdiadochokinesia. The lower limb examination showed generally brisk reflexes with downgoing plantar responses. The pulse was regular with normal heart sounds. The rest of the systemic examination was normal, beside consistently elevated blood pressure readings of ~180/110 mmHg.

She was admitted to hospital for blood pressure lowering and further investigations.

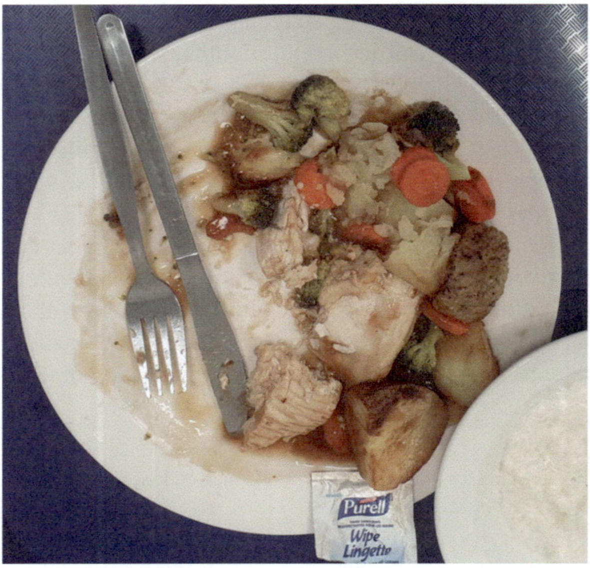

Fig. 2.1 Appearance of patient's dinner plate after she believed she had eaten it all, she has not attended to the left side confirming the examination finding of visual neglect

Investigations

Routine blood tests revealed mildly raised C-reactive protein (CRP) of 15 (normal range 0–5) with normal white cell and neutrophil count. Renal and liver function were also within normal limits. Extended blood test panel, including erythrocyte sedimentation rate, thyroid function tests, vitamin B12, folate, as well as infection and autoimmune screen, were all normal.

Computerised tomography (CT) performed on the day of the admission revealed extensive low-density change involving the white matter in both frontal, parietal and right temporal lobes with associated sulcal effacement. CT angiogram of the carotid and intracranial vessels showed mild atherosclerosis in the internal carotid artery with no other areas of stenosis. Subsequent MRI brain with contrast undertaken diffuse and confluent white matter abnormalities involving both frontal, temporal, parietal and occipital lobes seen on T2 and FLAIR imaging (Fig. 2.2). There were multiple associated areas of peripheral microbleeds on susceptibility weighted imaging (SWI), which co-localised to the areas of white matter signal change. There was no evidence of leptomeningeal enhancement.Lumbar puncture undertaken on this admission showed mildly raised protein (0.54 g/L, normal range 0.15–0.45 g/L), 18 red cells (normal range < 1) and < 1 white cell (normal range < 1), with normal CSF/serum glucose ratio. CSF gram stain, bacterial culture as well as viral PCR including HSV and VZV, were negative.

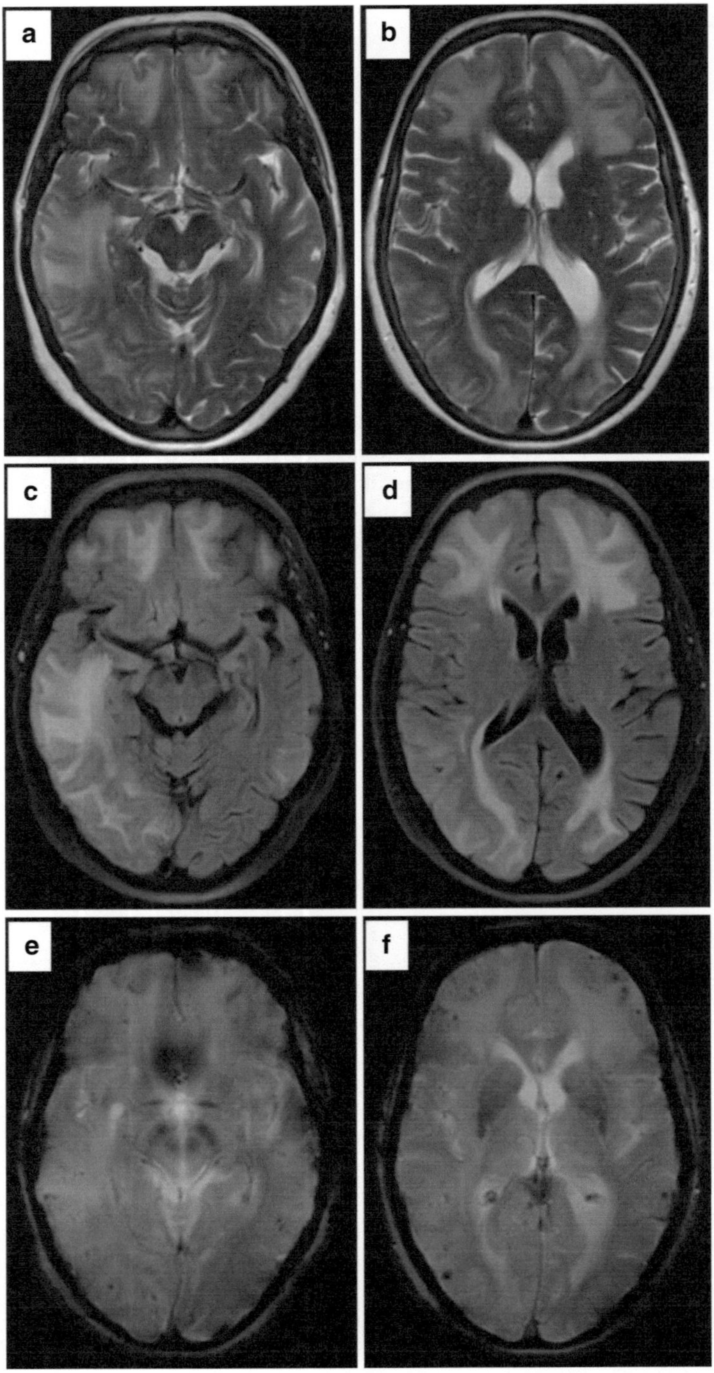

Fig. 2.2 MRI imaging performed on the hospital admission, with T2 (**a**, **b**) and FLAIR imaging (**c**, **d**) showing widespread subcortical white matter signal hyperintensity in the frontal, occipital and right temporal lobes, with multiple cortical microhaemorrhages seen on SWI imaging (**e**, **f**)

Discussion

In summary, the patient presented with a 6-month history of bitemporal headache, unsteadiness and multiple self-limiting episodes of encephalopathy, with recent unwitnessed collapse suggestive of possible seizure activity. Clinical examination revealed multifocal and widespread deficits pointing to diffuse frontal lobe dysfunction with pyramidal tract involvement as well as parietal lobe involvement with marked visual and sensory neglect. There was moderate hypertension on admission with mild elevation of CRP as well as CSF protein. MRI brain confirmed widespread asymmetrical white matter involvement in frontal, occipital, parietal and temporal lobes associated with multiple areas of cortical microbleeds with sparing of the deeper structures, including basal ganglia and the brainstem.

A wide differential diagnosis was considered on admission. An ischaemic aetiology was felt to be unlikely in view of a subacute presentation and the widespread white matter change seen on CT and MRI that were not restricted to a particular vascular territory. Posterior reversible encephalopathy syndrome (PRES) was considered a possibility, especially as there was evidence of untreated hypertension and symmetrical occipital and frontal lobe white matter involvement on imaging. However, relapsing course, prominent involvement of temporal lobe with widespread cortical microhaemorrhages were not consistent with the diagnosis [1]. Similarly, clinical history was not suggestive of autoimmune encephalitis, with no preceding symptoms suggestive of psychosis, pyrexia, autonomic disturbance or movement disorder seen in NMDA-R or LGI encephalitis, with subsequent negative serum antibody results. A possibility of CNS vasculopathy secondary to VZV infection was explored however there was no history of rash suggestive of shingles or other systemic symptoms of viral infection, with subsequent normal CSF white cell count, CSF VZV PCR and vessel imaging, which is abnormal in vast majority of patients with this condition [2]. Lastly, rare inflammatory conditions restricted to CNS with no systemic manifestations were considered, including primary angiitis of the CNS (PACNS). PACNS usually follows progressive and stepwise clinical course, with prominent symptoms of headache, cognitive impairment and focal neurological deficits that fits well with patient's clinical course. Typical imaging findings include multiple T2/FLAIR areas parenchymal change with leptomeningeal enhancement. Vessel imaging, including MRA or black blood MRI is abnormal in majority of patients with this condition, with areas of stenosis, occlusion, or wall enhancement [3]. However, evidence of multiple peripheral microbleeds would be atypical for this condition and strongly pointed to a related CNS inflammatory condition, cerebral amyloid angiopathy-related inflammation (CAAri), a rare subtype cerebral amyloid angiopathy (CAA) [4, 5]. CAAri usually presents with an acute encephalopathy with focal neurological deficits and typical brain abnormalities consisting of multiple confluent white matter hyperintensities coupled with areas of microhaemorrhage restricted to cerebral white matter which fits well with this patients' presentation. The diagnosis of probable CAAri in our patient was reached using clinicoradiological criteria [6] and treatment with a 3-day course of IV methylprednisolone was commenced after exclusion of an infectious cause, which was followed by high-dose daily steroid regime [6]. There was a rapid improvement in symptoms within days of introduction of steroid treatment, including marked improvement of confusion, sensory and visual neglect and left-sided weakness. She was discharged home with a tapering dose of oral steroid therapy and remains well, with no further clinical relapses 3 months after initial hospital admission.

Cerebral amyloid angiopathy (CAA) is a cerebrovascular disorder primarily affecting the elderly population and characterised by abnormal deposition of amyloid β (Aβ) in tunica media and adventitia of small to medium sized cerebral arteries and leptomeninges. As a result, the affected vessel walls undergo fibrinoid necrosis and microaneurysm formation, which in turn predisposes to microhaemorrhages, leukoencephalopathy and large lobar haemorrhages [7]. CAAri is a rare and increasingly recognised subtype of CAA characterised by marked inflammation and vasogenic oedema accompanying the Aβ deposition, often leading a much more aggressive clinical course [5]. Patients with CAAri most commonly present with an acute or subacute encephalopathy and focal neurological deficits, with prominent symptoms of headache and seizures. Rarely, the clinical course can be protracted or consist of series of self-limiting episodes, similarly to our case. Clinical examination is usually notable for multifocal neurological deficits that anatomically correspond to areas of subcortical inflammation seen on brain imaging.

Approximately half of patients with CAAri have mildly elevated CRP and ESR at presentation [8]. CSF examination is abnormal in majority of patients, most commonly showing lymphocytic pleocytosis and mild-to-moderate protein elevation [9]. Marked elevation of opening CSF pressure has also been reported [8].

MRI is abnormal in vast majority of patients and is often key to reaching the diagnosis, with T2 and FLAIR sequences showing extensive and asymmetrical white matter lesions corresponding to marked vasogenic oedema. The white matter changes can be multilobar and are associated with multiple microhaemorrhages present in cortical and subcortical areas, mirroring the Aβ deposition in small and medium-sized vessels. The brainstem, basal ganglia and deep white matter, which are the most common site for hypertensive microhaemorrhages, are usually spared [10]. Leptomeningeal enhancement is present in approximately half of all cases. The volume of T2/FLAIR hyperintensities has been shown to correlate with disease severity and can be used for monitoring of treatment response or clinical relapse [11]. Interestingly, the associated radiological changes associated with CAAri closely resemble amyloid-related imaging abnormalities (ARIA) seen in subset of patients who developed meningoencephalitis after treatment with monoclonal antibodies targeting Aβ in experimental Alzheimer's disease trials, suggesting a possible common autoimmune basis for both disorders. This is further supported by finding of CSF antibodies against Aβ that can be detected in patients with acute presentation of CAAri, with subsequent decline in titres after introduction of immunosuppression [12].

Tissue biopsy of affected cerebral and leptomeningeal vessels remains gold standard for the diagnosis of CAAri, usually showing vascular Aβ deposition with evidence of perivascular, transmural and intramural inflammation. However, in view of significant morbidity associated with brain biopsy and with increased recognition of typical MRI appearances of the disease on T2, FLAIR and SWI/GRE imaging, a set of pathologically-validated clinicoradiological criteria was created to allow a diagnosis of 'probable' and 'possible' CAAri with good sensitivity and specificity, which is now widely used in clinical practice [6]. Prompt and accurate diagnosis is crucial since patients with CAAri respond to appropriate immunosuppressive therapy, as demonstrated in a recent prospective study which recruited 113 participants with the disease [13]. Majority of patients in this study received 5 days of 1 g IV methylprednisolone course followed by high-dose oral steroid taper resulting in clinical recovery in 84% of patients, with similar rate of radiological improvement. Importantly, disease recurrence was much more likely if steroid treatment was stopped after IV course, favouring a longer course of immunosuppression. Wide range of other treatments have been trialled in patients with CAAri who either did not respond to steroid therapy or developed further clinical relapses, including cyclophosphamide, azathioprine and intravenous immunoglobulin (IVIG) [4].

Key Clinical Learning Points

- CAAri is a rare and increasingly recognised subtype of CAA, presenting as acute or subacute onset encephalopathy, headache, seizures and focal neurological signs.
- Brain biopsy remains gold standard for the diagnosis of CAAri, showing Aβ deposition in small and medium sized vessels accompanied by perivascular, intramural and transmural inflammation.
- Validated clinicoradiological criteria can be used in clinical practice to diagnose probable and possible CAAri, removing the need for brain biopsy in a subset of patients.
- The mainstay of treatment is immunosuppression with high-dose IV steroid therapy followed by slow oral taper, with clinical response to therapy expected first few weeks of therapy. Second line treatment options in cases of inadequate clinical response or relapse include cyclophosphamide, mycophenolate mofetil, azathioprine or IVIG.

Key Radiological Learning Points

- Typical T2/FLAIR MRI findings in patients with CAAri include extensive and asymmetrical white matter hyperintensities extending into the subcortical areas, coupled with multiple cerebral subcortical microbleeds and cortical superficial siderosis seen on GRE/SWI imaging
- Leptomeningeal contrast enhancement can also be seen in a subset of patients
- Serial MRI imaging can be used for monitoring of disease activity, with clinical relapses often being associated with recurrence of T2/FLAIR white matter hyperintensities seen during the initial presentation.

References

1. Bartynski WS, Boardman JF. Distinct imaging patterns and lesion distribution in posterior reversible encephalopathy syndrome. AJNR Am J Neuroradiol. 2007;28(7):1320–7.
2. Gilden D, Cohrs RJ, Mahalingam R, Nagel MA. Varicella zoster virus vasculopathies: diverse clinical manifestations, laboratory features, pathogenesis, and treatment. Lancet Neurol. 2009;8(8):731–40.
3. Sarti C, Picchioni A, Telese R, Pasi M, Failli Y, Pracucci G, et al. "When should primary angiitis of the central nervous system (PACNS) be suspected?": literature review and proposal of a preliminary screening algorithm. Neurol Sci. 2020;41(11):3135–48.
4. Kirshner HS, Bradshaw M. The inflammatory form of cerebral amyloid angiopathy or "cerebral amyloid angiopathy-related inflammation" (CAARI). Curr Neurol Neurosci Rep. 2015;15(8):54.
5. Chwalisz BK. Cerebral amyloid angiopathy and related inflammatory disorders. J Neurol Sci. 2021;424:117425.
6. Auriel E, Charidimou A, Gurol ME, Ni J, Van Etten ES, Martinez-Ramirez S, et al. Validation of clinicoradiological criteria for the diagnosis of cerebral amyloid angiopathy-related inflammation. JAMA Neurol. 2016;73(2):197–202.
7. Charidimou A, Gang Q, Werring DJ. Sporadic cerebral amyloid angiopathy revisited: recent insights into pathophysiology and clinical spectrum. J Neurol Neurosurg Psychiatry. 2012;83(2):124–37.
8. Chung KK, Anderson NE, Hutchinson D, Synek B, Barber PA. Cerebral amyloid angiopathy related inflammation: three case reports and a review. J Neurol Neurosurg Psychiatry. 2011;82(1):20–6.
9. Castro Caldas A, Silva C, Albuquerque L, Pimentel J, Silva V, Ferro JM. Cerebral amyloid angiopathy associated with inflammation: report of 3 cases and systematic review. J Stroke Cerebrovasc Dis. 2015;24(9):2039–48.
10. Martucci M, Sarria S, Toledo M, Coscojuela P, Vert C, Siurana S, et al. Cerebral amyloid angiopathy-related inflammation: imaging findings and clinical outcome. Neuroradiology. 2014;56(4):283–9.
11. Kinnecom C, Lev MH, Wendell L, Smith EE, Rosand J, Frosch MP, et al. Course of cerebral amyloid angiopathy-related inflammation. Neurology. 2007;68(17):1411–6.
12. Piazza F, Greenberg SM, Savoiardo M, Gardinetti M, Chiapparini L, Raicher I, et al. Anti-amyloid β autoantibodies in cerebral amyloid angiopathy-related inflammation: implications for amyloid-modifying therapies. Ann Neurol. 2013;73(4):449–58.
13. Antolini L, DiFrancesco JC, Zedde M, Basso G, Arighi A, Shima A, et al. Spontaneous ARIA-like events in cerebral amyloid angiopathy-related inflammation: a Multicenter prospective longitudinal cohort study. Neurology. 2021;97(18):e1809–e22.

Chapter 3
Running out of Steam

Edgar Chan and Richard Perry

Clinical History

A 53-year-old female executive secretary walked into A&E with her work colleague who reported that she had become confused. She is an avid runner and each morning before work she runs 5 miles around her neighbourhood. On the previous day, she had gone on her usual morning run and had returned home with a graze on her left cheek. When she was questioned by her partner, she could not remember what had happened or how she had sustained the injury. However, she was wearing a GPS fitness tracker at the time which tracked her route and heart rate (Fig. 3.1). The tracker showed that there was a sudden change in pace after about 4½ miles. Her partner reported that she appeared disorientated and confused for a few hours but she tried to carry on with her day nonetheless. She attempted to go to a Christmas party but lost her way travelling up and down the train line and could not reach her destination. She returned home and carried on with her usual activities. The next day she overslept, which is uncharacteristic, but she managed to get into work. Her colleagues noticed that she did not seem herself and suggested that she should go to hospital.

E. Chan (✉)
Department of Neuropsychology, The National Hospital for Neurology and Neurosurgery, Queen Square, London, UK

Stroke Research Centre, Institute of Neurology, UCL, London, UK
e-mail: edgar.chan1@nhs.net

R. Perry
Stroke Research Centre, Institute of Neurology, UCL, London, UK

Comprehensive Stroke Service, National Hospital for Neurology & Neurosurgery, UCL Hospitals NHS Foundation Trust, London, UK
e-mail: richard.perry2@nhs.net

S. K. Gill et al. (eds.), *Stroke Medicine*,
https://doi.org/10.1007/978-3-031-58188-5_3

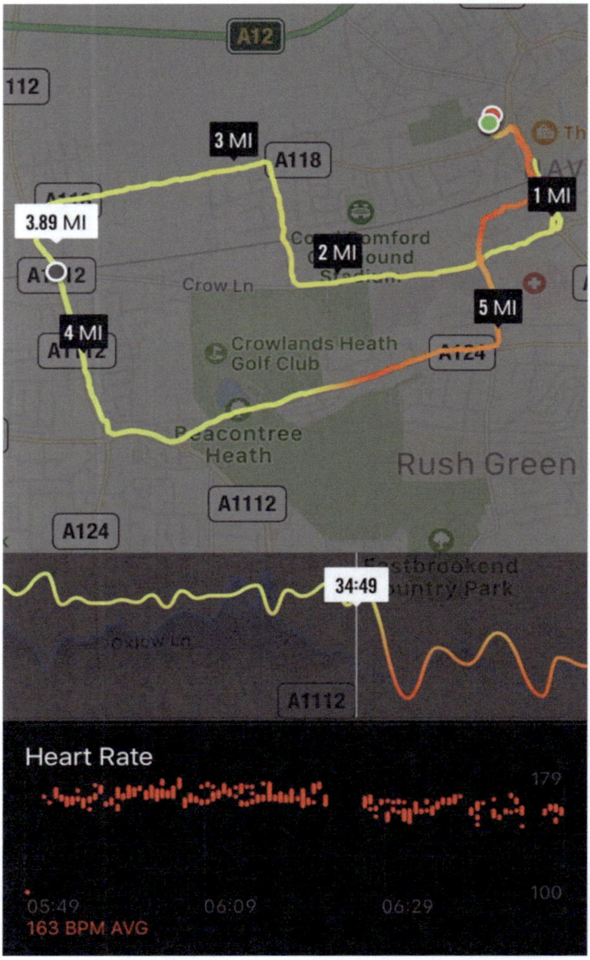

Fig. 3.1 Route of patient's run shown on GPS fitness tracker. The map shows the route that she took. Speed is colour-coded with green as the fastest pace and red as the slowest, on an arbitrary scale. A plot of speed and heart rate (bpm) against time is shown superimposed onto the lower part of the figure

Examination

On examination, there was a minor abrasion and swelling over the left cheek. Her Glasgow Coma Score (GCS) was 15/15, her blood pressure was 121/79 mmHg, and her heart rate was 52 bpm. She mobilised independently and had full limb power. There were no focal neurological signs. Her cardiovascular, respiratory and abdominal examinations were all normal. She was able to give a reasonable account of her history apart from the fact that she was not able to remember what had happened during her run the previous morning. She has no family history of ischaemic heart disease or stroke. She has never smoked or taken recreational drugs and she only drinks occasionally.

Investigations

An MRI of her head showed restricted diffusion on DWI in lenticulostriate regions bilaterally, likely extending into the body of the caudate nucleus particularly on the left (Fig. 3.2). There was also haemorrhagic transformation inferiorly involving both basal ganglia, again more extensive on the left.

Her blood results were unremarkable including normal lipids and HbA1c and a negative screen for antiphospholipid syndrome. Cardiac investigation revealed moderate mitral regurgitation, a patent foramen ovale with a very small shunt and Lambl's excrescences on her aortic valve. Rhythm monitoring by an implantable loop recorder was normal with no evidence of paroxysmal atrial fibrillation.

Functionally, her Barthel score was 20/20 indicating no loss of any basic functions. An initial assessment identified no requirement for physiotherapy or speech and language therapy. On a cognitive screening tool, the Montreal Cognitive Assessment (MoCA), she scored just below the normal range (22/30, normal range ≥ 26). The Occupational Therapist conducted a Multiple Errands Task and found evidence of poor navigation, poor organization skills and decreased processing speed. She also appeared apathetic and had limited insight into her cognitive difficulties. This observation was corroborated by the patient's daughter

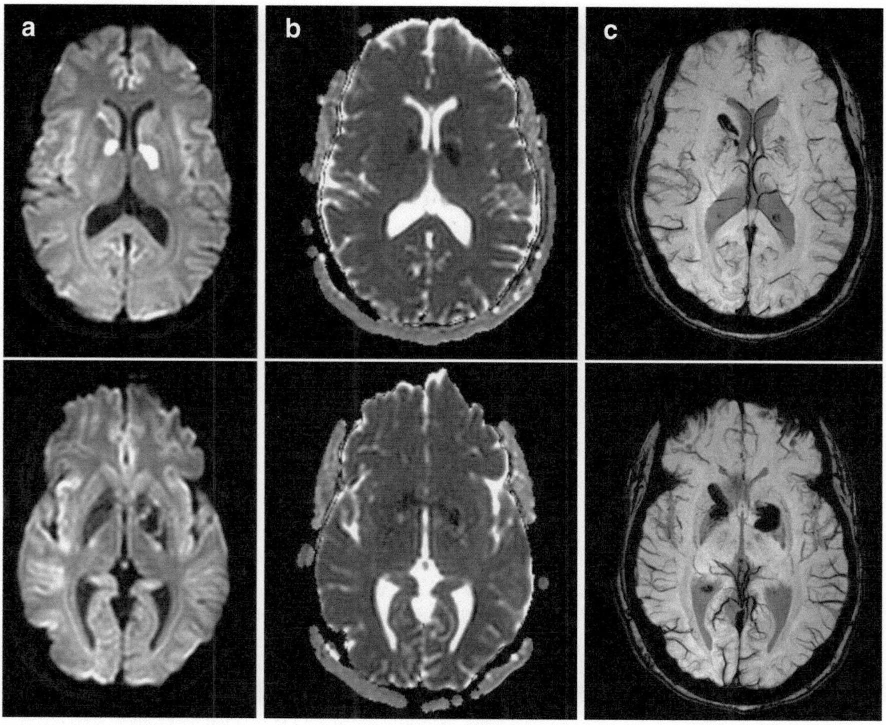

Fig. 3.2 MRI brain. (**a**) Axial DWI, (**b**) Axial ADC map, (**c**) Axial SWI. Images show, for two slices through the brain, areas of restricted diffusion (representing acute infarction) in the upper slice and areas of susceptibility artifact (representing haemorrhage) more prominent in the lower slice (shown in the lower row of images)

who commented that there had been a significant change in her mother's behaviour and personality; before this event she used to be highly motivated and a driven individual but now she seemed to be mainly nonchalant.

She was referred for a comprehensive neuropsychological assessment 6 days into her admission. A summary of her assessment scores are presented in Table 3.1.

Table 3.1 Summary of the neuropsychological assessment findings by cognitive domain with raw scores (percentile)

Premorbid functioning	
NART	102 (Average)
General intelligence	
WAIS-VIQ	85 (Low Average)
WAIS-PIQ	83 (Low Average)
Verbal Memory	
RMT-W	37/50 (<5)
AMIPB Story Immediate	23/56 (10–25)
AMIPB Story Delayed	16/56 (<10)
Visual Memory	
RMT-F	43/50 (25–50)
AMIPB Figure Immediate	59/80 (50)
AMIPB Figure Delayed	49/80 (25–50)
Naming	
GNT	21/30 (50–75)
Visuo-perceptual functions	
VOSP-OD	17/20 (>5)
VOSP-PD	20/20 (>5)
Frontal Executive functions	
CETA	11 (<5)
BADS Zoo Map	Poor
BADS Key Search	Intact
Stroop	109 (72)
Fluency S	15 (34)
Speed of processing	
SDMT	47 (51)
Mood	
HADS—Anxiety	0 (normal)
HADS—Depression	2 (normal)
Apathy	
Lille Apathy Rating Scale	
Self-report	−8 (severe apathy)
Partner rating	+10 (severe apathy)

NART National Adult Reading Test, *WAIS* Wechsler Adult Intelligence Test, *VIQ* Verbal Intelligence Quotient, *PIQ* Performance Intelligence Quotient, *RMT* Recognition Memory Test, *W* Words, *F* Faces, *AMIPB* Adult Memory and Information Processing Battery, *GNT* Graded Naming Test, *VOSP* Visual Object and Space Perception, *OD* Object Decision, *PD* Position Discrimination, *CET A* Cognitive Estimation Test Form A, *BADS* Behavioural Assessment of the Dysexecutive Syndrome, *SDMT* Symbol Digit Modalities Test, *HADS* Hospital Anxiety and Depression Scale

Assessment revealed significant decline in her general intellect which was in the low average range. Examination of separate cognitive domains revealed difficulties with verbal recall and recognition memory, poor complex reasoning and problem solving. In contrast, visual memory, language abilities, visuo-perceptual functions and processing speed were all broadly intact. She denied any low mood or anxiety concerns. Notably however, scores on the Lille Apathy Rating Scale from her own self-report and her partner's observations were both in the severely apathetic range (−8 and +10 respectively; score range [−36 (no apathy) to +36 (extreme apathy)]). Her partner scored her 18 points higher suggesting some degree of reduced insight into her own behavioural changes.

Clinical Progress

When she was discharged home, formal therapies assessments of her needs suggested that she did not require any carer support, yet even a month after discharge her partner reported significant concerns. She continued to behave in a child-like manner, spending much of her time watching television, going out for runs without informing anyone, laughing problems away and not taking things seriously. Given her cognitive and behavioural changes, she was referred to a tertiary Vocational Rehabilitation team to support her return to work. She was prescribed a dopamine agonist for treatment of apathy, she was started on aspirin 75 mg daily after clopidogrel caused itching and she remains under cardiological follow-up.

Discussion

Traditionally, stroke affecting the basal ganglia is associated with changes to motor function. However, basal ganglia strokes can also lead to significant cognitive and behavioural changes that can have a profound impact on recovery and outcomes.

The basal ganglia (BG) are a set of deep grey matter nuclei consisting of the striatum (caudate nucleus, putamen, nucleus accumbens and olfactory tubercle), the globus pallidus, the ventral pallidum, the subthalamic nucleus, and the substantia nigra. The basal ganglia receive inputs from all cortical regions and are a part of a complex network of parallel pathways to motor and non-motor areas of the cerebral cortex [1, 2].There are five defined frontal-subcortical circuits that link the frontal cortex to the basal ganglia and thalamus [3, 4]. In addition, these circuits receive and integrate input from temporal, parietal and limbic brain regions. Damage to the basal ganglia can therefore lead to a host of cognitive and behavioural changes following disruption to these circuits. In this patient's case, lesions to the basal ganglia bilaterally led to a significant decline in general intellect, verbal memory impairment, executive dysfunction and apathy.

Cognitive impairment is common after basal ganglia strokes. Compared to neurologically intact participants, patients with basal ganglia stroke have been found to perform more poorly across most neuropsychological domains [5]. Although cortical strokes are often thought to lead to greater impairment than subcortical strokes, this may be an artefact, in that cortical strokes usually involve larger vascular territories. Once lesion volume is taken into account, cognitive performance between those with cortical or subcortical strokes is relatively comparable across cognitive domains [6]. Damage to the right basal ganglia tend to result in greater executive and visuo-spatial impairments [7, 8], while damage to left basal ganglia result in greater language and memory impairments [7, 9].Our patient had lesions to the basal ganglia bilaterally, but more extensive in the left hemisphere which likely led to greater damage to left-lateralised circuits. This might help explain our patient's selective memory impairment for verbal but not visual material, as material-specific memory processes are known to be lateralized based on the hemisphere of language dominance [10].

In addition to cognitive changes, lesions in the basal ganglia can also lead to apathy. Prevalence of apathy in stroke is around one third [11], with studies reporting ranges from 19% up to 55% [12]. Apathy can co-occur with depression, but is dissociable in terms of the neurobiology, symptomatology and time-course. Apathy is defined clinically as a quantitative reduction of goal-directed activity in comparison to previous level of functioning [13]. The reduction can be in behaviour and/or cognition, spontaneous or reactive emotions, or social interactions. It has been recently proposed that apathy might be best understood in the context of a three-part model of motivated/goal-directed behaviour [14] consisting of a valuation system that computes the subjective value of a task, a mediating system that integrates reinforcers with motor systems to act on a goal and lastly a motor system that actions the goal/behaviour.

Apathy can result from stroke damage across many different brain regions because goal-directed activity is supported by a large-scale brain network [15]. While lesions to peripheral nodes of the network such as premotor or parietal regions may result in apathy through indirect processes of diaschisis and transneuronal degeneration, focal lesions in critical nodes such as the basal ganglia, anterior cingulate or orbitofrontal regions lead to immediate network failure and apathy. Damage to the basal ganglia directly disrupts the frontal-subcortical and limbic-subcortical circuits involved in goal-directed behaviour leading to apathy [16]. Apathy is more common after bilateral basal ganglia strokes but has also been found following unilateral strokes [e.g. 17]. In keeping with this, a study that compared the regional cerebral blood flow of stroke patients with and without apathy, those with apathy demonstrated significantly worse perfusion to the basal ganglia bilaterally [18]. Furthermore, lesions only to the left basal ganglia were also found to be associated with bilateral basal ganglia hypo-perfusion and apathy.

Post-stroke apathy is associated with worse patient outcomes. Mayo and colleagues [12] looked at the extent to which apathy changes over the first year after stroke and its impact on recovery. Of a group of first-ever stroke patients (n = 408), 50% had no apathy while 33% had mild and 3% had severe apathy. Results showed that even mild apathy had a strong negative association with recovery, with poor physical function, physical health, participation and perceived health outcomes. A meta-review of studies examining post-stroke apathy found that apathy was associated with worse cognitive functioning, increased disability and poorer rehabilitation outcomes [11]. Pharmacological treatment for apathy following stroke still lacks sufficient high-quality evidence, but medications targeting dopamine receptors such as ropinirole, a selective D2/D3 agonists, seem to show strong promise [19].

In summary, stroke affecting the basal ganglia can lead to cognitive difficulties and behavioural changes. Impaired cognition after stroke can have a significant impact on recovery and increase the level of functional dependence of the patient [20, 21]. Accurate assessment of cognitive functions can help to predict length of stay and functional outcome, leading to better rehabilitation planning [22–24]. Even in patients without evidence of physical disability or any obvious functional deficits, clinicians should carefully consider and examine for more subtle cognitive and/or behavioural changes following stroke. Simple cognitive screening measures such as the MoCA are quick to administer and may provide some information about possible underlying deficits. However, intact performance on cognitive screening tools might not always be a valid marker of intact cognition. Screens such as the MoCA often underestimate impairment as they do not cover all the relevant cognitive domains that might be affected after stroke and they often do not adequately tap into right hemisphere deficits [25, 26]. In these cases, a comprehensive neuropsychological assessment by a clinical neuropsychologist is often most useful to help discern any cognitive or behavioural changes following stroke and provide a useful formulation from which rehabilitation and recovery can be planned.

Key Clinical Learning Points

- Stroke in the basal ganglia can have no motor consequences but lead to significant cognitive and behavioural impairments.
- Cognitive impairment can occur in any domain, but executive difficulties are most common.
- Apathy is also common and is defined as a reduction in goal-directed activity (behaviour, emotion or social).
- Cognitive and behavioural impairments are primarily due to disruption of frontal-subcortical and limbic-subcortical circuits.
- Cognitive screening and neuropsychological assessment is prudent after stroke.

References

1. Nelson AB, Kreitzer AC. Reassessing models of basal ganglia function and dysfunction. Annu Rev Neurosci. 2014;37:117–35.
2. Middleton FA, Strick PL. Basal ganglia output and cognition: evidence from anatomical, behavioral, and clinical studies. Brain Cogn. 2000;42(2):183–200.

3. Mega MS, Cummings JL. Frontal-subcortical circuits and neuropsychiatric disorders. J Neuropsychiatry Clin Neurosci. 1994;6(4):358–70.
4. Tekin S, Cummings JL. Frontal–subcortical neuronal circuits and clinical neuropsychiatry: an update. J Psychosom Res. 2002;53(2):647–54.
5. Hochstenbach J, van Spaendonck KP, Cools AR, Horstink MW, Mulder T. Cognitive deficits following stroke in the basal ganglia. Clin Rehabil. 1998;12(6):514–20.
6. Turunen KE, Kauranen TV, Laari SP, Mustanoja SM, Tatlisumak T, Poutiainen ET. Cognitive deficits after subcortical infarction are comparable with deficits after cortical infarction. Eur J Neurol. 2013;20(2):286–92.
7. Su CY, Chen HM, Kwan AL, Lin YH, Guo NW. Neuropsychological impairment after hemorrhagic stroke in basal ganglia. Arch Clin Neuropsychol. 2007;22(4):465–74.
8. Arsalidou M, Duerden EG, Taylor MJ. The centre of the brain: topographical model of motor, cognitive, affective, and somatosensory functions of the basal ganglia. Hum Brain Mapp. 2013;34(11):3031–54.
9. Kim SH, Park KH, Sung YH, Lee YB, Park HM, Shin DJ. Dementia mimicking a sudden cognitive and behavioral change induced by left globus pallidus infarction: review of two cases. J Neurol Sci. 2008;272(1–2):178–82.
10. Milner B. Memory and the medial temporal regions of the brain. Biol Mem. 1970;23:31–59.
11. Van Dalen JW, van Charante EP, Nederkoorn PJ, van Gool WA, Richard E. Poststroke apathy. Stroke. 2013;44(3):851–60.
12. Mayo NE, Fellows LK, Scott SC, Cameron J, Wood-Dauphinee S. A longitudinal view of apathy and its impact after stroke. Stroke. 2009;40(10):3299–307.
13. Robert P, Lanctôt KL, Agüera-Ortiz L, Aalten P, Bremond F, Defrancesco M, Hanon C, David R, Dubois B, Dujardin K, Husain M. Is it time to revise the diagnostic criteria for apathy in brain disorders? The 2018 international consensus group. Eur Psychiatry. 2018;54:71–6.
14. Le Heron C, Holroyd CB, Salamone J, Husain M. Brain mechanisms underlying apathy. J Neurol Neurosurg Psychiatry. 2019;90(3):302–12.
15. Tay J, Lisiecka-Ford DM, Hollocks MJ, Tuladhar AM, Barrick TR, Forster A, O'Sullivan MJ, Husain M, de Leeuw FE, Morris RG, Markus HS. Network neuroscience of apathy in cerebrovascular disease. Prog Neurobiol. 2020;188:101785.
16. Levy R, Dubois B. Apathy and the functional anatomy of the prefrontal cortex–basal ganglia circuits. Cereb Cortex. 2006;16(7):916–28.
17. Benke T, Delazer M, Bartha L, Auer A. Basal ganglia lesions and the theory of fronto-subcortical loops: neuropsychological findings in two patients with left caudate lesions. Neurocase. 2003;9(1):70–85.
18. Onoda K, Kuroda Y, Yamamoto Y, Abe S, Oguro H, Nagai A, Bokura H, Yamaguchi S. Post-stroke apathy and hypoperfusion in basal ganglia: SPECT study. Cerebrovasc Dis. 2011;31(1):6–11.
19. Chong TJ, Husain M. The role of dopamine in the pathophysiology and treatment of apathy. Prog Brain Res. 2016;229:389–426.
20. Cumming TB, Marshall RS, Lazar RM. Stroke, cognitive deficits, and rehabilitation: still an incomplete picture. Int J Stroke. 2013;8(1):38–45.
21. Umarova RM, Nitschke K, Kaller CP, Klöppel S, Beume L, Mader I, Martin M, Hennig J, Weiller C. Predictors and signatures of recovery from neglect in acute stroke. Ann Neurol. 2016;79(4):673–86.
22. Galski T, Bruno RL, Zorowitz R, Walker J. Predicting length of stay, functional outcome, and aftercare in the rehabilitation of stroke patients. The dominant role of higher-order cognition. Stroke. 1993;24(12):1794–800.
23. Park YH, Jang JW, Park SY, Wang MJ, Lim JS, Baek MJ, Kim BJ, Han MK, Bae HJ, Ahn S, Kim S. Executive function as a strong predictor of recovery from disability in patients with acute stroke: a preliminary study. J Stroke Cerebrovasc Dis. 2015;24(3):554–61.

24. Mole JA, Demeyere N. The relationship between early post-stroke cognition and longer term activities and participation: a systematic review. Neuropsychol Rehabil. 2020;30(2):346–70.
25. Chan E, Khan S, Oliver R, Gill SK, Werring DJ, Cipolotti L. Underestimation of cognitive impairments by the Montreal Cognitive Assessment (MoCA) in an acute stroke unit population. J Neurol Sci. 2014;343(1–2):176–9.
26. Chan E, Altendorff S, Healy C, Werring DJ, Cipolotti L. The test accuracy of the Montreal Cognitive Assessment (MoCA) by stroke lateralisation. J Neurol Sci. 2017;373:100–4.

Chapter 4
Cerebral Cavernous Malformations

Anna Sadnicka and Sumanjit K. Gill

Clinical History

A 77 year old retired man presented with chest pain to accident and emergency. The chest pain was of sudden onset, central, sharp and radiated to the back between the shoulder blades. He had a previously history of ischaemic heart disease with coronary artery bypass grafting performed 20 years ago. Three years prior to the current presentation non ST elevation myocardial infarction required intervention to both native vessels and his vein graft. Shortly after a permanent pacemaker was inserted due to atrial fibrillation and complete heart block. He had little chest discomfort on exertion, a reasonable exercise tolerance and mild left ventricular impairment. He was on secondary prevention with both Clopidogrel 75 mg od and Rivoraxaban 20 mg od. Other medications included Bisoprolol 5 mg od, Ramipril 5 mg od and Rosuvastatin 10 mg od.

A. Sadnicka (✉)
Royal Free Hospital, London, UK

Motor Control and Neuromodulation Lab, St George's University of London, London, UK

Movement and Clinical Neurosciences, University College London, London, UK
e-mail: anna.sadnicka@nhs.net

S. K. Gill
Institute of Neurology, UCL, National Hospital for Neurology and Neurosurgery, London, UK
e-mail: Sumanjit.Gill@uclh.nhs.uk

S. K. Gill et al. (eds.), *Stroke Medicine*,
https://doi.org/10.1007/978-3-031-58188-5_4

Examination

He was hypertensive with a blood pressure of 220/110 mmHg with an irregular heart rate 72 beats per minute. A systemic examination was otherwise normal.

Investigations and Clinical Progress

His 12 L ECG and troponin results did not support the diagnosis of an ischaemic acute coronary syndrome. CT angiogram of the aortic arch did not reveal any evidence of dissection. In view of his uncontrolled high blood pressure a CT head was also performed. The CT head revealed multiple subcortical foci throughout the brain including the cerebellar hemispheres, right frontal and temporal lobes (Fig. 4.1). It was commented that these were suspicious for metastases yet the cystic component within the right cerebellar lesion was atypical. In view of his blood pressure and the abnormal scan findings the anticoagulation and anti platelets were stopped. His blood pressure was reduced with oral agents over the next 3 days and his chest pain resolved completely. An MRI Brain with contrast revealed multiple supra- and infra-tentorial lesions of variable size were seen. On susceptibility weighted imaging these lesions had the appearance of multiple cerebral cavernous malformations (CCMs) (Fig. 4.2). There was no evidence of leak from any of lesions. Once his blood pressure was maintained at <135/85 mmHg both this anti platelet and oral anticoagulant were restarted after discussion of risks and benefits with the patients. He was referred for genetic counselling and was found to be heterozygous for the CCM2 gene.

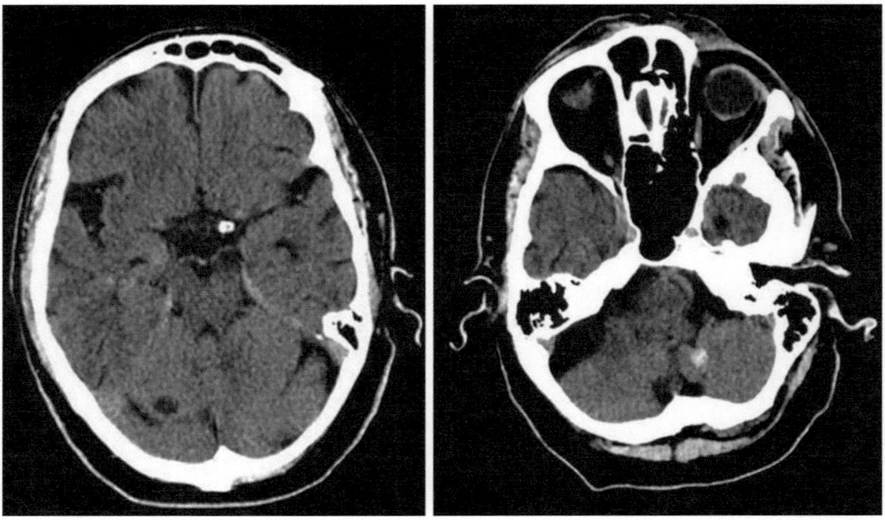

Figs. 4.1 Axial non contrast CT Head images showing cystic lesion in right cerebellar lesion (left hand image) and hyperdense lesion in left cerebellar hemisphere (right hand image)

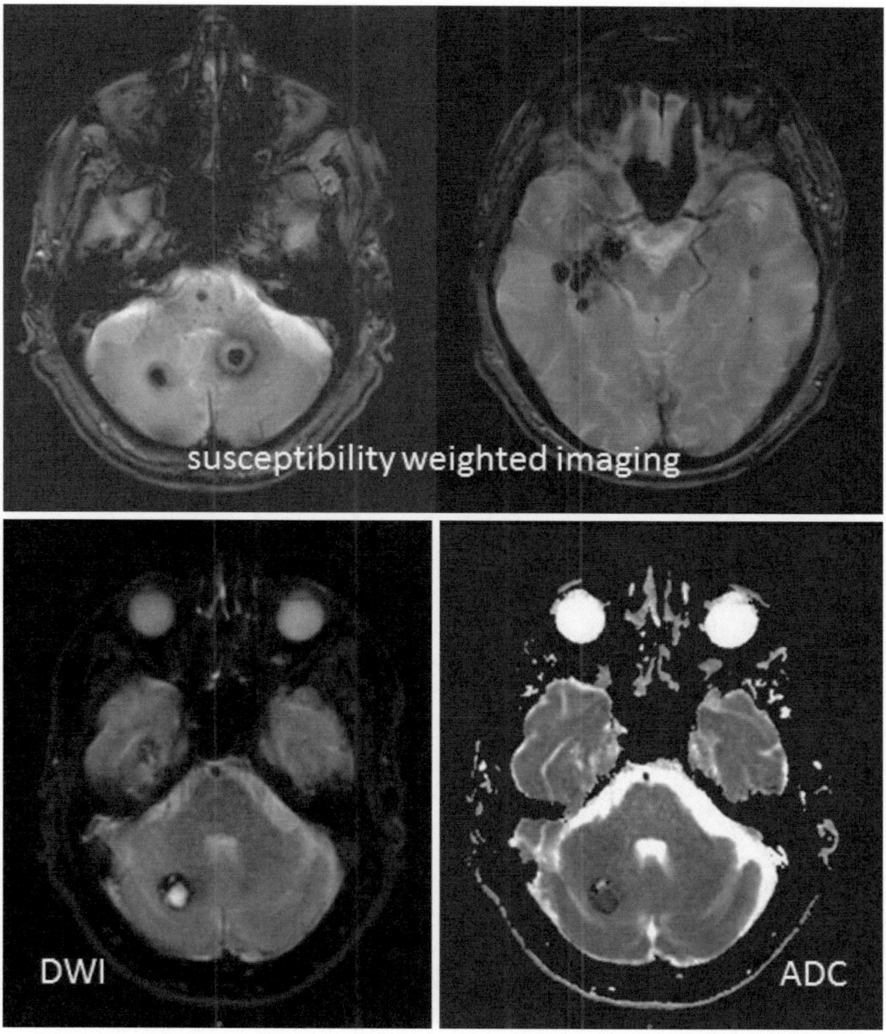

Fig. 4.2 Axial MRI images showing infra- and supra-tentorial lesions on susceptibility weighted imaging and diffusion weighted imaging

Discussion

CCMs have been reported to be the second most common vascular malformation of the central nervous system after developmental venous anomalies [1]. Disease prevalence is estimated at 0.15% to 0.5% [1]. The majority of CCM cases comprises a single lesion and are called sporadic CCMs and are often asymptomatic and nonhereditary. Approximately 20% of cases present with multiple CCMs, and many of these have a positive family history consistent with autosomal dominant inheritance. The diagnosis of familial CCM can be confirmed by genetic testing for mutations in three genes: CCM1 (KRIT1), CCM2 (MGC4607), or CCM3 (PDCD10) [2]. Research suggests that each of these genes are part of a greater signalling pathway that regulates cell proliferation, network formation, and growth in the endothelial layer and have a common direct interaction with a heterotrimeric adaptor complex (CCM complex) [2]. Microscopically CCMs are made up of multiple mulberry-like distended caverns of dilated thin-walled capillaries without the normal intervening brain parenchymal architecture. Often, individual cavernomas are surrounded by hemosiderin representing remote oozing due to the abnormal capillaries [1]. CCM is also referred to in the literature as cavernous angioma, hemangioma, or cavernoma. They most often present with headaches or seizures and less frequently with 'leak'.

Anticoagulation in Patients with Cavernomas

In this case, CCMs were clinical silent with no history of focal neurological deficits, no seizures and no history of symptomatic intracranial haemorrhage. However, the CCMs raised an interesting clinical debate surrounding his anticoagulation. His relative risk of future stroke was high due to his ongoing atrial fibrillation, age, hypertension and prior cardiac vascular disease. Indeed, approximately a quarter of patients with CCMs have an indication for antithrombotic (anticoagulant or antiplatelet) therapy for the prevention of occlusive vascular disease. Yet, in the past decisions have been made based on common sense that anticoagulation should be withheld for fear of increasing the risk of intracranial haemorrhage in adults with CCMs.

A recent systematic reappraisal of evidence has forced a major rethink of such caution. The evidence for whether anticoagulation can be safely given in CCMs has been reviewed and a population based cohort study published within the same report [3]. Interestingly, antithrombotic therapy was associated with a *lower* risk of intracranial haemorrhage in a meta-analysis of six comparative cohort studies of patients with CCMs with no inconsistency between their findings (Fig. 4.3) [3]. In the population based cohort study, antithrombotic therapy use in patients with CCMs was similarly associated with a lower risk of intracranial haemorrhage (Fig. 4.4) and a lower risk of focal neurological deficit due to any cause [3]. These findings were also consistent with previous studies that examined antiplatelet therapy for patients with CCMs. These findings therefore provided reassurance about safety for clinical practice and the authors suggested that their findings require further investigation in a randomised controlled trial [3].

The association between antithrombotic therapy and a lower risk of intracranial haemorrhage from a CCM is consistent with the hypothesis that these events might be triggered by thrombus formation in the dilated caverns of CCMs in which blood flow is slow, or thrombus in an associated venous malformation [3]. A similar pathophysiological mechanism underlies haemorrhagic infarcts in patients with cerebral venous thrombosis which is treated with anticoagulation to improve

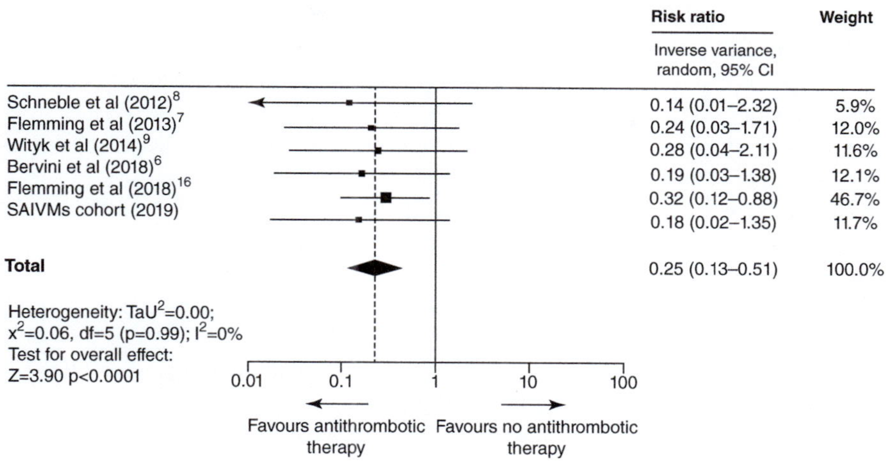

Fig. 4.3 Meta-analysis of the association between antithrombotic therapy use and the risk of intracranial haemorrhage from cerebral cavernous malformations in cohort studies. SAIVMS=Scottish Audit of Intracranial Vascular Malformations. Reproduced from Zuurbier et al. [3]

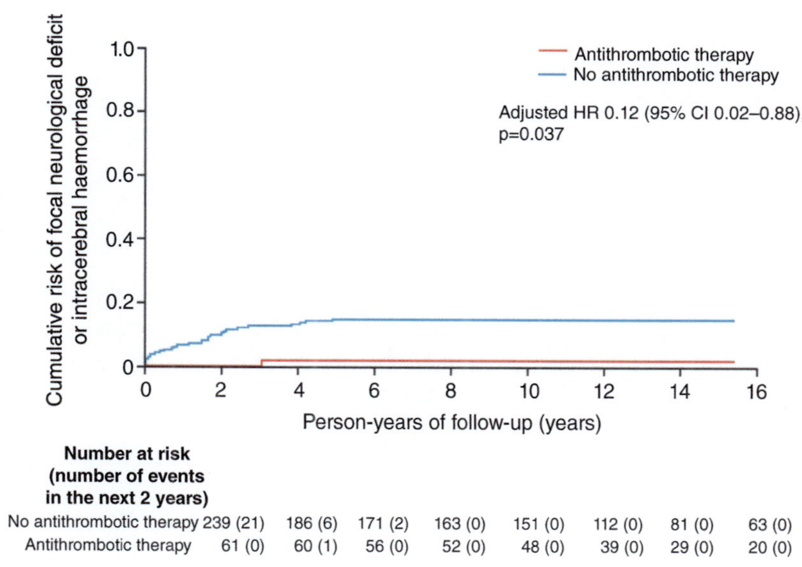

Fig. 4.4 Kaplan-Meier plot. Risk of first intracranial haemorrhage or persistent or progressive focal neurological deficit due to cerebral cavernous malformations according to antithrombotic therapy use during 15 years of follow-up in the Scottish Audit of Intracranial Vascular Malformations. Reproduced from Zuurbier et al. [3] under Creative Commons CC-BY License

outcome and reduce the risk of recurrence, regardless of the presence of haemorrhagic infarction [3]. This is the reasoning that was used to restart his anticoagulation, after a discussion of risks and benefits with the patient and strong advice to monitor his blood pressure frequently.

Key Clinical Learning Points

- CCM is also referred to in the literature as cavernous angioma, hemangioma, or cavernoma
- A single or multiple cavernomas can present with seizures or headaches in addition to an intracerebral haemorrhage
- Around a quarter of patients with CCMs have an indication for antithrombotic (anticoagulant or antiplatelet) therapy for the prevention of occlusive vascular disease [3].
- The addition of anticoagulation therapy needs to be considered on a case by case basis.
- Multiple CCM can be familial with mutations in a number of genes including KRIT1, MGC4607 and PDCD10 [2]

Key Radiological Learning Points

- CCM can be difficult to see on CT. If large, they usually appear as regions of hyper-density resembling blood products and speckles of calcification. If there has been a recent bleed then the lesion will be conspicuous and may be surrounded by oedema.
- MRI is the imaging modality of choice and lesions often demonstrate a characteristic popcorn or berry appearance with a rim of signal loss due to hemosiderin.
- Gradient echo or susceptibility sequences may reveal smaller CCMs not visible on conventional MRI sequences, particularly in association with familial CCM.
- The radiological differential is numerous and includes cerebral amyloid angiopathy, chronic hypertensive encephalopathy (more common in the basal ganglia) and haemorrhagic metastasis. Calcified lesions such as old neurocystericercosis or other infections (e.g. tuberculoma) should also be considered.
- CCMs are angiographically occult and do not demonstrate arteriovenous shunting

References

1. Akers A, Al-Shahi Salman R, Awad AI, Dahlem K, Flemming K, Hart B, Kim H, Jusue-Torres I, Kondziolka D, Lee C, Morrison L, Rigamonti D, Rebeiz T, Tournier-Lasserve E, Waggoner D, Whitehead K. Synopsis of guidelines for the clinical management of cerebral cavernous malformations: consensus recommendations based on systematic literature review by the Angioma Alliance Scientific Advisory Board Clinical Experts Panel. Neurosurgery. 2017;80(5):665–80.

2. Zafar A, Quadri SA, Farooqui M, Ikram A, Robinson M, Hart BL, Mabray MC, Vigil C, Tang AT, Kahn ML, Yonas H, Lawton MT, Kim H, Morrison L. Familial cerebral cavernous malformations. Stroke. 2019;50(5):1294–301.
3. Zuurbier SM, Hickman CR, Tolias CS, et al. Long-term antithrombotic therapy and risk of intracranial haemorrhage from cerebral cavernous malformations: a population-based cohort study, systematic review, and meta-analysis. Lancet Neurol. 2019;18(10):935–41. https://doi.org/10.1016/S1474-4422(19)30231-5.

Chapter 5
Migrainous Stroke: When Headache Presents with Persistent Visual Symptoms

FIzzah Ali and Sumanjit K. Gill

Clinical History

A 40 year old right-handed animal trainer presented to the emergency department after waking with a moderately severe, pressure-like headache affecting the left orbit and forehead. The initial headache lasted 20 min, it was exacerbated over the next 2 days by coughing and movement of the head. Her symptoms were not associated with nausea, vomiting, photophobia, photophobia or osmophobia.

She had a background of migraines affecting different locations of her head, and these had been triggered by stressful circumstances such as exams. These had not been associated with visual symptoms. On this occasion, as she had prepared her son for his school day, she noticed parts of her mobile phone screen to be missing. There was no headache this time or any of her other migranous features such as nausea or photophobia.

Two days later her visual symptom had shown significant resolution, with persisting blurring in the right eye between '12 and 3 o'clock'.

She continued to make an excellent recovery and 1 month later had a small residual homonymous right upper quadrantanopia.

F. Ali
Royal Free Hospital, London, UK
e-mail: fizzah.ali@nhs.net

S. K. Gill (✉)
Institute of Neurology, UCL, National Hospital for Neurology and Neurosurgery, London, UK
e-mail: Sumanjit.Gill@uclh.nhs.uk

S. K. Gill et al. (eds.), *Stroke Medicine*,
https://doi.org/10.1007/978-3-031-58188-5_5

Examination

Cranial nerve examination revealed a persisting right upper quadrantanopia. The rest of her neurological examination was normal.

Investigations

Factor VIII was raised with a mildly elevated d-dimer and fibrinogen at the time of presentation. Total cholesterol was also slightly raised. ECG was normal. Following the initial CT imaging, MRI brain showed restricted diffusion consistent with acute infarction in the medial aspect of the left occipital lobe (Fig. 5.1), with corresponding FLAIR hyperintensity (Fig. 5.2).

A full stroke workup was requested with a bubble echocardiogram and 72 h tape (these were all normal).

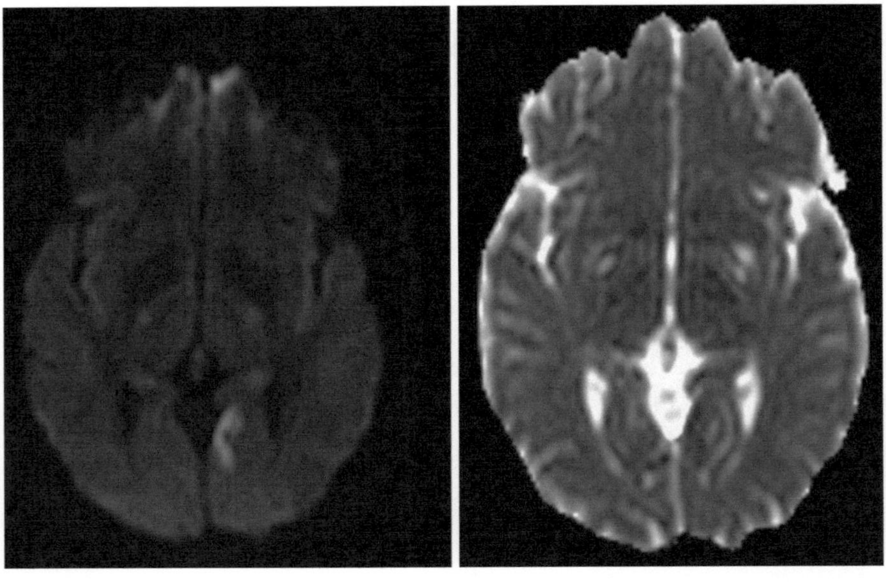

Fig. 5.1 A matched defect seen on B1000 and ADC map showing an acute infarct in the medial occipital lobe

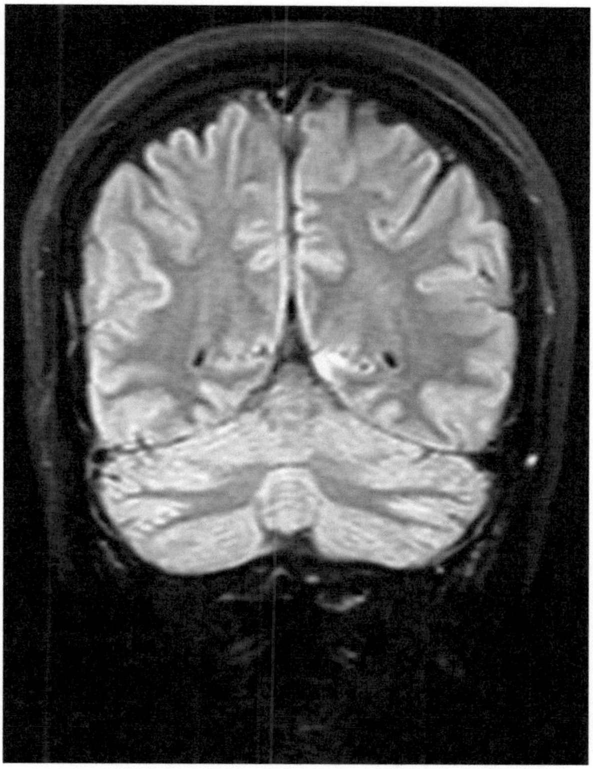

Fig. 5.2 FLAIR image showing infarct which was initially seen on DWI

Discussion

Migraine and stroke vary in aspects of their clinical presentation, for example age at onset and gender preponderance, as well as clinical management. Yet, recent years have seen an expansion in the literature supporting an association between migraine and stroke that is not yet clearly understood [1]. Headache without migranous features is also associated with stroke and can be at onset or persisting [2]. An underlying vascular disease may cause both the migraine with aura and ischaemic stroke or it might be that ischaemic stroke itself triggers a migraine with aura. The distinction between the two maybe due to differences in aetiology.

A number of studies have demonstrated an association between migraine with aura and an up to two fold increased risk of stroke [3–7]. This is particularly emphasised in the case of migraine with aura, where the relative risk of ischaemic stroke is twice compared to those without migraine. This association between migraine and stroke is stronger for women particularly thoseunder the age of 45 years old [3]. Smoking and oral contraceptive use also add additive risk for ischaemic stroke. The risk is increased in those individuals with a higher frequency of migraine [8, 9] and those with active rather than a history of migraine [10] In addition to be more complex than initially understood, the association between migraine and stroke risk is bi-directional. Cerebrovascular events, including ischaemic stroke, can precipitate a migraine-like episode that may or may not be accompanied by aura. This presents an additional diagnostic challenge, and in this instance a stroke may be interpreted to be migraine with prolonged or persisting aura symptoms [11]. A more widespread use of MRI imaging in stroke and TIA patients will hopefully lead to some clarity about the distinction between the migranous episodes which are associated with ischaemic stroke and those which are not.

The aetiological link between migraine and stroke is not clearly delineated, and a number of pathophysiological mechanisms have been cited. Cortical spreading depression can be considered as a ripple of sustained depolarisation that advances over the cerebral cortex which then completely recovers, and it is believed to be a key mechanism in the pathophysiology of migraine [12]. This activation of neurones is associated with a state of short-lasting hyperperfusion, the subsequent neuronal suppression brings a more sustained period of hypoperfusion which is well above the critical blood flow thresholds which cause ischaemia [13] It might be that in the genetic syndromes which lead to migranous stroke i.e. CADASIL the episodes of hypoperfusion do enter into the critical range to cause ischaemia.

Other factors which have been posed as potential aetiological links relate to alterations in endothelial and arterial function, although the underlying evidence for this is inconsistent [1]. A shared genetic susceptibility may also play a role in the occurrence of migraine and ischaemic stroke. This genetic overlap is evidenced though genome-wide analysis studies, [14] as well as a host of rare neurological conditions which typically display both migraine and stroke as characteristic features. These include cerebral autosomal dominant arteriopathy with subcortical infarcts and leukoencephalopathy (CADASIL), as well as mitochondrial encephalomyopathy, lactic acidoses and stroke-like episodes (MELAS).

The International Classification of Headache Disorders version 3 (ICHD-3) diagnostic criteria outlines migranous infarction as a condition occurring in an individual with migraine with aura. The sufferer will experience their typical attack with one or more aura symptoms being prolonged over 60 minutes. This corresponds with cerebral ischaemia in the relevant area and can be seen on neuroimaging [15]. In keeping with this case presentation, migrainous infarction is most commonly noted in the territory of the posterior circulation. Moreover, the reduction in cerebral blood flow that is associated with visual aura is most commonly noted in the posterior circulation [16, 17]. Migrainous infarction is rare, with the incidence being 0.2–0.5% of all cerebral ischaemia causes, [17, 18] and it carries a favourable prognosis in terms of neurological recovery [19].

Diagnostically, there are a number of key indicators which should generate suspicion and therefore further investigation of a cerebral infarction in a patient seemingly presenting with migraine. These include the presence of:

- Prolonged aura (greater than 1 h), as described in the International Classification of Headache Disorders version 3 (ICHD-3) diagnostic criteria
- Negative symptoms, such as a scotoma or field loss, as in the illustrating case, rather than photopsia

- Fixed, non-evolving features otherwise typical of migraine aura
- Significant increase in aura frequency or significant change in aura type
- First occurrence of migraine aura at an older age (for example, greater than 50 years old)

The management of migraine with aura includes the use of acute treatments such as non-steroidal anti-inflammatory drugs. Despite the historical reluctance to use triptans in migraine with aura, there does not appear to be an association with triptan use in those with migraine with aura, and stroke [20] Conversely, considering the prevention of stroke in patients with migraine with aura, modifiable risk factors such as smoking cessation and avoidance of the combined oral contraceptive pill is advised. The use of anti-platelets in patients with migraine with aura should be employed in the presence of established vascular disease, also employing statins and anti-hypertensives to manage vascular risk factors where necessary.

Key Clinical Learning Points

- The risk of ischaemic stroke in people with migraine with aura is twice compared to people without migraine.
- Migranous infarction is a recognized vascular event and is included in the International Classification of Headache Disorders. A significant increase in aura frequency or type, or first episode of migraine aura at an older age should all be considered red flags for migranous infarction.
- Genetic syndromes which causes both cerebral ischaemia and migraine are sometimes encountered in clinical practice CADASIL, CARASIL being more frequently seen than MELAS

Key Radiological Learning Points

- White matter hyper-intensities found in the deep or peri-ventricular white matter are noted in patients with migraine. These are not known to be a risk factor for ischaemic stroke [21, 22].
- Migrainous infarction is most commonly noted in the territory of the posterior circulation.

References

1. Oie LR, Kurth T, Gulati S, Dodick DW. Migraine and risk of stroke. J Neurol Neurosurg Psychiatry. 2020;91(6):593–604.
2. Harriott AM, Karakaya F, Ayata C. Headache after ischemic stroke: a systematic review and meta-analysis. Neurology. 2020;94(1):e75–86.

3. Etminan M, Takkouche B, Isorna FC, et al. Risk of ischaemic stroke in people with migraine: systematic review and meta-analysis of observational studies. BMJ. 2005;330:63.
4. Schürks M, Rist PM, Bigal ME, et al. Migraine and cardiovascular disease: systematic review and meta-analysis. BMJ. 2009;339:b3914.
5. Spector JT, Kahn SR, Jones MR, et al. Migraine headache and ischemic stroke risk: an updated meta-analysis. Am J Med. 2010;123:612–24.
6. Hu X, Zhou Y, Zhao H, et al. Migraine and the risk of stroke: an updated meta-analysis of prospective cohort studies. Neurol Sci. 2017;38:33–40.
7. Mahmoud AN, Mentias A, Elgendy AY, et al. Migraine and the risk of cardiovascular and cerebrovascular events: a meta-analysis of 16 cohort studies including 1 152 407 subjects. BMJ Open. 2018;8:e020498.
8. MacClellan LR, Giles W, Cole J, et al. Probable migraine with visual aura and risk of ischemic stroke: the stroke prevention in young women study. Stroke. 2007;38:2438–45.
9. Kurth T, Schürks M, Logroscino G, et al. Migraine frequency and risk of cardiovascular disease in women. Neurology. 2009;73:581–8.
10. Kurth T, Gaziano JM, Cook NR, et al. Migraine and risk of cardiovascular disease in women. JAMA. 2006;296:283–91.
11. Kurth T, Diener H-C. Migraine and stroke: perspectives for stroke physicians. Stroke. 2012;43:3421–6.
12. Ayata C, Lauritzen M, Depression S. Spreading depression, spreading depolarizations, and the cerebral vasculature. Physiol Rev. 2015;95:953–93.
13. Kurth T, Chabriat H, Bousser M-G. Migraine and stroke: a complex association with clinical implications. Lancet Neurol. 2012;11:92–100.
14. Winsvold BS, Bettella F, Witoelar A, et al. Shared genetic risk between migraine and coronary artery disease: a genome-wide analysis of common variants. PLoS One. 2017;12:e0185663.
15. Headache Classification Committee of the International Headache Society (IHS) The International classification of headache disorders, 3rd edition. Cephalalgia. 2018;38:1–211.
16. Kruit MC, Launer LJ, Ferrari MD, van Buchem MA. Infarcts in the posterior circulation territory in migraine. The population-based MRI CAMERA study. Brain. 2005;128(Pt 9):2068–77.
17. Wolf ME, Szabo K, Griebe M, et al. Clinical and MRI characteristics of acute migrainous infarction. Neurology. 2011;76:1911–7.
18. Sochurkova D, Moreau T, Lemesle M, Menassa M, Giroud M, Dumas R. Migraine history and migraine-induced stroke in the Dijon stroke registry. Neuroepidemiology. 1999;18(2):85–91.
19. Laurell K, Artto V, Bendtsen L, et al. Migrainous infarction: a Nordic multicenter study. Eur J Neurol. 2011;18(10):1220–6.
20. Arboix A, Massons J, Garcia-Eroles L, Oliveres M, Balcells M, Targa C. Migrainous cerebral infarction in the Sagrat Cor Hospital of Barcelona stroke registry. Cephalalgia. 2003;23(5):389–94.
21. Hedman C, Andersen AR, Andersson PG, et al. Symptoms of classic migraine attacks: modifications brought about by metoprolol. Cephalalgia. 1988;8:279–84.Lupus erythematosus: a case-control study. Cephalalgia. 2011;31:401–8.
22. Cheng CY, Cheng HM, Chen SP, Chung CP, Lin YY, Hu HH, Chen CH, Wang SJ. White matter hyperintensities in migraine: clinical significance and central pulsatile hemodynamic correlates. Cephalalgia. 2018;38(7):1225–36.

Chapter 6
A Case of Primary Post-Stroke Fatigue: Origins in Abnormal Sensorimotor Neural Network Activity

William De Doncker and Annapoorna Kuppuswamy

Clinical History

A 60-year-old, right-handed, female was admitted to University College London Hospital on the 22/07/2016 at the age of 54. She presented with mild left-sided upper motor neuron facial weakness. She had difficulties finding the right words despite no problem with speech production.

Examination

On admission, she had a Glasgow Coma Scale (GCS) of 15/15, normal visual fields, and muscle power of 5/5 throughout. Her pulse was 80 beats per minute, with a blood pressure of 158/96 mmHg and a temperature of 36.8 °C. Her fasting glucose was 5.5 mmol/l with a known vascular risk factor for stroke, raised cholesterol. She scored a 2 on the National Institute of Health Stroke Scale (NIHSS), which is indicative of a minor stroke. CT was unremarkable. MRI revealed a focus of restricted diffusion in the right external capsule just superior to the insular cortex, consistent with an acute focal infarct. Minor findings included mild chronic small vessel disease, indicated by minor background deep white matter and periventricular high signal on T2/FLAIR. There was no acute haemorrhage or hydrocephalus, and the ventricles were of normal size and configuration.

Upon discharge from University College London Hospital on the 24/07/2016 she was eating and drinking normally and was fully ambulant and walking unaided. She

W. De Doncker · A. Kuppuswamy (✉)
Department of Clinical and Movement Neuroscience, Institute of Neurology, University College London, London, UK
e-mail: william.doncker.11@ucl.ac.uk; a.kuppuswamy@ucl.ac.uk

S. K. Gill et al. (eds.), *Stroke Medicine*,
https://doi.org/10.1007/978-3-031-58188-5_6

was prescribed conventional blood thinners and high dose statins (Clopidogrel 75 mg once a day and Atorvastatin 40 mg once a day). She was then followed up in an outpatient clinic on the 17/10/2016 where her examination was normal, and was subsequently discharged.

Investigations

Our patient was identified as someone who suffered from post-stroke fatigue by the Effort Lab research team on the 16/05/2019. As there was no immediately obvious reason for her fatigue, she was selected for further investigations to investigate the cause of her fatigue.

Post-stroke fatigue that persists longer than / develops after 3 months post-stroke is not uncommon with a prevalence rate of up to 85% [1]. There are no established causes of chronic post-stroke fatigue. In the Effort Lab, to identify potential causes, we first perform a basic test battery of motor, cognitive and mood related tests to identify if fatigue is a primary or secondary manifestation.

Motor Tests

To ensure minimal physical impairment, she performed a grip strength test, the Nine Hole Peg Test (NHPT) and the Action Research Arm Test (ARAT), testing grip strength, manual dexterity, and gross upper limb function respectively [2, 3]. Her scores for each of the test are found in Table 6.1.

Cognitive Tests

To ensure minimal cognitive impairment, AO performed the Symbol Digits Modalities Test (SDMT), a primary measure of information processing speed, but also tests attention and memory [4]. In the coding section of the test, AO completed 63 symbols in 90 s, while in the copying section of the test, she completed 117

Table 6.1 Motor function and impairment scores of AO

Test	Affected hand	Unaffected hand	$\frac{\text{Affected Hand}}{\text{Unaffected Hand}} \times 100$
Grip Strength	13.16 kg	13.90 kg	94.72%
NHPT	11.75 seconds	11.17 s	95.06%
ARAT	57	57	100%

symbols in 60 s. Her overall SDMT score (number of correct responses per second for coding/ number of correct responses per second for copying) was 0.915, where anything below 2 is considered not excessively delayed.

Questionnaires for Mood and Fatigue

Depression and anxiety were assessed using the Hospital Anxiety and Depression Scale (HADS), a 14-item questionnaire with a depression and anxiety subscale were participants are asked to rate the degree to which the agree with a statement ranging from 0 (strongly disagree) to 3 (strongly agree). The total score for each subscale is calculated by adding up the score across the items. Our patient scored 6/21 for the Anxiety subscale and 8/21 for the Depression subscale.

Two measures of trait fatigue were used to quantify post-stroke fatigue. The Fatigue Severity Scale-7 (FSS-7), a 7-item instrument where each item is scored on a scale from 1 to 7, with 1 being strong disagreement and 7 being highest agreement [5]. The average score of the 7 statement scores represents the total fatigue score. It is generally agreed that anyone who scores greater than 4 suffers from fatigue and those greater than 5 present with severe fatigue [6]. She scored 5.14/7. The second measure of fatigue was the Neurological Fatigue Index—Stroke: a stroke specific fatigue 12 item inventory covering both physical and cognitive aspects of fatigue [7], with each item having a minimum score of 0 and a maximum score of 3. AO scored on average 1.83/3.

The motor, cognitive and questionnaire scores at the point of entry into the Effort Lab suggested that AO suffered from severe fatigue, despite good, symmetrical motor function, normal cognitive function and in the absence of anxiety and depression. Therefore, we concluded that AO presented with primary fatigue, and her fatigue was not secondary to motor, cognitive or mood related disorder. Although we did not test for other possible causes of fatigue such as metabolic disorders, or any other undiagnosed non-neurological disease, there were no other presenting symptoms to suspect any known aetiology of fatigue.

Detailed Examination of Sensorimotor Networks

Fatigue in the chronic phase of stroke has been proposed to be a disorder of network level dysfunction, specifically the sensorimotor networks [8–10]. Our patient performed a number of tests to understand if there has been any alterations in how sensory information (proprioceptive and visual) is being processed, whether such altered processing might affect how sensory input is perceived (greater effort perception in relation to physical and cognitive tasks) and whether temporary modulation of sensorimotor networks reduce fatigue?

AO visited the Effort Lab on several occasions over 2.5 years since her first referral, for various tests. In every visit, the FSS-7 measure was performed to check the fluctuation of fatigue over time (Fig. 6.1).

Resting Motor Thresholds

Despite good motor function, a stroke results in changes within sensorimotor networks [11]. A measure of motor network function, is the excitability of the motor cortex at rest often measured using non-invasive brain stimulation techniques such as Transcranial Magnetic Stimulation [12]. We measured the resting motor threshold (RMT), a measure of motor cortex excitability, in both hemispheres. RMT on the right (affected) hemisphere was 80% of maximum stimulator output (MSO) and RMT on the left (unaffected) hemisphere was 72% MSO. We recently showed that higher RMTs (lower motor cortex excitability) is associated with greater post-stroke fatigue [13]. Although there are no normative values for RMT in the healthy population, on average, 45%-55% MSO is considered a normal threshold range for motor cortex excitability in healthy humans [14]. Our patient presented with higher than normal threshold, specifically on her affected hemisphere, suggesting a possible reconfiguration of sensorimotor networks as the basis of her high levels of fatigue.

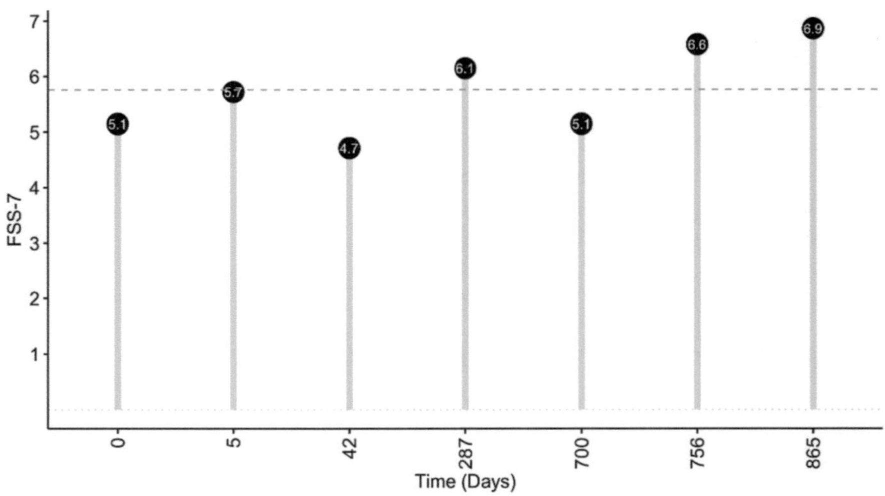

Fig. 6.1 In the x-axis the time points at which FSS-7 was administered is shown in days, with 0 being the day of admission to Effort Lab on the 16th of May 2019. The y-axis is the FSS-7 scale score. The dotted horizontal line shows the average fatigue over 865 days

Effort Perception

A significant feature of post-stroke fatigue is the report of excessive effort needed to complete simple daily activities, such as brushing teeth, taking a shower, preparing a meal etc. Some patients attribute this to greater concentration required to perform activities, and others attribute it to the physical effort needed to complete the tasks. Physical effort perception is heightened in post-stroke fatigue, specifically in relation to low force muscle contractions. We tested effort perception in a hand-grip task at 3 different force levels, 20% of maximal voluntary force (MVF), 40% MVF and 60% MVF. Figure 6.2 shows our patient's effort perception scores in the grip force task. We show that in the low force condition (20% MVF) there is an effect of fatigue on effort perception, however, in medium and high forces (40% and 60% MVF) there was no significant relationship [15].

Processing of Distractors

Stroke survivors with fatigue often report being overwhelmed by sensory stimuli, such as, finding lights being overly bright, or sounds being overly loud, and inability to filter out irrelevant conversations in a crowded space such as a pub. A selective

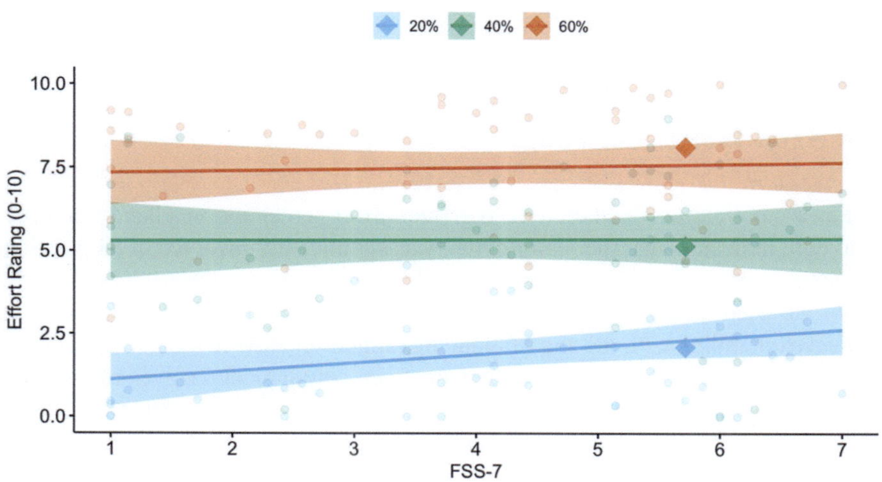

Fig. 6.2 The x-axis shows the FSS-7 scores of individual participants and y-axis shows the perceived effort rating on a VAS scale of 1-10. This plot shows data from a cohort of 57 stroke survivors with varying levels of fatigue and their associated effort levels for 20% MVF (blue dots), 40% MVF (green dots) and 60% MVF (red dots). AO's scores in the three effort levels is shown in large filled diamonds

attention visual task with and without distractors, and simultaneous EEG, was used to investigate if, in our patient, there was a greater processing of distractors as suggested by self-report. The task involved responding to a target stimulus within a stream of consecutively presented target and non-target stimuli. The attentional load of the task was increased by increasing the visual features of the target. For example, in the low load condition, she had to press a button every time she saw a red cross, whereas in the high load condition, she had to press a button not just based on the colour of the target but also the orientation of the target, such as, a red cross but only when it is inverted and not straight. The distractor was a flickering (10 Hz) checkerboard that surrounded the stimulus stream. The oscillating frequency of the distractor induces a 10 Hz power in the visual cortex of the EEG recording and is a measure of distractor processing. Normally, with increasing load, the distractors are processed less as the task at hand requires greater attention (perceptual load theory [16]) and the expectation was that, in those with high fatigue increasing load does not have an effect on distractor processing (no change in induced 10 Hz power with increasing load). Behaviourally, both reaction time and accuracy was expected to be modulated by fatigue. In Fig. 6.3, we show her responses to the visual selective attention task. AO showed a significant reduction in accuracy and response time of responses in the high load condition with distractors. In the EEG results, the induced 10 Hz power in the high load condition did not reduce in line with increasing load. This suggests that the distractor was being processed at the expense of the target stimuli. Other high fatigue patients also showed a similar profile unlike those with low fatigue.

Effect of Anodal Transcranial Direct Current Stimulation (tDCS) on Post-Stroke Fatigue

Reduced motor cortex excitability and greater effort perception in a hand grip task, were both indicators that the motor cortex was significantly involved in fatigue that our patient reported. She was enrolled into an experimental interventional study where we used anodal tDCS, an established non-invasive technique to modulate cortical excitability, with the aim of reducing fatigue severity. In the random allocation of participant to the real or the sham treatment, our patient received real anodal tDCS at 2 mA for 40 min in two sessions in a single day. The electrode configuration was a bilateral M1 configuration with extra-chephalic cathode placement. For further details of the study please see De Doncker et al., 2021 [17]. After having received anodal tDCS the FSS-7 score dropped from 5.71/7 to 4.14/7 one week after the stimulation session. A month later, FSS-7 remained reduced at 4.71/7. The resting motor thresholds on the affected side dropped from 80% MSO to 76% MSO, while there was no change immediately after stimulation of the RMT on the unaffected side. At one-week post-stimulation, RMT of the affected side went back up

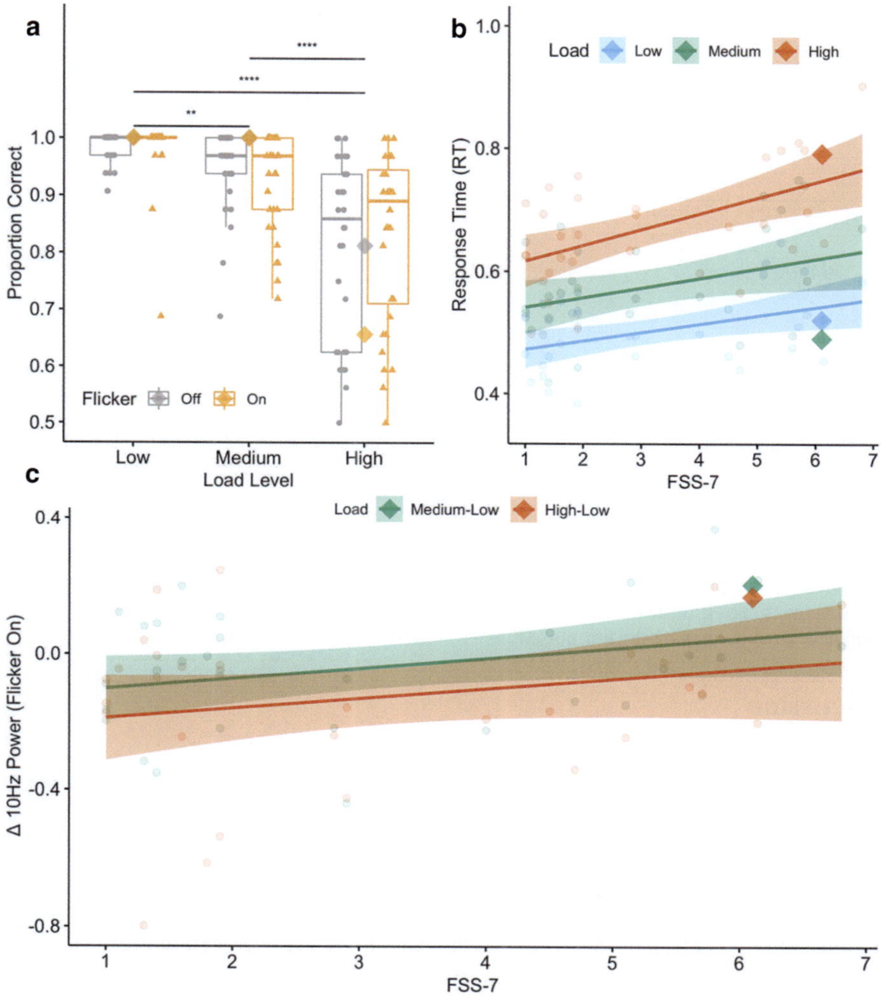

Fig. 6.3 (**a**) The response accuracy (proportion correct—y-axis) is shown for all three load conditions (x-axis) in the presence (ochre) or absence (grey) of a flickering distractor. Proportion correct was significantly lower with increasing load, with no effect of flicker. (**b**) Response Time (y-axis) is shown to increase significantly with increase in fatigue levels (FSS-7, x-axis) in the flicker ON condition. (**c**) The decrease in 10 Hz power (Δ10Hz power) from medium to low (green) and high to low (red) load is correlated to fatigue levels (FSS-7), the higher the fatigue, the smaller is the decrease in distractor related power as load increases whether from low to medium or from low to high. Our patient's scores in all panels are shown as large, filled diamonds

to 80% MSO while the RMT of the unaffected side dropped to 68% MSO. A month later, RMT of the unaffected side dropped further to 66% MSO, and RMT of the affected side climbed up to 84% MSO. Perceived effort also showed a drop at the week time point, with the effect wearing out by the month time point (Fig. 6.4).

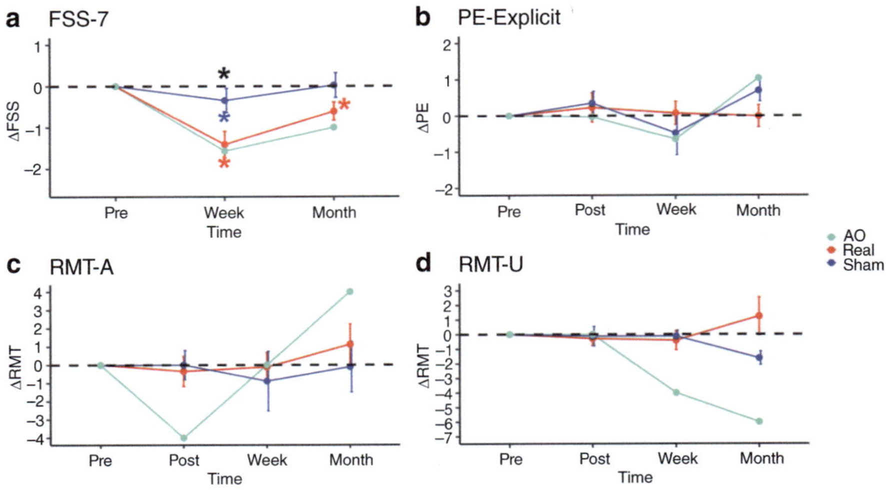

Fig. 6.4 Changes in trait fatigue (**a**), explicit perceived effort (**b**), resting motor threshold of the affected and unaffected hemisphere (**c**, **d**) compared to baseline (pre stimulation time point) across the different time points for both the real (red) and sham (blue) stimulation group. Error bars represent standard error of the means. Significance levels are indicated by * ($p < 0.05$). AO's scores in all panels are indicated by the turquoise line

Discussion

In our case, a 60-year-old female with minimal physical and cognitive impairment, and no signs of anxiety or depression presented with severe post-stroke fatigue 3 years after her stroke. Our investigation of the sensorimotor network shows that fatigue might be driven by altered motor control that was reflected in changes in biomarkers of motor function i.e. motor cortex excitability and motor perception (increase in perception of effort for a motor task). We also showed that an intervention aimed at increasing motor cortex excitability resulted in a significant drop in fatigue levels a week post-intervention which was maintained at a month post-intervention. We suggest that in stroke survivors who present with high levels of post-stroke fatigue, where there is no obvious cause, altered sensorimotor network function could explain high levels of fatigue. A possible effective intervention is non-invasive brain stimulation. We also propose that reduced excitability may reflect a reduced capacity to attenuate incoming sensory information from contraction muscles (poor sensory attenuation) which might then explain why a low force muscle contraction is experienced as being more effortful, which is reflected in the perceived exertion score. For a more detailed discussion of the sensory attenuation hypothesis of pathological fatigue please refer to Kuppuswamy, 2017 and 2021 [8, 9].

Key Clinical Learning Points

- Post-stroke fatigue (PSF) occurs in young strokes (<60 years).
- Stroke survivors with PSF often have good motor and cognitive function.
- Stroke survivors with PSF do not always suffer from anxiety or depression
- PSF can persists for more than 5 years in some stroke survivors
- PSF is relatively stable over time, especially in the chronic phase (>1 year)

Key Behavioural and Neurophysiological Learning Points

- Stroke survivors with PSF perceive a given muscle contraction to be more effortful than someone without PSF.
- Stroke survivors with PSF exhibit slowed reaction times.
- Stroke survivors with PSF have low motor cortical excitability.
- With greater PSF, there is higher processing of task-irrelevant sensory stimuli.
- Increasing motor cortex excitability can significantly reduce fatigue levels.

References

1. Cumming TB, Packer M, Kramer SF, English C. The prevalence of fatigue after stroke: a systematic review and meta-analysis. Int J Stroke. 2016;11(9):968–77.
2. Kellor M, Frost J, Silberberg N, Iversen I, Cummings R. Hand strength and dexterity. Am J Occup Ther. 1971;25(2):77–83.
3. Nijland R, van Wegen E, Verbunt J, van Wijk R, van Kordelaar J, Kwakkel G. A comparison of two validated tests for upper limb function after stroke: the Wolf Motor function test and the action research arm test. J Rehabil Med. 2010;42(7):694–6.
4. Costa SL, Genova HM, DeLuca J, Chiaravalloti ND. Information processing speed in multiple sclerosis: past, present, and future. Mult Scler. 2017;23(6):772–89.
5. Johansson S, Kottorp A, Lee KA, Gay CL, Lerdal A. Can the fatigue severity scale 7-item version be used across different patient populations as a generic fatigue measure—a comparative study using a Rasch model approach. Health Qual Life Outcomes. 2014;12:24.
6. Valko PO, Bassetti CL, Bloch KE, Held U, Baumann CR. Validation of the fatigue severity scale in a Swiss cohort. Sleep. 2008;31(11):1601–7.
7. Mills RJ, Pallant JF, Koufali M, Sharma A, Day S, Tennant A, et al. Validation of the neurological fatigue index for stroke (NFI-stroke). Health Qual Life Outcomes. 2012;10:51.
8. Kuppuswamy A. The fatigue conundrum. Brain. 2017;140(8):2240–5.
9. Kuppuswamy A. The neurobiology of pathological fatigue: new models, new questions. Neuroscientist. 2021:1073858420985447.
10. De Doncker W, Dantzer R, Ormstad H, Kuppuswamy A. Mechanisms of poststroke fatigue. J Neurol Neurosurg Psychiatry. 2018;89(3):287–93.
11. McDonnell MN, Stinear CM. TMS measures of motor cortex function after stroke: a meta-analysis. Brain Stimul. 2017;10(4):721–34.
12. Terao Y, Ugawa Y. Basic mechanisms of TMS. J Clin Neurophysiol. 2002;19(4):322–43.

13. Kuppuswamy A, Clark EV, Turner IF, Rothwell JC, Ward NS. Post-stroke fatigue: a deficit in corticomotor excitability? Brain. 2015;138(Pt 1):136–48.
14. Wassermann EM. Variation in the response to transcranial magnetic brain stimulation in the general population. Clin Neurophysiol. 2002;113(7):1165–71.
15. Doncker WD, Charles L, Ondobaka S, Kuppuswamy A. Exploring the relationship between effort perception and poststroke fatigue. Neurology. 2020;95(24):e3321–e30.
16. Lavie N. Perceptual load as a necessary condition for selective attention. J Exp Psychol Hum Percept Perform. 1995;21(3):451–68.
17. De Doncker W, Ondobaka S, Kuppuswamy A. Effect of transcranial direct current stimulation on post-stroke fatigue. J Neurol. 2021;17

Chapter 7
Stroke and Endocarditis

Talal Al-Mayhani, Robert Simister, and Sumanjit K. Gill

A 39-year-old right-handed woman complained of lethargy, chest pain and dyspnoea, for 1 week. She was then found unconscious in the street by her partner, with signs of cocaine and buprenorphine overdose, and was brought to the hospital. Her past medical history included alcohol dependence, intravenous substance abuse, hepatitis C, multiple DVTs, iron deficiency anaemia, recurrent folliculitis and staphylococcal groin abscesses.

Examination and Localization

On arrival to the emergency department, she was pyrexic at 37.9 °C with a reduced level of consciousness—Glasgow coma score of 11/15. Chest auscultation revealed notable diastolic murmur. Showing no signs of improvement after administration of Naloxone, she became combative, and new symptoms developed with reduced movements in the right hemibody. The neurological assessment revealed weakness

T. Al-Mayhani (✉)
Comprehensive Stroke Unit, National Hospital for Neurology and Neurosurgery, Queen Square, London, UK

R. Simister
Comprehensive Stroke Service, The National Hospital for Neurology and Neurosurgery, UCLH Foundation Trust, Stroke Research Centre, London, UK

S. K. Gill
Institute of Neurology, UCL, National Hospital for Neurology and Neurosurgery, London, UK

S. K. Gill et al. (eds.), *Stroke Medicine*,
https://doi.org/10.1007/978-3-031-58188-5_7

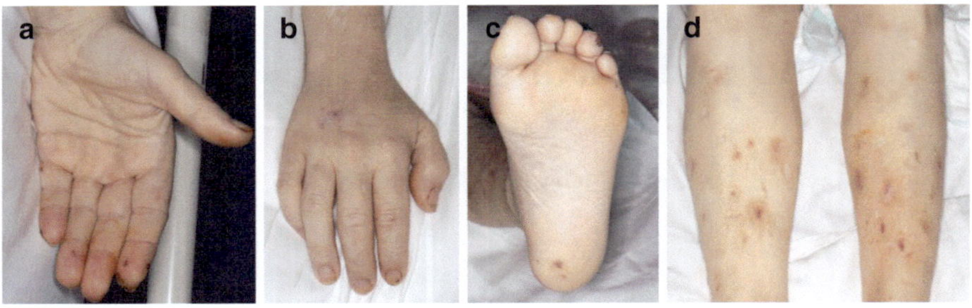

Fig. 7.1 widespread skin lesions. (**a**) Osler nodes in the left finger tips. (**b**) subungual splinter hemorrhages in the right hand. (**c**) Janeway lesions on the sole of the foot (**d**) erythema nodosum on shins

in the right side of the face, sparing the forehead, possible neglect to the right and no spontaneous movements in the right upper or lower limb. There were widespread skin lesions (Fig. 7.1).

Investigations and Management

The blood tests were deranged with haemoglobin 72 g/L, white cell count 25 × 10 * 9/L (predominantly neutrophils), c-reactive protein 191 mg/L, urea 17 mg/dL. The 12 L ECG showed sinus tachycardia with ST segment elevation. The patient was commenced on empirical antibiotics (Vancomycin, Rifampicin and Linezolid) for suspected endocarditis after blood cultures were taken.

The plain CT head scan showed bilateral multifocal areas of low attenuation in both hemispheres, raising suspicion of acute infarcts (Fig. 7.2a). Bedside echocardiogram showed significant tricuspid and aortic valvular disease: thickened tricuspid valve with moderate tricuspid regurgitation, a thickened aortic valve with mobile structures attached to it and torrential aortic regurgitation.

She underwent emergency tissue aortic valve replacement with aortic root patch repair. During the operation pyo-pericardium was detected and drained and a left ventricular thrombus was found.

She was commenced on anticoagulation with low molecular weight heparin (LMWH) that was switched later to Warfarin, given the left ventricular thrombus and the high risk of further thrombotic events.

MRI head with contrast 10 days later showed multifocal infarcts, haemorrhages and ring enhancing lesions, indicating abscesses forming within the embolic infarcts (Fig. 7.2b–f).

The CT chest, abdomen and pelvis revealed intra-abdominal and splenic abscesses, and the CT angiogram revealed multiple mycotic aneurysms in the splenic, renal and intracranial arteries.

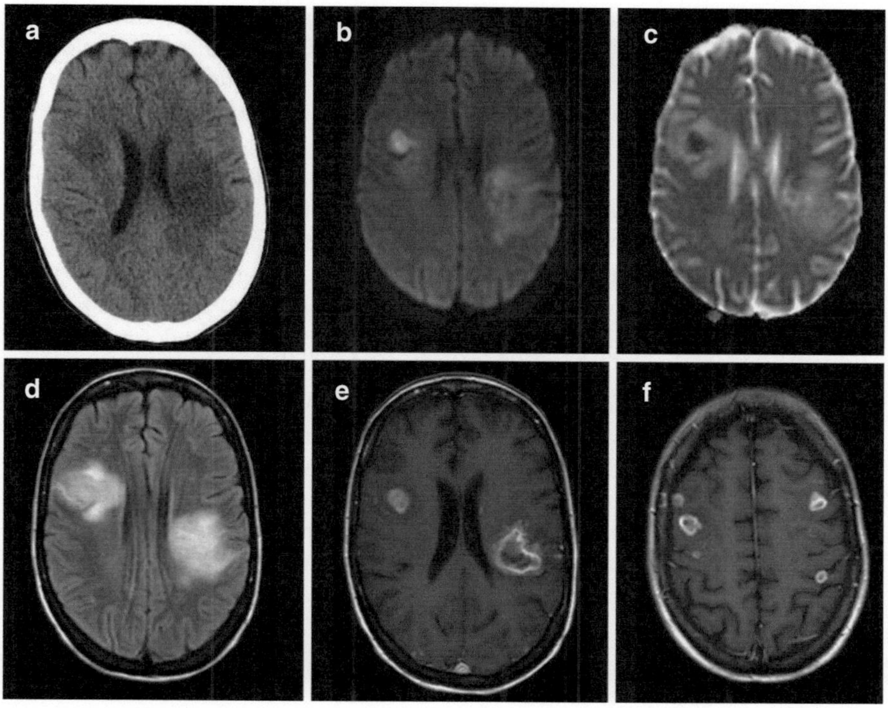

Fig. 7.2 (**a**) axial CT head with no contrast showing multifocal parenchymal hypodensities and raising suspicion of ischemic lesions. (**b, c**) axial MRI head DWI and ADC sequences showing foci of restricted diffusion in the right frontal lobe, and to less extent in the left centrum semiovale, indicating ischaemic lesions. (**d**) axial MRI head T2-weighted image showing high intensity areas. (**e, f**) axial MRI head T1-weighted images with contrast showing multifocal ring enhancing lesions, some of the them are inside the lesions with restricted diffusion, indicating septic infarcts

The patient admission was complicated by seizures, and Levetiracetam was started with complete seizure cessation.

She responded well to antibiotics with resolution of abscesses. Her level of function continued to improve and she was discharged after a period of rehabilitation. At the point of discharge she was able to communicate and swallow normally and mobilise indoors using a frame, outdoors with a wheelchair. She achieved complete cessation of drug and alcohol use.

Discussion

Classically, endocarditis presents with fever, new cardiac murmur and raised inflammatory markers. The presentation can be insidious and a high index of suspicion should be exercised in immunocompromised or patients considered at higher risk of developing infective endocarditis [1]. The higher risk group includes patients with exogenous implants i.e. intravenous catheters, cardiac implantable devices, valvular heart disease, prosthetic valves and cardiomyopathies, noting that rheumatic fever is still one of the leading risk factors of endocarditis in the developing countries. Intravenous substance abuse, as in the case presented here is a major risk factor in the developed world.

The vast majority of cases are caused by bacteria staphylococcus aureus (70% of cases), streptococcus and enterococcus are among the most common pathogens. Less common bacterial causes can also be encountered in the appropriate context, such as brucella and the HACEK complex (haemophilus, aggregiatibacter, cardiobacterium, eikinella, kingella). Fungi (candida and aspergillus) and rickettsia (coxiella burnetti) should also be suspected in blood culture negative endocarditis.

Importantly, non-infective, endocarditis may develop in context of rheumatological and autoimmune diseases (as in anti-phospholipids syndrome, and lupus' Libman-Sacks endocarditis), inflammatory conditions (Loeffler eosinophilia) or malignancy (marantic endocarditis). This still promotes a thrombogenic state [1].

As illustrated in the case above, infective endocarditis is a well-reported complication of intravenous substance abuse, due to combination of non-hygienic paraphernalia, use of dirty needles and contaminated injected materials.

When endocarditis occurs as a complication of intravenous substance abuse, the neurological involvement is over-represented [2]. It is therefore recommended to perform neuroimaging in all patients with endocarditis, regardless of the presence or absence of the neurological symptoms or signs.

The neurological manifestations of endocarditis have usually septic embolic basis, leading to direct occlusion of the small arteries, or infection of the wall of blood vessels (by damaging the vasa vasorum rather than the endothelia) with subsequent formation of mycotic aneurysm, rupture and haemorrhage or direct invasion of the parenchyma. Cerebral microbleeds are found in 60% of patients and in those with a subacute onset can be a useful clue [3]. In addition to septic emboli, endocarditis in patients with substance abuse may also develop neurological complications due to the type of the drug (vasculitis and, sympathomimetics resulting in vasospasm and intracranial bleeding), or the filler substances (starch and talc may cause direct arterial occlusions).

Clinically, the cerebral involvement by multifocal septic emboli may be subtle with headache, change in mentation and clouded consciousness, and encephalopathic or neuropsychiatric features without focal deficits. These symptoms can also be multifactorial in context of pyrexia and cardiac failure leading to delirium or hypotension and hypoperfusion.

Endocarditis symptoms may also include seizures, infarction of the spinal cord, neuropathies (cranial and peripheral), discitis, spondylitis and epidural collections [4, 5].

Ischaemic events due to the septic emboli is perhaps the most common neurological complication encountered in endocarditis patients, and the middle cerebral artery territory is the most commonly involved. Higher rate of haemorrhagic transformation has been noted. Septic infarcts can also be seen when abscesses develop within the site of ischaemic stroke [1].

Subarachnoid and, more commonly, intracerebral haemorrhages, can be encountered due to the haematological disturbance associated with systemic illness (such as thrombocytopenia and DIC), but more directly to rupture of necrotic intracranial vessels, haemorrhagic transformation of infarcts or mycotic aneurysms leak or rupture [1].

The incidence of clinically detectable mycotic aneurysms (or more accurately infectious aneurysms) is reported around 2–9% of infective endocarditis cases [6], although the rate is much higher in postmortem studies. In those cases where aneurysm is identified they are multiple in 20% [6].

In 2015, the American Heart Association and American College of Cardiology (AHA/ACC) published a statement that summarized the treatment guidelines [7]. The ongoing risk of septic emboli causing spongy necrotic ischaemic lesions with a propensity to bleed in association with intracerebral haemorrhage and aneurysms vulnerable to rupture mean that this group of patients must be carefully managed. Antibiotics remains the mainstay of treatment, as the risk of new septic emboli is reduced to 15% and 4%, in the first and second week after initiating the antibiotics, respectively [4]. Thrombectomy can be offered in case of ischaemic stroke but thrombolytic therapy cannot—the risk of intracranial bleed is too high. Emergency cardiothoracic surgery is indicated in case of severe cardiac dysfunction, significant vegetations and high risk of septic emboli such decisions are usually taken after careful MDT discussion taking into account their degree of neurological deficit.

However, anticoagulation can be offered on case-by-case basis, for instance, to patients with prosthetic valves, or high thrombotic risk due to cardiac pathologies such as large intraventricular thrombus (as in our case).

About a third of the mycotic aneurysms regress completely with antibiotics [7], others remain unchanged, while a small proportion may form or even rupture years after full recovery from endocarditis. Serial angiography is therefore recommended, although there are no clear guidelines regarding the long-term follow up. Rarely, radiological intravascular intervention or surgical clipping would be offered in selected cases of mycotic aneurysms so all must be discussed with neurosurgery.

The prognosis remains guarded in general. Although it varies between studies, the mortality is significant with estimated overall figure of 20–40% [8]. Having neurological complications double the mortality rate in endocarditis patients. Notably, the rate is even much higher in patients with substance abuse, partly due to the higher incidence of neurological involvement, and partly due to the generally poor health baseline, alcohol dependence, malnutrition and HIV status [9].

Key Clinical Learning Points

- Careful history should be taken in all stroke patients to identify any known risk factors such as cardiac or dental procedures and substance misuse.
- All patients who present with stroke should have their temperature checked and a full examination for vasculitic stigmata (Janeway lesions, Roth spots and Oslers nodes)

- The management of endocarditis requires a multidisciplinary input by infectious disease, microbiology, neurology/stroke medicine, neurosurgery, cardiology, cardiothoracic surgery, psychiatry and rehabilitation teams, communication is key
- The risk of intracerebral haemorrhage is high and thrombolysis is contraindicated and anti platelets or anti coagulation are used with caution.

Key Radiological Learning Points

- Imaging of organs other than the heart and brain (CT chest, abdomen and pelvis with contrast) is necessary to look for septic emboli or seeded infection in the form of abscess.
- CTA or MRA of the intra and extracranial vessels will demonstrate any mycotic aneurysms which will contribute to the risk of haemorrhage.
- MRI with blood sensitive sequences i.e. susceptibility weighted imaging will demonstrate microbleeds/larger areas of haemorrhages.

References

1. Rajani R, Klein J. Infective endocarditis : a contemporary update. Clin Med (Lond). 2020;20(1):31–5.
2. Pruitt A. 114 Endocarditis (Infective and. Neurological Therapeutics: Principles and Practice. 2006 Apr 20;1:1393.
3. Jiad E, Gill SK, Krutikov M, et al. When the heart rules the head: ischaemic stroke and intracerebral haemorrhage complicating infective endocarditis. Pract Neurol. 2017;17:28–34.
4. Rizzi M, Ravasio V, et al. Investigators of the Italian Study on Endocarditis. Predicting the occurrence of embolic events: an analysis of 1456 episodes of infective endocarditis from the Italian Study on Endocarditis (SEI). BMC Infect Dis. 2014;14:230.
5. Habib G, Erba PA, Lung B, et al. EURO-ENDO Investigators. Clinical presentation, aetiology and outcome of infective endocarditis. Results of the ESC-EORP EURO-ENDO (European infective endocarditis) registry: a prospective cohort study. Eur Heart J. 2019;40(39):3222–32.
6. Hui FK, Bain M, et al. Mycotic aneurysm detection rates with cerebral angiography in patients with infective endocarditis. J Neurointerv Surg. 2015;7(6):449–52.
7. Baddour LM, Wilson WR. Infective endocarditis in adults: diagnosis, antimicrobial therapy, and management of complications: a scientific statement for healthcare professionals from the American Heart Association. Circulation. 2015;132:1435–86.
8. Abegaz TM, Bhagavathula AS, et al. Short- and long-term outcomes in infective endocarditis patients: a systematic review and meta-analysis. BMC Cardiovasc Disord. 2017;17:291.
9. Brown PD, Levine DP. Infective endocarditis in the injection drug user. Infect Dis Clin N Am. 2002;16(3):645–65.

Chapter 8
Sudden Onset Focal Neurology: A Cardiac Cause

Benjamin Sacks, Sanjay Budhdeo, Timothy Prossor, Vishal Vyas, and Salman Haider

Clinical History

An 86 year old woman was referred to the Emergency Stroke Unit with aphasia, anisocoria and dizziness. Her husband reported that for the past few days she had been more withdrawn and verbalising less than usual. The patient did not report any sensory disturbance or visual impairment. She had a past medical history of type 2 diabetes mellitus, hypertension, hypercholesterolaemia, cholecystectomy and previous breast cancer, for which she had received a mastectomy 12 years prior. She was a non-smoker and did not drink alcohol. She lived with her husband and was normally independent in all activities of daily living.

B. Sacks (✉) · T. Prossor · S. Haider
Department of Stroke Medicine, National Hospital for Neurology & Neurosurgery, London, UK
e-mail: benjamin.sacks@ucl.ac.uk; timothy.prossor@nhs.net; salman.haider@nhs.net

S. Budhdeo
Department of Stroke Medicine, National Hospital for Neurology & Neurosurgery, London, UK

Department of Clinical and Movement Neuroscience, University College London, London, UK
e-mail: sanjay.budhdeo@nhs.net

V. Vyas
Department of Cardiology, St Bartholomew's Hospital, Barts Health NHS Trust, London, UK
e-mail: vishal.vyas@nhs.net

S. K. Gill et al. (eds.), *Stroke Medicine*,
https://doi.org/10.1007/978-3-031-58188-5_8

Examination

On initial assessment by the paramedics she was noted to be tachypnoeic, diaphoretic and found to be in atrial fibrillation on her electrocardiogram (ECG) with a ventricular rate of 76 bpm. Examination revealed a left-sided facial droop and anisocoria . On arrival in the emergency stroke unit she was found to have a dense right-sided weakness, expressive aphasia and significant anisocoria. She scored 15 on the National Institute of Health Stroke Scale. Her neurological symptoms were fluctuant, with intermittent episodes of aphasia, anisocoria and hemiplegia.

Investigations

At the time of admission, routine blood tests including C-reactive protein, renal function, liver function and ammonia levels were all within normal range. Her white cell count was raised at 14×10^9 (neutrophilia) and her lactate was 2.6 mmol/L on a venous blood gas. Her capillary blood glucose was 15.3 mmol/L. Computed tomography (CT) of her head demonstrated no acute intracranial pathology. CT angiography of her intracranial vessels was performed and did not identify any proximal arterial occlusion or background steno-occlusive disease. As she was only 3 h from symptom onset and the diagnosis remained unclear, she had an MRI scan with abbreviated sequences to assess her suitability for thrombolysis. This demonstrated no matched diffusion weighted imaging (DWI) and apparent diffusion coefficient (ADC) changes, essentially ruling out acute stroke.

Clinical Narrative

Shortly after presentation, the patient had a progressive, rapid decline in consciousness. Within minutes, she had a GCS of 3 with agonal breathing, pallor and no detectable peripheral or central puse. On commencing chest compressions her consciousness returned within 1 min; cardiac monitoring subsequently demonstrated atrial fibrillation that spontaneously terminated before treatment could be administered. She went on to have further episodes of loss of consciousness lasting 2–3 min, followed by short-lasting atrial fibrillation, which spontaneously reverted to sinus rhythm. In between episodes, she was in sinus rhythm.

Her neurology continued to fluctuate with variable pupil size and reactivity, improvement in aphasia and near-complete resolution of her right sided weakness. She was reacting to threat bilaterally, had full range of eye movements, intact and equal facial sensation to pinprick, intact and equal facial movements, normal power of sternocleidomastoid and trapezius, with a central position of her tongue and uvula. Her left and right upper and lower limb power was 4/5 between episodes of dense right sided weakness. She had symmetrical and equal reflexes throughout the upper and lower limbs, along with downgoing plantars bilaterally. She was transferred to the intensive care unit for cardiac monitoring.

She had serial ECGs, initially demonstrating borderline first degree heart block with a PR interval of 200 ms and prolonged QTc at 494 ms (Fig. 8.1). During subsequent episodes of loss of consciousness, her ECGs demonstrated recurrent third degree atrioventricular (AV) block with ventricular standstill as evidenced by P waves without any corresponding QRS complexes (Fig. 8.2), followed by a short period of sinus tachycardia transitioning into complete heart block with a narrow complex ventricular escape rhythm (Fig. 8.3).

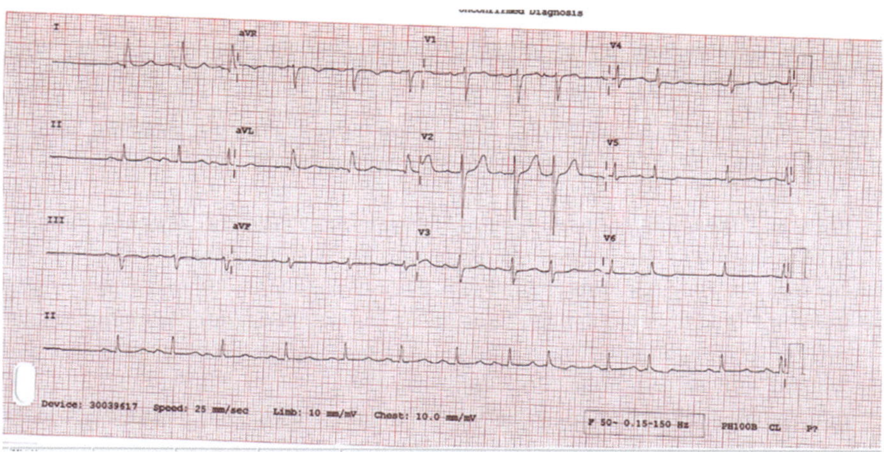

Fig. 8.1 Baseline ECG demonstrating sinus rhythm with first degree atrioventricular block and prolonged QTc

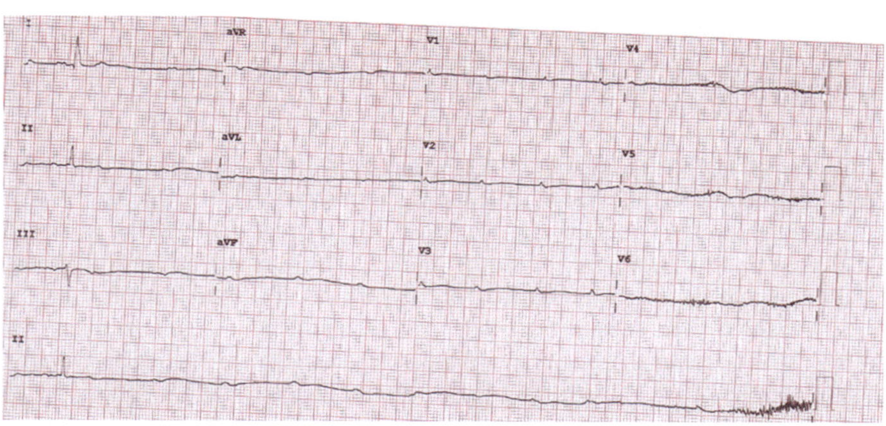

Fig. 8.2 ECG during an episode of loss of consciousness. Third degree atrioventricular block. P waves are visible with no evidence of ventricular conduction

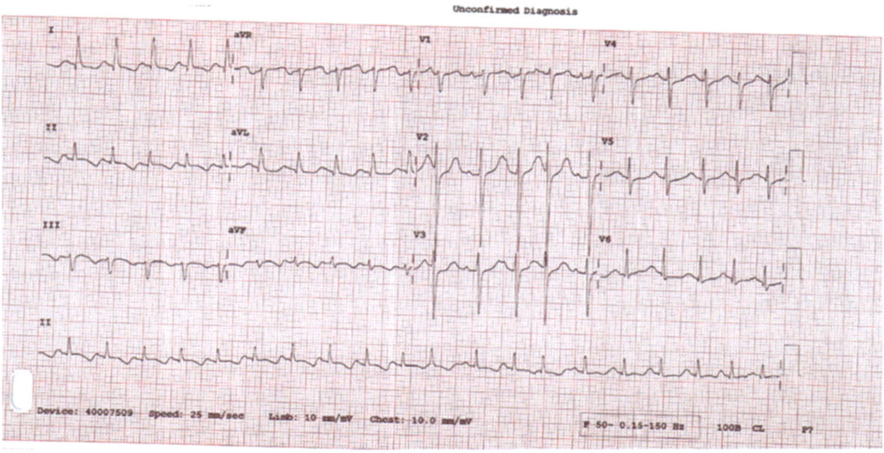

Fig. 8.3 ECG following episode of loss of consciousness. Sinus tachycardia transitions into third degree atrioventricular block with narrow complex ventricular escape

In view of the complete heart block with ventricular standstill, she was immediately discussed with the local cardiology unit at St Bartholomew's Hospital for emergency transfer. An isoprenaline infusion was commenced and transfer was arranged for emergency pacing. She went on to have a dual-chamber pacemaker inserted at the St Bartholomew's Hospital cardiac electrophysiology unit and was discharged without complication the following day.

Her neurological presentation was felt to be secondary to transient cerebral ischaemia secondary to short episodes of ventricular standstill associated with her third degree AV block leading to loss of sufficient cardiac output.

Case Discussion

Stroke Mimics

Ischaemic strokes are a common cause of severe mortality and morbidity. Due to the time-dependent nature of the available recanalisation options, the rapid assessment of stroke syndromes is paramount. However, due to the variable nature of stroke syndromes and the potential for stroke mimics, misdiagnosis remains common. Stroke assessment tools are designed to prevent missed strokes and therefore have a higher sensitivity than specificity, compounding the problem of stroke mimicry [1]. Around 26% of patients presenting with a suspected stroke are subsequently found to have a stroke mimic [2]. In a retrospective review of nearly 78,000 stroke patients across the United States, 3.5% of patients that received intravenous thrombolysis ended up with a non-stroke diagnosis. Patients with stroke mimics have a lower risk of symptomatic intracranial haemorrhage than stroke patients [3].

Stroke Mimic Aetiologies

The most common differential diagnoses of suspected stroke are seizures, syncope, sepsis, space occupying lesions, metabolic disturbance, migraine and functional disorders (see Fig. 8.4) [2]. Neurological conditions comprise the bulk of stroke mimics, the commonest being seizures, migraine and middle ear conditions, in descending order of incidence. Cardiovascular pathology is implicated in 11% of SMs and psychiatric conditions in 10%. It is worth noting that nearly one third of SM cases remain without a formal diagnosis [3].

Management of Conduction Block

Bradyarrhythmias are the most likely dysrhythmia to present with focal neurology. Third degree AV block is the most severe form of bradyarrhythmia and, with ventricular standstill, is a class I indication for emergency pacing. Prompt recognition of this potentially fatal but treatable condition is vital [4]. The acute management involves positive chronotropes, such as isoprenaline, to increase the heart rate and restore blood pressure. Of note, intermittent tachyarrhythmias are a recognized phenomenon and are usually reactive. Restoration of normal heart rate should prevent reactive tachyarrhythmias and they are not a contraindication to cautious isoprenaline administration. If there is no response to pharmacological therapy then emergency transcutaneous pacing is indicated, however this is only an interim measure to aid the transfer of patients to a cardiac centre with capability for emergency permanent pacemaker (PPM) insertion. Third degree AV block, even without ventricular standstill, still requires close cardiac monitoring and urgent PPM implantation.

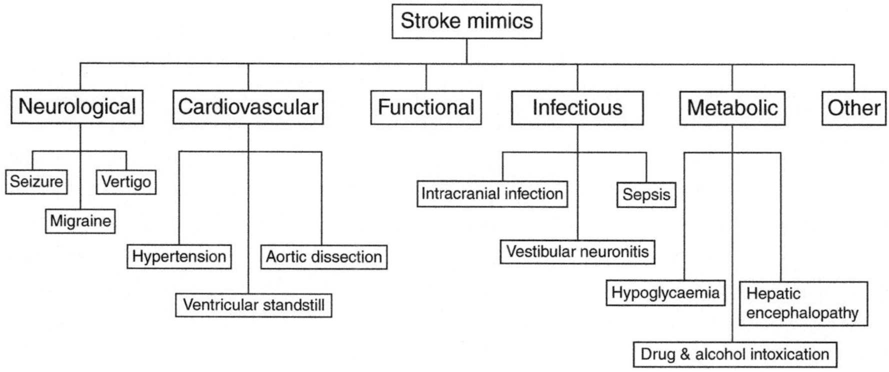

Fig. 8.4 Common differential diagnoses for suspected strokes

The most common cause of advanced AV block in the elderly is degenerative changes of the cardiac conduction system, and this is likely the aetiology in the case described above. Aside from ischaemia-related AV block, in younger patients, infiltrative conditions such as sarcoidosis and amyloidosis or cardiomyopathies such as hypertrophic cardiomyopathy and arrhythmogenic right ventricular cardiomyopathy should be considered [5]. Structural imaging of the heart with cardiac magnetic resonance imaging and echocardiography can assist in this diagnosis. In an otherwise well young person with no evidence of pre-existing structural heart disease, those with a history of tick bites, erythema migrans or symptoms of neuroborreliosis, borrelia serology [6] should be sent and antibiotic treatment commenced.

Conduction Block with Focal Neurology

During periods of systemic hypotension, focal neurology is a previously described but frequently overlooked phenomenon [7]. We hypothesise that the focal neurological deficits in this case were due to transient cerebral hypoperfusion secondary to ventricular pauses in the context of intermittent, third degree AV conduction block. Third degree AV block with ventricular standstill is more commonly associated with symptoms of global cerebral hypoperfusion such as dizziness, syncope and visual loss, however it may present with focal neurology [8, 9]. In a review of 290 patients with cardiac arrhythmias requiring pacemaker insertion, 81% reported general neurological symptoms such as syncope, pre-syncope, dizziness and seizures; 1% had focal neurological symptoms, including three cases of fluctuant dysphasia with hemiparesis, as in the case described above [10]. Focal neurological symptoms have also been observed in the context of pacemaker malfunctions [11]. In all of these cases, as in ours, treatment of the underlying bradyarrhythmia led to resolution of the neurology.

In patients with underlying cerebrovascular disease, systemic hypotension is thought to preferentially affect the cerebral tissue supplied by stenotic vessels, resulting in focal neurological deficits. This case serves as a reminder that, in the absence of steno-occlusive disease, focal neurology can still be a presenting symptom of cardiac arrhythmia. The heterogeneous, fluctuant neurological deficits that we observed are likely due to a lack of territory-specific regions of vulnerability.

The described association should be borne in mind whenever assessing a patient with sudden onset focal neurology, normal intracranial vessels and an abnormal ECG. This is especially relevant given the high incidence of cardiovascular comorbidities in the stroke patient population. In a patient with known structural heart disease, intermittent unexplained focal neurology should prompt consideration of transient cardiac output loss. If a patient has a pacemaker in-situ and develops acute, unexplained neurology, pacemaker dysfunction should be considered.

Key Learning Points

- Focal neurology may be a presenting symptom in patients with cardiac conduction block.
- A broad differential diagnosis should always be considered, taking into account stroke mimic syndromes.
- Patients with pacemakers and new onset focal neurology require investigation for pacemaker dysfunction.
- Conduction block with ventricular standstill is an indication for emergency pacing.

References

1. Rudd M, Buck D, Ford GA, Price CI. A systematic review of stroke recognition instruments in hospital and prehospital settings. Emerg Med J. 2016;33:818–22.
2. Gibson LM, Whiteley W. The differential diagnosis of suspected stroke: a systematic review. J R Coll Physicians Edinb. 2013;43:114–8.
3. Xian Y, Federspiel JJ, Cox M, Hernandez AF, Kosinski AS, Bettger JP, et al. Use of intravenous tissue plasminogen activator in patients without a stroke (stroke mimics): findings from the get with the guidelines stroke registry. Stroke. 2016;47:AWMP34.
4. McClelland G, Rodgers H, Flynn D, Price CI. The frequency, characteristics and aetiology of stroke mimic presentations. Eur J Emerg Med. 2019;26(1):2–8. https://doi.org/10.1097/MEJ.0000000000000550.
5. Barra SN, Providência R, Paiva L, Nascimento J, Marques AL. A review on advanced atrioventricular block in young or middle-aged adults. Pacing Clin Electrophysiol. 2012;35(11):1395–405. https://doi.org/10.1111/j.1540-8159.2012.03489.
6. Scheffold N, Herkommer B, Kandolf R, May AE. Lyme carditis—diagnosis, treatment and prognosis. Dtsch Arztebl Int. 2015;112(12):202–8. https://doi.org/10.3238/arztebl.2015.0202.
7. Ryan DJ, Harbison JA, Meaney JF, Rice CP, King-Kallimanis B, Kenny RA. Syncope causes transient focal neurological symptoms. QJM. 2015;108(9):711–8. https://doi.org/10.1093/qjmed/hcv005.
8. de Bono DP, Warlow CP, Hyman NM. Cardiac rhythm abnormalities in patients presenting with transient non-focal neurological symptoms: a diagnostic grey area? Br Med J (Clin Res Ed). 1982;284:1437. https://doi.org/10.1136/bmj.284.6327.1437.
9. Pilling JB, Nanton MA. Progressive external ophthalmoplegia and heart block. Br Med J. 1974;1(5906):492–3. https://doi.org/10.1136/bmj.1.5906.492.
10. Gregoratos D, Cheitlin M, Conill A, et al. ACC/AHA guidelines for implantation of cardiac pacemakers and antiarrhythmia devices: executive summary. 1998;97:1325–35. https://doi.org/10.1161/01.CIR.97.13.1325.
11. Reed RL, Siekert RG, Merideth J. Rarity of transient focal cerebral ischemia in cardiac dysrhythmia. JAMA. 1973;223(8):893–5. https://doi.org/10.1001/jama.1973.03220080025006.

Chapter 9
An Unusual Case of Paradoxical Embolus

Sandeep Singh, Sumanjit K. Gill, and Nicholas Losseff

Clinical History

A 62-year-old gentleman was electively admitted for laparoscopic robotic prostatectomy, to treat localized prostate carcinoma. He had no other past medical history. His pre-operative assessment was unremarkable and the only investigations performed were a routine set of blood tests, which were normal, and a 12-lead ECG which showed him to be in sinus rhythm with left axis deviation but no hypertrophy. The surgery (during which he was in lithotomy in the Trendelenberg position i.e. lying supine with his feet 30 degrees higher than the head) was uneventful. He was transferred back to the ward but around 8 h later was noted to be still drowsy, a state originally ascribed to the general anesthetic, which had been administered earlier.

Examination

He was drowsy but opened his eyes to pain. He was not vocalising. He had a gaze preference towards the right side. He had left hemiparesis and neglect. There was an extensor plantar response on the left side, the right plantar response was flexor. His blood pressure was 150/70 mmHg and his pulse was regular.

S. Singh
The Royal Free Hospital, London, UK
e-mail: sandeep.singh22@nhs.net

S. K. Gill (✉)
Institute of Neurology, UCL, National Hospital for Neurology and Neurosurgery, London, UK

N. Losseff
National Hospital for Neurology and Neurosurgery, London, UK
e-mail: nicholas.losseff@uclh.nhs.uk

S. K. Gill et al. (eds.), *Stroke Medicine*,
https://doi.org/10.1007/978-3-031-58188-5_9

Investigations and Clinical Progress

CT (Fig. 9.1) confirmed the clinical suspicion of a right middle cerebral artery territory infarct. There was a visible thrombus in the right middle cerebral artery but he was out of the time window for either thrombolysis or endovascular treatment, and of course, he had also just undergone major surgery. A subsequent MRI is shown in Fig. 9.2. Further investigation for possible causes of his stroke included a 24 hours tape that showed occasional ventricular ectopics but no arrhythmia. MRA of the neck and intracranial vessels was normal. His fasting glucose was normal and his total cholesterol 4.4 mmol/L. A bubble echocardiogram showed a patent foramen ovale (PFO) on Valsalva and there was a highly mobile intra-arterial septum.

He recovered rapidly despite the radiological appearances of a large infarct. When discharged a week later he was independently mobile and his cognition was intact. There was some persisting upper limb weakness for which he continued to have physiotherapy in the community.

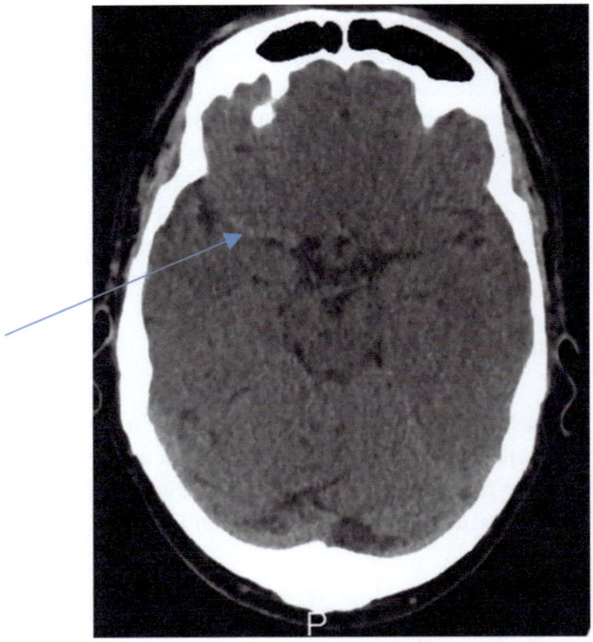

Fig. 9.1 Unenhanced CT scan—hyper-dense clot is visible in the right middle cerebral artery

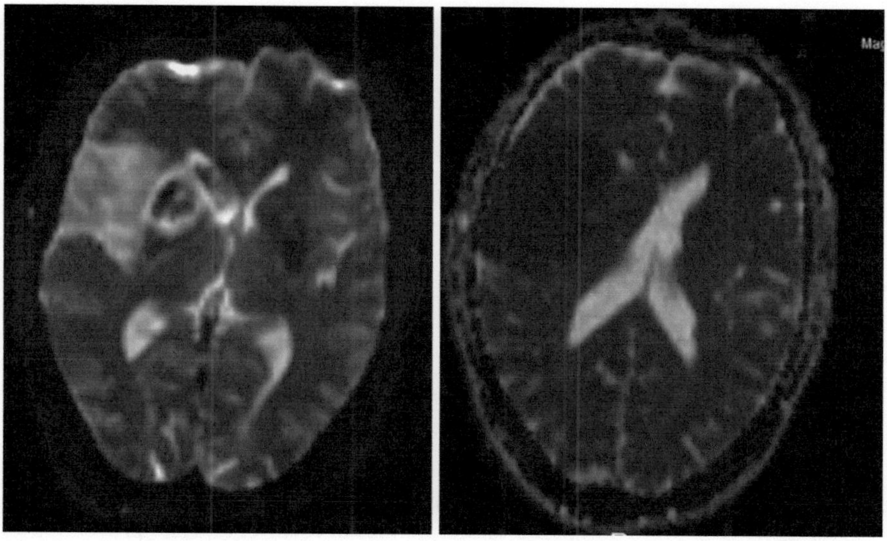

Fig. 9.2 Axial diffusion weighted imaging: B1000 DWI (*left*) and ADC map (*right*) show matched defect in the right middle cerebral artery territory indicating an acute infarct

Discussion

Mechanisms for stroke in those with PFO include paradoxical embolus from the deep veins, thrombus generated by cardiac arrhythmia or local formation of thrombus within the PFO, which is a tunnel rather than a hole between the atria. Paradoxical embolus is also associated with atrial septal defects, ventricular septal defects and pulmonary arteriovenous fistulae. In the adult population, PFO prevalence has been noted to be around 20–25% and nearly 40–50% of patients with cryptogenic stroke have a PFO [1, 2]. This overlap means that PFO can be incidental finding and a careful case analysis has to be performed in order to clarify the aetiology. A RoPE score is helpful in discussions about the aetiology of cryptogenic stroke in the presence of PFO as it has been found to correlate with the probability that the stroke is causally related to PFO [3].

The presence of PFO has been linked to the increased risk of recurrent stroke. A study by Mas et al. showed patients with PFO alone had a recurrent stroke risk of 2.3% (95% CI 0.3%–4.3%) whereas 15.2% (95% CI 1.8%–28.6%) among patients with both PFO and atrial septal aneurysm [3]. The presence of PFO and atrial septal aneurysm together was significantly associated with recurrent stroke, whereas isolated PFO was not [4]. Therefore, closure of a PFO percutaneously to reduce the risk of recurrent stroke, owing to paradoxical embolism, has been considered a possible treatment option.

Possible treatment strategies are that of closure (either open or percutaneous), antiplatelet therapy or anticoagulation. A meta-analysis comprising of 10,327 patients from 48 observational studies compared the rate of recurrent neurological events among patient with cryptogenic stroke or transient ischemic attack (TIA) and concomitant PFO [5]. They found 6.3 times increased rate of neurological events in patients with medical management group compared to the ones who underwent transcatheter closure. Despite this cases are considered on a case by case basis by a multidisciplinary group of radiologists, cardiologists and stroke physicians as there is the potential for complications in addition to uncertainty about stroke causation.

Anticoagulant Vs Antiplatelet Therapy

In those who are not suitable for PFO closure it is still worth exploring the relative of benefits of anticoagulation vs anti platelets. A meta-analysis of five randomized controlled trials included 1565 patients [5] to compare the risk/benefits of anticoagulation over antiplatelet in patients with PFO associated stroke. They found there was no net benefit associated with anticoagulation (OR = 0.66, 95% CI 0.41–1.07, p heterogeneity = 0.46) compared to antiplatelet in recurrent stroke prevention in patients with PFO. In addition, a non-significant increased risk of major bleeding (OR = 1.64, 95% CI 0.79–3.43, *p* heterogeneity = 0.57) in anticoagulation arm was reported compared to the antiplatelet group. However, a significant reduction (OR = 0.22, 95% CI 0.06–0.8, *p* heterogeneity = 0.88) in recurrent stroke risk with anticoagulation was noticed in patients with high RoPE score raising the question of whether this could be an alternative in those not suitable for closure [6]. This is not accepted clinical practice where the focus remains on managing modifiable vascular risk factors.

PFO Closure

Early RCTs failed to show any significant benefit of percutaneous closure of PFO in secondary prevention of cryptogenic stroke. However, the CLOSE trial [7], REDUCE trial [8] and long term data from the RESPECT trial [9] were more positive. PFO closure is not overall a win-win situation, complications include pericardial effusion, air embolism and device embolus. A major concern with closure of PFO is the induction of atrial fibrillation (AF) episodes which in turn increases risk of recurrent stroke. A Bayesian Network Meta-analysis (NMA) of six RCTs estimated the risk-effectiveness balance [10]. This meta-analysis showed PFO closure was associated with increased AF episodes compared to medical treatment but the number of strokes saved was still in favour of PFO closure providing some reassurance.

There is also debate about how the outcome of PFO closure is influenced by the type of device used. The answer to this question comes from a meta analysis which favours PFO closure in preventing subsequent neurological events over medical treatment but shows that no one device is better than another in secondary stroke

Table 9.1 RoPE score to calculate probability of causality of PFO and stroke. A RoPE of more than 6 is considered highly likely to be associated with stroke due to PFO [3]

RoPE score calculator		
Characteristic	Points	RoPE score
No history of hypertension	1	
No history of diabetes	1	
No history of stroke/tia	1	
Non smoker	1	
Cortical infarct	1	
Age (years)		
18–29	5	
30–39	4	
40–49	3	
50–59	2	
60–69	1	
≥70	0	
Total Score		

prevention [11]. In terms of cost effectiveness [12] it was found that PFO closure was associated with an improved quality of life and is cost-effective compared to medical treatment.

In clinical practice, each case is considered by a multidisciplinary team including both stroke physicians and cardiologists with decision-making based upon consid-

Key Clinical Learning Points

- PFO can be an incidental finding in cryptogenic stroke and the RoPE helps to establish likelihood of causality of stroke
- Presence of Atrial septal abnormality (septal aneurysm) is associated with a higher risk of recurrent stroke
- Data from RCTs favours percutaneous PFO closure over medical management for secondary stroke prevention in selected patients where there is certainty about causation

Key Radiological Learning Points

- Cardioembolic infarcts are usually cortical infarcts, they can affect multiple arterial territories and be bilateral
- A hyperdense middle cerebral artery can be seen on plain CT and is indicative of clot of significant size lodged in the artery

ering all other risk factors for stroke and imaging review. The RoPE score [3] is used to grade the likelihood of causality (Table 9.1).

References

1. Hara H, Virmani R, Ladich E, Mackey-Bojack S, Titus J, Reisman M, et al. Patent foramen ovale: current pathology, pathophysiology, and clinical status. J Am Coll Cardiol. 2005;46(9):1768–76.
2. Lechat P, Mas JL, Lascault G, Loron P, Theard M, Klimczac M, et al. Prevalence of patent foramen ovale in patients with stroke. N Engl J Med. 1988;318(18):1148–52.
3. Kent DM, Ruthazer R, Weimar C, Mas JL, Serena J, Homma S, Di Angelantonio E, Di Tullio MR, Lutz JS, Elkind MS, et al. An index to identify stroke-related vs incidental patent foramen ovale in cryptogenic stroke. Neurology. 2013;81:619–25. https://doi.org/10.1212/WNL.0b013e3182a08d59.
4. Mas JL, Arquizan C, Lamy C, Zuber M, Cabanes L, Derumeaux G, et al. Recurrent cerebrovascular events associated with patent foramen ovale, atrial septal aneurysm, or both. N Engl J Med. 2001;345(24):1740–6.
5. Agarwal S, Bajaj NS, Kumbhani DJ, Tuzcu EM, Kapadia SR. Meta-analysis of transcatheter closure versus medical therapy for patent foramen ovale in prevention of recurrent neurological events after presumed paradoxical embolism. J Am Coll Cardiol Intv. 2012;5(7):777–89.
6. Romoli M, Giannandrea D, Eusebi P, Cupini LM, Ricci S, Calabresi P. Aspirin or anticoagulation after cryptogenic stroke with patent foramen ovale: systematic review and meta-analysis of randomized controlled trials. Neurol Sci. 2020;41(10):2819–24.
7. Mas JL, Derumeaux G, Guillon B, Massardier E, Hosseini H, Mechtouff L, et al. Patent foramen closure or anticoagulation vs. antiplatelets after stroke. NEJM. 2017;377:1011–21. https://doi.org/10.1056/NEJMoa1705915.
8. Sondergaard L, Kasner SE, Rhodes JF, Anderson G, Iversen H, et al. Patent foramen Ovale closure of antiplatelet therapy for cryptogenic stroke. NEJM. 2017;377:1033–42.
9. Saver JL, Carroll JD, Thaler DE, Smalling RW, MacDonald LA, et al. Long term outcomes of patent foramen ovale closure or medical therapy after stroke. NEJM. 2017;377:1022–32.
10. Varotto L, Bregolin G, Paccanaro M, De Boni A, Bonanno C, Perini F. Network meta-analysis on patent foramen ovale: is a stroke or atrial fibrillation worse? Neurol Sci. 2021;42(1):101–9.
11. Varotto L, Bregolin G, Paccanaro M, De Boni A, Bonanno C, Perini F. The closure of patent foramen ovale in preventing subsequent neurological events: a Bayesian network meta-analysis to identify the best device. Cerebrovasc Dis. 2020;49(2):124–34.
12. Leppert MH, Poisson SN, Carroll JD, Thaler DE, Kim CH, Orjuela KD, et al. Cost-effectiveness of patent foramen ovale closure versus medical therapy for secondary stroke prevention. Stroke. 2018;49(6):1443–50.

Chapter 10
Stroke Associated with an Atrial Myxoma

Adnan Hammad and Sumanjit K. Gill

Clinical History

A 49-year-old gentleman presented to the emergency department with a 4 day history of worsening headache and binocular blurred vision. The headache was right sided, temporal, and sudden in onset. There was no photophobia, neck stiffness, vomiting or preceding head injury. Vision gradually deteriorated bilaterally, and he became unable to read and was having difficulty recognising people's faces. There was no associated ocular pain. He had no limb weakness nor any peripheral sensory disturbances.

His past medical history included Type II diabetes mellitus, hypercholesterolaemia, and depression. He had smoked 20 cigarettes a day for the preceding 11 years, and was binge drinking up to 15 pints of beer at weekends.

He was initially thought to have giant cell arteritis (GCA) and was referred to ophthalmology. However, after a thorough ophthalmological assessment, it was suspected that he may have suffered a stroke and he was referred back to the emergency department for further assessment.

A. Hammad (✉)
Neurology Department, Royal Free Hospital, London, UK

Royal Victoria Hospital, Belfast, UK
e-mail: adnan.hammad@nhs.net

S. K. Gill
Institute of Neurology, UCL, National Hospital for Neurology and Neurosurgery, London, UK

S. K. Gill et al. (eds.), *Stroke Medicine*,
https://doi.org/10.1007/978-3-031-58188-5_10

Examination

The patient's vital signs were all normal. General examination was unremarkable. His Glasgow Coma Scale (GCS) score was 15. The temporal arteries were non-tender and pulsatile bilaterally. Visual acuity was 3/9 unmasked bilaterally. Visual fields were grossly intact bilaterally. There was full range of movement in both eyes with no evidence of nystagmus. Pupils were equal and reactive to light and accommodation. The other cranial nerves were intact. Tone, reflexes, power and coordination were normal in all four limbs. Sensory examination did not reveal any abnormalities in any of the patient's limbs.

Investigations

Routine bloods were unremarkable, except for a slightly raised C-reactive protein (CRP) of 7. An ECG demonstrated sinus rhythm. An urgent CT head was performed, which identified a subacute infarct in the right occipital lobe (Fig. 10.1). An MRI head performed the following day confirmed this, in addition to revealing a further smaller area of signal alteration with restricted diffusion in the left posterior frontal lobe and white matter lesions in the deep white matter of the right periventricular posterior parietal lobe. In view of the different vascular territories implicated, the aetiology was thought to be most likely embolic.

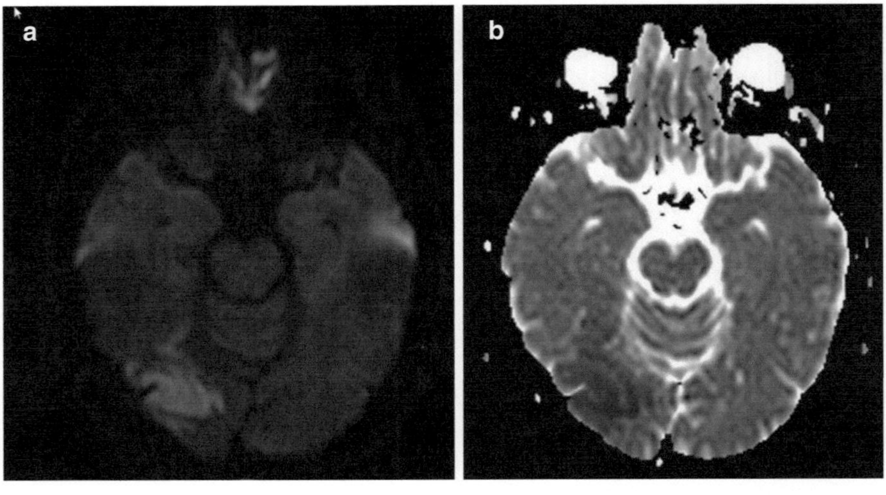

Fig. 10.1 Diffusion weighted images confirming an acute infarct in the right occipital lobe—high signal on B1000 images (**a**) matched by restricted diffusion on ADC map (**b**)

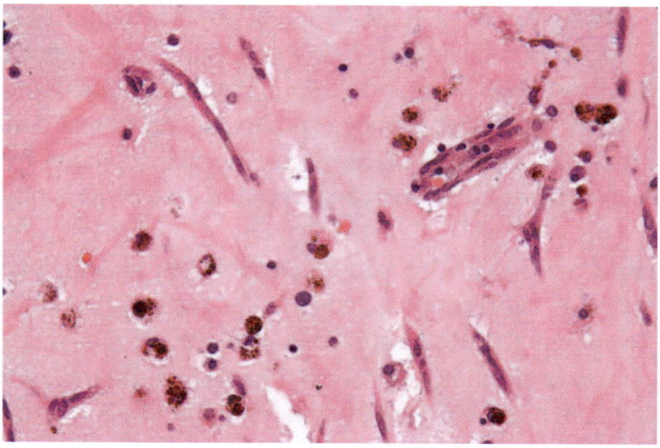

Fig. 10.2 High magnification micrograph of an atrial myxoma . Features: Hypocellular myxoid polypoid mass with cells that are: perivascular, finely vacuolated with eosinophilic cytoplasm, elongated in shape, can be mononuclear or multinucleated. May contain macrophages, other inflammatory cells. May be covered with endothelium. (Wikipedia 2023)

He subsequently had an ultrasound (US) doppler of his carotids, which did not demonstrate any significant stenoses within the common, internal or external carotids. A transthoracic echocardiogram (TTE) showed a large multilobular mobile mass in the left atrium (LA), which occupied >50% of the LA cavity. In view of this, the patient was transferred to another centre for further characterisation and management of this mass. The mass was finally identified as an atrial myxoma, which was successfully resected, its benign nature confirmed on histopathology (Fig. 10.2).

Discussion

Cardioembolic stroke accounts for 14–30% of all ischaemic strokes, and is associated with both early and late recurrence [1]. Major aetiologies predisposing to cerebral emboli include atrial fibrillation (AF), infective endocarditis, valvular heart disease, myocardial infarction (MI) and atrial myxoma [2]. AF is the most common underlying cause of cerebral emboli, accounting for approximately 45% of cardiogenic cerebral emboli [3]. These strokes can be recognised clinically by a step wise neurological deterioration (as ischaemic lesions accrue) and strokes of varying ages in differing vascular territories seen on imaging.

Cardiac myxoma is the most prevalent primary cardiac tumour, but is a rare though important cause of cardiogenic cerebral emboli, particularly in younger patient [4]. It is a benign tumour of mesenchymal origin, which is histologically made up of scattered cells embedded in a mucopolysaccharide stroma [5]. Cardiac myxomas have a female preponderance (2:1 female to male ratio) and most commonly present between the ages of 30 and 60 [6]. The majority of cardiac myxomas are seen in the atria, with around 75% being found in the left atrium [6]. Atrial myxomas are mostly sporadic (around 90%) [7], with the remaining 10% or so of cases occurring in the context of Carney complex, an autosomal dominant disease, caused by mutations in the PRKAR1α gene, and characterised by a number of benign tumours, also affecting the endocrine system, as well as spotty skin pigmentation [8].

Atrial myxomas are classically said to present with at least one of a triad of symptoms: obstructive, constitutional and embolic, the most common of which are constitutional symptoms [7]. Routine bloods often reveal non-specific abnormalities, which may include anaemia, thrombocytopaenia, raised inflammatory markers (such as CRP and ESR), and elevated immunoglobulin levels [5, 9]. Unfortunately, a diagnosis of atrial myxoma can often be elusive, especially in the presence of non-specific systemic symptoms [10]. The delay in diagnosis from the onset of symptoms has been reported to range from 1 to 126 months [11]. A delayed diagnosis may result in stroke progression, with the eventual development of multi-infarct dementia [12], in addition to the occurrence of peripheral embolic events. Therefore, recognition of the clinical features of cardioembolic stroke secondary to atrial myxoma is vital.

Transoesophageal echocardiography (TOE) is the gold standard for diagnosing atrial myxomas, and has been reported to have a 100% sensitivity for the detection of atrial myxomas [13]. Further information that may be required for subsequent surgical resection may be obtained by cardiac MRI, which can delineate the size, degree of mobility and attachment of the tumour [14].

Once a diagnosis of atrial myxoma has been made, immediate resection should be undertaken [15]. Surgical resection has been shown to have excellent outcomes in patients with benign cardiac tumours, including atrial myxomas [16]. Recurrence rate is around 1–3%, usually secondary to incomplete resection [7].

Key Clinical Learning Points

- Cardioembolic stroke aetiologies should be considered in patients who present with a step wise neurological deterioration.
- While AF, MI and valvular heart disease are more common underlying causes of cardioembolic stroke, atrial myxoma should be considered in younger patients presenting with features of cardioembolic stroke.
- Atrial myxoma can be challenging to diagnose, however it tends to present with at least one of three categories of phenomena: obstructive, constitutional and embolic.
- Once identified the myxoma should be resected as soon as possible.

Key Radiological Learning Points

- If atrial myxoma is suspected, the patient should undergo echocardiography, with TOE being preferred to TTE. Cardiac MRI may further characterise the lesion, which may be useful for subsequent surgery.
- Cardioembolic strokes cause strokes which are seen in multiple vascular territories in both hemispheres on imaging
- MRI imaging is useful to identify ischaemic lesions as cardioembolic strokes can often be small and cortical and not visible on CT imaging

References

1. Arboix A, Alió J. Cardioembolic stroke: clinical features, specific cardiac disorders and prognosis. Curr Cardiol Rev. 2010;6(3):150–61.
2. Vahedi K, Amarenco P. Cardiac causes of stroke. Curr Treat Options Neurol. 2000;2(4):305–18.
3. Yuan S-M, Humuruola G. Stroke of a cardiac myxoma origin. Rev Bras Cir Cardiovasc. 2015;30(2):225–34.
4. Sanya EO, Kolo PM, Adamu UG, Opadijo OG, Wahab KW, Mustapha AF, et al. Intracardiac tumor: a risk factor for stroke in the young—a case report. Niger J Clin Pract. 2008;11(1):81–4.
5. Akhtar J, Wasay M, Rauf J. Atrial myxoma: a rare cause of cardioembolic stroke. BMJ Case Rep. [Internet]. 2012 [cited 2021 Jun 9]. 2012;
6. Reynen K. Cardiac myxomas. N Engl J Med. 1995;333(24):1610–7.
7. McCarthy PM, Piehler JM, Schaff HV, Pluth JR, Orszulak TA, Vidaillet HJ, et al. The significance of multiple, recurrent, and 'complex' cardiac myxomas. J Thorac Cardiovasc Surg. 1986;91(3):389–96.
8. Kirschner LS, Carney JA, Pack SD, Taymans SE, Giatzakis C, Cho YS, et al. Mutations of the gene encoding the protein kinase A type I-alpha regulatory subunit in patients with the Carney complex. Nat Genet. 2000;26(1):89–92.
9. Mendoza CE, Rosado MF, Bernal L. The role of interleukin-6 in cases of cardiac myxoma: clinical features, immunologic abnormalities, and a possible role in recurrence. Tex Heart Inst J. 2001;28(1):3–7.
10. Aziz F, Zaeem M. Atrial myxoma presenting as acute stroke: a case report and review of literature. Greener J Med Sci. 2013;3(5):171–3.
11. MacGowan SW, Sidhu P, Aherne T, Luke D, Wood AE, Neligan MC, et al. Atrial myxoma: national incidence, diagnosis and surgical management. Ir J Med Sci. 1993;162(6):223–6.
12. Hutton JT. Atrial myxoma as a cause of progressive dementia. Arch Neurol. 1981;38(8):533.
13. Engberding R, Daniel WG, Erbel R, Kasper W, Lestuzzi C, Curtius JM, et al. Diagnosis of heart tumours by transoesophageal echocardiography: a multicentre study in 154 patients. European Cooperative Study Group. Eur Heart J. 1993;14(9):1223–8.
14. Abbas A, Garfath-Cox KAG, Brown IW, Shambrook JS, Peebles CR, Harden SP. Cardiac MR assessment of cardiac myxomas. Br J Radiol. 2015;88:1045. [Internet] [cited 2021 Jun 10]
15. Keeling IM, Oberwalder P, Anelli-Monti M, Schuchlenz H, Demel U, Tilz GP, et al. Cardiac myxomas: 24 years of experience in 49 patients. Eur J Cardiothorac Surg. 2002;22(6):971–7.
16. Bakaeen FG, Reardon MJ, Coselli JS, Miller CC, Howell JF, Lawrie GM, et al. Surgical outcome in 85 patients with primary cardiac tumors. Am J Surg. 2003;186(6):641–7.

Chapter 11
Antiphospholipid Syndrome and Stroke: Diagnosis and Management

Prabal Mittal, Maria Efthymiou, Zara Sayar, and Hannah Cohen

Abbreviations

aCL	Anticardiolipin antibodies
AIS	Acute ischaemic stroke
aPL	Antiphospholipid antibodies
APS	Antiphospholipid syndrome
aß2GP1	Anti-beta2 glycoprotein 1 antibodies
DOAC	Direct oral anticoagulant
INR	International Normalised Ratio
LA	Lupus anticoagulant
TIA	Transient ischaemic attack

P. Mittal (✉) · H. Cohen
Department of Haematology, University College London Hospitals NHS Foundation Trust, London, UK

Haemostasis Research Unit, Department of Haematology, University College London, London, UK
e-mail: prabal.mittal@nhs.net; hannah.cohen@ucl.ac.uk

M. Efthymiou
Haemostasis Research Unit, Department of Haematology, University College London, London, UK
e-mail: maria.efthymiou@nhs.net; m.efthymiou@ucl.ac.uk

Z. Sayar
Department of Haematology, University College London Hospitals NHS Foundation Trust, London, UK

Department of Haematology, Whittington Health NHS Trust, London, UK
e-mail: zara.sayar@nhs.net

S. K. Gill et al. (eds.), *Stroke Medicine*,
https://doi.org/10.1007/978-3-031-58188-5_11

Case Presentation

A 40-year-old right-handed man woke with headache, dysphasia and right-hand weakness. He had no past medical history or regular medications. He was a non-smoker, did not drink alcohol or use recreational drugs. There was no family history of venous thromboembolic events (VTE), premature myocardial infarction or stroke. At presentation, he was hypertensive (BP 185/105 mmHg) and in sinus rhythm. Body mass index was 35. Neurological assessment showed right arm pronator drift and markedly reduced power, along with dysphasia. The rest of the examination was unremarkable.

Magnetic resonance imaging (MRI) of the head revealed acute left middle cerebral artery (MCA) territory infarcts. CT angiogram (CTA) of brain and neck vessels showed no evidence of atherosclerotic stenosis, thrombus or dissection. Initial blood work-up revealed mild thrombocytopenia: platelet count 84–108 × 10^9/L (NR: 150–400 × 10^9/L), total cholesterol 4.1 mmol/L (NR: 2.5–5.0 mmol/L), with LDL 2.5 mmol/L (NR: 0–3.5 mmol/L).

Initial treatment was aspirin 300 mg once daily (OD) for 2 weeks, followed by clopidogrel 75 mg OD. Amlodipine and atorvastatin were also commenced. One month after the initial stroke, he re-presented with acute left upper limb weakness and mild dysarthria. A repeat MRI head revealed multiple acute infarcts in the right hemisphere and multiple FLAIR hyperintensities within the deep white matter, considered of likely ischaemic origin (Fig. 11.1). Antiphospholipid antibody (aPL) screening revealed triple aPL-positivity: positive lupus anticoagulant (LA), high titre IgG anticardiolipin (aCL) (>100 GPLU/mL; NR: 0–12 GPLU/mL) and

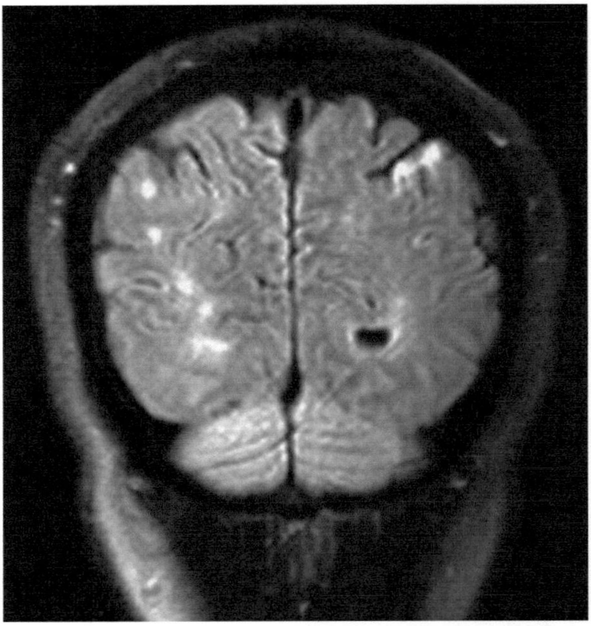

Fig. 11.1 MRI head image; FLAIR sequence showing bilateral MCA infarcts and white matter hyperintensities consistent with small vessel disease. *MRI* magnetic resonance imaging, *MCA* middle cerebral artery, *FLAIR* fluid attenuated inversion recovery

anti-beta2 glycoprotein 1 (aß2GP1) (>100 GPLU/mL; NR: 0–10 U/mL) antibodies. This suggested an underlying diagnosis of thrombotic antiphospholipid syndrome (APS) and prompted a transition of antithrombotic therapy from clopidogrel to high-intensity warfarin (International Normalised Ratio [INR] target 3.5, range 3.0–4.0). His aPL profile remained triple-positive after a 12-week interval and beyond, confirming a diagnosis of thrombotic APS.

There were no further arterial thrombotic events. However, at 21–26 months follow-up, he suffered a series of unprovoked VTE, comprising three right lower limb deep venous thromboses (DVTs) and one segmental pulmonary embolism (PE), despite anticoagulation. These events prompted sequential modifications to anticoagulation management, including transitions to low-molecular-weight heparin (standard therapeutic dose, followed by 20% dose increase) and subsequently therapeutic dose fondaparinux. As his APS was following an aggressive anticoagulant-refractory course, immunosuppression with rituximab was added. No further large vessel thrombotic events occurred over several years follow-up, however, interval MRI imaging suggested an increasing burden of ischaemic brain lesions.

Discussion

APS is a systemic autoimmune disease, characterised by vascular thrombosis and/or obstetric morbidity, in the setting of persistent antiphospholipid antibodies (aPL) [1]. Obstetric manifestations comprise recurrent early miscarriage, late pregnancy loss, stillbirth and placental insufficiency. Thrombotic disease may involve any vascular territory—arterial, venous or microvascular—and is further complicated by an increased risk of recurrent events, including breakthrough events on antithrombotic therapy. With the relatively young age of affected individuals (mean age at diagnosis of around 50 years [2]), the potential for long-term morbidity and adverse impact on quality-of-life is considerable. APS may occur in conjunction with other autoimmune diseases, most often systemic lupus erythematosus (SLE), where it may exacerbate disease severity [3].

APS-Associated Cerebrovascular Ischaemic Disorders

Acute ischaemic stroke (AIS) or transient ischaemic attack (TIA) are the most frequent arterial manifestations of APS, with approximately 20% of patients with APS suffering a stroke over 10 years [4]. In individuals aged below 50 years, a systematic review suggested that 17% of strokes and 12% of TIA are associated with aPL [5].

The most common mechanism of APS-associated stroke is thought to be in-situ thrombosis, whilst embolism from valvular heart lesions (Liebman-Sacks endocarditis) and extracranial carotid artery lesions is also described [6]. A range of infarct sizes—large, small and lacunar—are seen [6], and the middle cerebral artery region appears to be frequently involved [7]. Catastrophic antiphospholipid syndrome

(CAPS), a rare life-threatening manifestation characterized by fulminant multifocal thrombosis, is frequently associated with brain involvement including AIS [8].

Outside of acute cerebrovascular events, a spectrum of chronic brain lesions, including white matter hyperintensities (WMH), cortical atrophy and silent infarcts, are found in patients with APS and may have important neurocognitive sequalae [6, 9]. Cognitive impairment appears to be common in APS patients and is associated with WMH and cerebral infarcts [9].

Diagnostic Evaluation

International consensus classification criteria for APS [1], although developed mainly for research purposes, form the basis of current diagnostic guidance. The key to diagnosis is coexistence of an appropriate clinical event with evidence of persistent antiphospholipid antibodies (aPL), detected on two or more consecutive occasions, at least 12 weeks apart. Clinical and laboratory data require expert evaluation, ideally within a multidisciplinary team setting.

Antiphospholipid Antibody Laboratory Testing

The relationship between age and aPL frequency and clinical significance is not fully defined. The prevalence of incidental autoantibodies including aPL increases with age, as does the constitutional risk of thrombosis [2]. Nonetheless, late-onset APS may occur and could be associated with a higher rate of arterial thrombosis [10]. As a pragmatic approach, current guidance recommends routine screening for aPL in younger patients (<50 years) with stroke [11, 12]. In older patients, aPL testing may be considered on a case-by-case basis, considering factors such as a history of autoimmune disease, venous thromboembolism or obstetric morbidity, and the presence or not of an alternative stroke aetiology.

All three criteria aPL—LA, and IgG and IgM anticardiolipin (aCL) and anti-beta 2 glycoprotein 1 (aß2GP1) antibodies—should be included in diagnostic aPL testing [11]. Establishing persistence of aPL positivity beyond 12 weeks is essential to optimise diagnostic specificity, given the potential for confounders and sources of interference. Transient aPL can develop in association with other processes, notably viral and bacterial infections (e.g. hepatitis B/C; syphilis), and in this context are more likely epiphenomenal than pathogenic.

LA detection, based on in vitro prolongation of phospholipid-dependent clotting assays, is susceptible to interference from anticoagulant therapy. It is important to provide the laboratory with information about anticoagulant therapy, as this will influence assay methodology. Acute phase reactants can also disrupt LA assessment (e.g. raised factor VIII may cause false negatives; raised C-reactive protein may cause false positives) [11], and may therefore affect the reliability of testing in situations such as the early post-thrombotic period, pregnancy and intercurrent illness.

Moderate-to-high titre aCL and aß2GP1 antibodies, defined by a cut-off of >40 units/mL or > 99th centile of a normal reference population, are viewed as clinically relevant for thrombosis [1]. Low titre aPL may be associated with obstetric morbidity [13]. In contrast to IgG aPL, the diagnostic value of IgM aPL in thrombotic APS is uncertain, owing to limited clinical data.

The optimal timing of aPL testing after a thrombotic event is undefined. Although LA testing may be less reliable in the early post-thrombotic phase, a triple-positive aPL profile, as in our patient, is likely to be persistent and thus clinically meaningful [14]. It is unknown whether early anticoagulation (prior to demonstrating aPL persistence beyond 12 weeks) influences disease outcomes, but as exemplified in this case, early testing provides a useful opportunity to identify APS patients.

Risk Stratification

This patient exhibited several established biomarkers for the prediction of higher thrombotic risk associated with APS. Triple aPL-positivity is associated with the highest risk of thrombosis, both for first events in asymptomatic carriers (cumulative 10-year incidence 37% in a prospective study [15]) and recurrent events in established APS patients [16]. Thrombocytopenia occurs in 16–53% of APS patients, typically at a mild-to-moderate level (50–150 platelets/L), and is associated with a two- to four-fold increase in thrombosis risk [17]. Conventional cardiovascular risk factors likely potentiate risk in arterial APS patients; the adjusted Global Antiphospholipid Syndrome Score (aGAPSS), combining aPL phenotype with arterial hypertension and hyperlipidaemia, may help to predict risk of recurrent arterial thrombosis [18].

Management

A multidisciplinary team approach, including neurology, haematology, and rheumatology input, can aid optimal management.

Antithrombotic Treatment

The mainstay of APS-associated AIS/TIA treatment is anticoagulation with warfarin or other VKA. Recommended antithrombotic options for the treatment of initial ischaemic stroke in patients with APS include a VKA at target INR range 2.0–3.0, with or without LDA, or target INR range of 3.0–4.0, taking into account bleeding risk factors [19–21]. Surveillance brain MRI could be considered to guide ongoing treatment. In a retrospective study, serial MRI showed new brain lesions, mainly ischaemic, in approximately 45% of patients, despite antithrombotic treatment.

Patients treated with high-intensity warfarin appeared less likely to develop ischaemic lesions [22].

The role of dual antiplatelet therapy (DAPT) and combined anticoagulant-antiplatelet therapy in APS-associated arterial thrombosis is of interest, with a meta-analysis suggesting potential benefit (DAPT vs single antiplatelet therapy, and combined VKA-antiplatelet vs VKA alone), albeit from evidence of limited quality [23]. An ISTH (International Society of Haemostasis and Thrombosis) Registry for arterial APS patients treated with these regimens is ongoing (https://www.isth.org/news/567340/SSC-Subcommittee-Share-New-Registry-on-Treatment-Regimens-for-Patients-With-Arterial-APS.htm).

Current guidance [19, 20, 24] recommend against using DOACs in arterial APS patients, based on unfavourable trial data. A meta-analysis [25] of four RCTs concluded that DOAC treatment was associated with an increased risk of subsequent arterial thrombosis compared to warfarin, particularly in patients with triple-aPL positivity and/or previous arterial thrombosis, though subsequent VTE risk was not significantly higher. The RISAPS (Rivaroxaban in Stroke Patients with APS) trial aims to assess the efficacy of high-intensity rivaroxaban 15 mg twice-daily (rather than the standard 20 mg daily dose), to match our current approach of high-intensity warfarin, target INR 3.5 (range 3.0–4.0) in patients with APS and previous ischaemic stroke or other ischaemic brain injury (ClinicalTrials.gov Identifier: NCT03684564).

Supportive Management Conventional cardiovascular risk factors require close monitoring and optimization. Specialist heamatology input should be sought to negotiate situations of increased thrombotic risk, such as surgery and pregnancy. Oestrogen-containing hormonal preparations should be avoided [26]. Adjunctive treatments include vitamin D, hydroxychloroquine and statins [26, 27].

Anticoagulant-refractory APS Management of breakthrough thrombosis in APS patients on standard-intensity warfarin is largely empirical. Options include escalating to high-intensity warfarin, addition of an antiplatelet agent, or changing anticoagulation to low-molecular-weight heparin or fondaparinux [27]. Immunomodulatory treatments such as rituximab and IVIg have also been used [27].

Clinical Learning Points

- Testing for aPL should be considered in individuals with AIS/TIA, particularly those under the age of 50, and/or with a history of autoimmune disease, venous thromboembolism or obstetric morbidity.
- aPL testing should include all three criteria aPL: LA, IgG and IgM aCL and aß2GP1, with repeat testing after at least 12 weeks to establish persistence.

- For LA testing, it is important to provide the laboratory with information about anticoagulant therapy, as this will influence assay methodology.
- A multidisciplinary team approach, including neurology, haematology, and rheumatology input, can aid optimal management.
- Recommended options for the treatment of initial APS-associated ischaemic stroke include a vitamin K antagonist at target INR range 2.0–3.0, with or without low dose aspirin, or target INR range of 3.0–4.0. DOAC use should be confined to clinical studies.
- Specialist heamatology input should be sought to negotiate situations of increased thrombotic risk, such as surgery and pregnancy.

Key Radiological Learning Points

- AIS caused by APS in not a radiological diagnosis and can cause a range of sizes of infarct in single or multiple territories
- APS is more frequently associated with AIS in the in middle cerebral artery territory
- CAPS can cause multifocal acute ischaemic stroke in multiple territories
- MRI in a patient with APS may show 'silent' disease which is a risk for cognitive impairment: white matter hypertensities, cortical atrophy, mature ischaemic stroke

References

1. Miyakis S, Lockshin MD, Atsumi T, et al. International consensus statement on an update of the classification criteria for definite antiphospholipid syndrome (APS). J Thromb Haemost. 2006;4(2):295–306.
2. Dabit JY, Valenzuela-Almada MO, Vallejo-Ramos S, et al. Epidemiology of antiphospholipid syndrome in the general population. Curr Rheumatol Rep. 2021;23(12):85.
3. Ruiz-Irastorza G, Egurbide MV, Ugalde J, et al. High impact of antiphospholipid syndrome on irreversible organ damage and survival of patients with systemic lupus erythematosus. Arch Intern Med. 2004;164(1):77–82.
4. Cervera R, Serrano R, Pons-Estel GJ, et al. Morbidity and mortality in the antiphospholipid syndrome during a 10-year period: a multicentre prospective study of 1000 patients. Ann Rheum Dis. 2015;74(6):1011–8.
5. Sciascia S, Sanna G, Khamashta MA, et al. The estimated frequency of antiphospholipid antibodies in young adults with cerebrovascular events: a systematic review. Ann Rheum Dis. 2015;74(11):2028–33.
6. Ricarte IF, Dutra LA, Abrantes FF, et al. Neurologic manifestations of antiphospholipid syndrome. Lupus. 2018;27(9):1404–14.
7. Miesbach W, Gilzinger A, Gökpinar B, et al. Prevalence of antiphospholipid antibodies in patients with neurological symptoms. Clin Neurol Neurosurg. 2006;108(2):135–42.
8. Cervera R, Rodríguez-Pintó I, Legault K, Erkan D. 16th international congress on antiphospholipid antibodies task force report on catastrophic antiphospholipid syndrome. Lupus. 2020;29(12):1594–600.

9. Donnellan C, Cohen H, Werring DJ. Cognitive dysfunction and associated neuroimaging biomarkers in antiphospholipid syndrome: a systematic review. Rheumatology (Oxford). 2021;61(1):24–41.
10. Grimaud F, Yelnik C, Pineton de Chambrun M, et al. Clinical and immunological features of antiphospholipid syndrome in the elderly: a retrospective national multicentre study. Rheumatology (Oxford). 2019;58(6):1006–10.
11. Devreese KMJ, Groot PG, Laat B, et al. Guidance from the scientific and standardization committee for lupus anticoagulant/antiphospholipid antibodies of the international society on thrombosis and haemostasis: update of the guidelines for lupus anticoagulant detection and interpretation. J Thromb Haemost. 2020;18(11):2828–39.
12. Royal College of Physicians Intercollegiate Stroke Working Party 2016. National Clinical Guideline for Stroke. https://www.rcplondon.ac.uk/guidelines-policy/stroke-guidelines
13. Arachchillage DR, Machin SJ, Mackie IJ, Cohen H. Diagnosis and management of non-criteria obstetric antiphospholipid syndrome. Thromb Haemost. 2015;113(1):13–9. https://doi.org/10.1160/TH14-05-0416. Epub 2014 Oct 16
14. Pengo V, Ruffatti A, Del Ross T, et al. Confirmation of initial antiphospholipid antibody positivity depends on the antiphospholipid antibody profile. J Thromb Haemost. 2013;11(8):1527–31.
15. Pengo V, Ruffatti A, Legnani C, et al. Incidence of a first thromboembolic event in asymptomatic carriers of high-risk antiphospholipid antibody profile: a multicenter prospective study. Blood. 2011;118(17):4714–8.
16. Pengo V, Ruffatti A, Legnani C, et al. Clinical course of high-risk patients diagnosed with antiphospholipid syndrome. J Thromb Haemost. 2010;8(2):237–42.
17. Vreede AP, Bockenstedt PL, McCune WJ, Knight JS. Cryptic conspirators: a conversation about thrombocytopenia and antiphospholipid syndrome. Curr Opin Rheumatol. 2019;31(3):231–40.
18. Radin M, Sciascia S, Erkan D, et al.; APS ACTION. The adjusted global antiphospholipid syndrome score (aGAPSS) and the risk of recurrent thrombosis: Results from the APS ACTION cohort. Semin Arthritis Rheum. 2019;49(3):464–8. https://doi.org/10.1016/j.semarthrit.2019.04.009.
19. Tektonidou MG, Andreoli L, Limper M, et al. EULAR recommendations for the management of antiphospholipid syndrome in adults. Ann Rheum Dis. 2019;78(10):1296–304.
20. Cohen H, Cuadrado MJ, Erkan D, et al. 16th international congress on antiphospholipid antibodies task force report on antiphospholipid syndrome treatment trends. Lupus. 2020;29(12):1571–93.
21. Tektonidou MG, Andreoli L, Limper M, Tincani A, Ward MM. Management of thrombotic and obstetric antiphospholipid syndrome: a systematic literature review informing the EULAR recommendations for the management of antiphospholipid syndrome in adults. RMD Open. 2019;5(1):e000924.
22. Efthymiou M, SvrKova P, Moll R, et al. Progression of ischaemic and haemorrhagic brain lesions on MRI in APS patients on antithrombotic therapy [abstract]. Res Pract Thromb Haemost. 2021;5(Suppl 2) https://abstracts.isth.org/abstract/progression-of-ischaemic-and-haemorrhagic-brain-lesions-on-mri-in-aps-patients-on-antithrombotic-therapy
23. Aibar J, Schulman S. Arterial thrombosis in patients with antiphospholipid syndrome: a review and meta-analysis. Semin Thromb Hemost. 2021; s-0041-1725057
24. Zuily S, Cohen H, Isenberg D, et al. Use of direct oral anticoagulants in patients with thrombotic antiphospholipid syndrome: guidance from the scientific and standardization Committee of the International Society on thrombosis and haemostasis. J Thromb Haemost. 2020;18(9):2126–37.
25. Dufrost V, Wahl D, Zuily S. Direct oral anticoagulants in antiphospholipid syndrome: meta-analysis of randomized controlled trials. Autoimmun Rev. 2021;20(1):102711.
26. Sayar Z, Moll R, Isenberg D, Cohen H. Thrombotic antiphospholipid syndrome: a practical guide to diagnosis and management. Thromb Res. 2021;198:213–21.
27. Cohen H, Isenberg DA. How I treat anticoagulant-refractory thrombotic antiphospholipid syndrome. Blood. 2021;137(3):299–309.

Chapter 12
A Progressive Headache

Fiona Humphries and Matthew Adams

History

A 34-year-old right-handed female presented to the Accident and Emergency Department with a five-day history of a headache. The headache began at her right temple and spread to involve the whole right side of her head and was associated with nausea, vomiting and dizziness. The pain radiated down to the right side of her neck but there was no neck stiffness or photophobia. Neurological examination was normal as were full blood count, renal profile and a plain CT head. The headache improved with simple analgesics and she was discharged with a diagnosis of likely migraine. Three days later she represented with new photophobia and a significantly worsening headache with cough and sneeze induced vomiting suggestive of raised intracranial pressure. She gave a past medical history of having started the combined oral contraceptive pill a few months prior to the headache, and previous cholecystitis.

F. Humphries (✉)
Stroke Medicine and Geriatric Medicine, UCLH Stroke Services, The National Hospital for Neurology and Neurosurgery, London, UK

Medicine for the Elderly, London, UK
e-mail: f.humphries@nhs.net

M. Adams
Lysholm Department of Neuroradiology, National Hospital for Neurology and Neurosurgery, London, UK
e-mail: matthew.adams9@nhs.net

S. K. Gill et al. (eds.), *Stroke Medicine*,
https://doi.org/10.1007/978-3-031-58188-5_12

Examination

She was slightly drowsy with a GCS of 14/15 but orientated. Her temperature was 36.2 °C, blood pressure 130/86 mmHg and her pulse was 57 beats per minute and regular. There were no rashes but there was photophobia and neck stiffness suggestive of meningism. Her pupils were equal and reactive, there was no conjunctival injection, and the cranial nerves were intact. Strength, sensation and reflexes were normal throughout upper and lower limbs bilaterally and plantar responses were flexor. Fundoscopy was normal, as was the general examination.

Investigations

Blood samples sent on arrival in the emergency department showed white blood cells 15.0 × 10^9/L, CRP 23.4 mg/L, and normal renal and liver profiles. A lumbar puncture was performed with normal CSF protein, glucose, white blood cell count, and gram stain and CSF culture were both negative. No significant red blood cell pigments were detected in the CSF and bilirubin and oxyhaemoglobin were not increased. Repeat CT head which was 5 days after her first scan demonstrated hyperattenuation of the transverse sinus (Fig. 12.1), the straight sinus (Fig. 12.2),

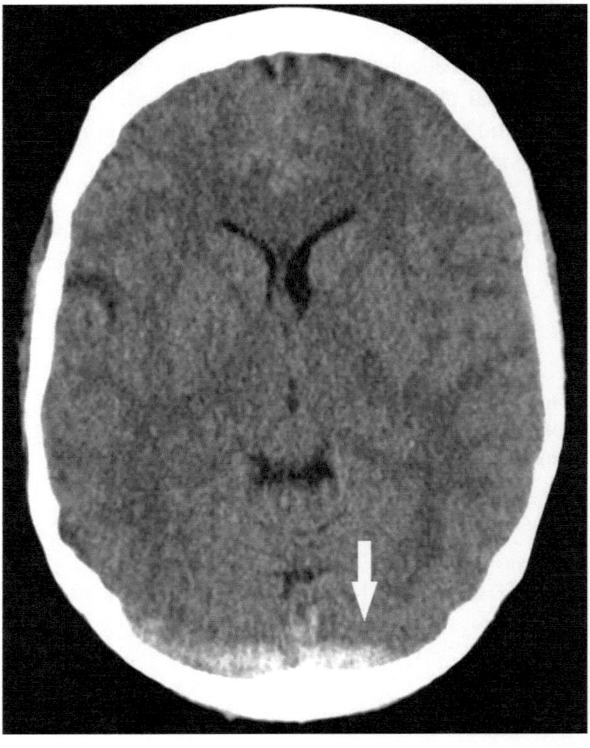

Fig. 12.1 CT showing high attenuation thrombus within the transverse sinus (white arrow)

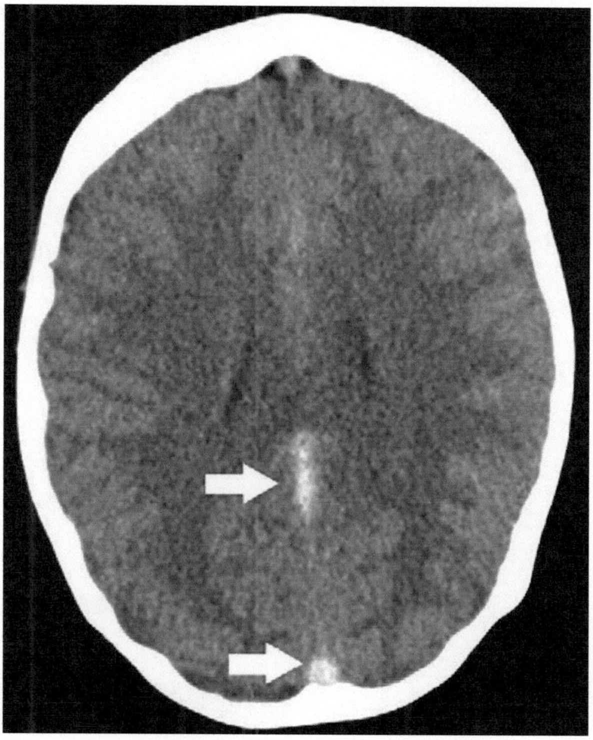

Fig. 12.2 CT showing hyperattenuation in the straight and superior sagittal sinuses (white arrows)

the superior sagittal sinus and numerous cortical veins (Fig. 12.3) with widespread effacement of the sulci and evidence of cerebral swelling (Figs. 12.1 and 12.2). CT venogram (CTV) confirmed extensive thrombus throughout the cerebral venous system involving superior sagittal sinus, the straight sinus, the transverse sinuses and the right sigmoid sinus (Figs. 12.4 and 12.5).

A diagnosis of extensive cerebral venous thrombosis was made and she was anticoagulated with treatment dose low molecular weight heparin. The oral contraceptive pill was stopped and subsequent thrombophilia screen was negative. She made a full recovery with no significant neurology, although serial CT venography demonstrated venous sinus stenosis so she is being treated with long term anticoagulation.

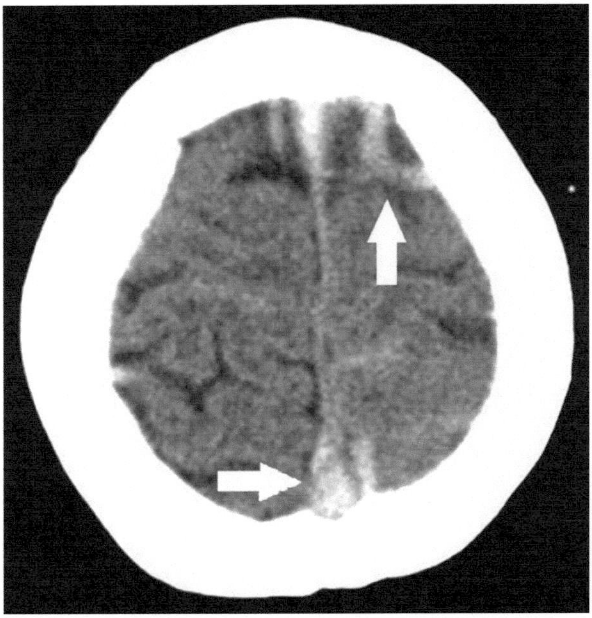

Fig. 12.3 CT showing thrombus in superior sagittal sinus and hyperattenuation of cortical veins

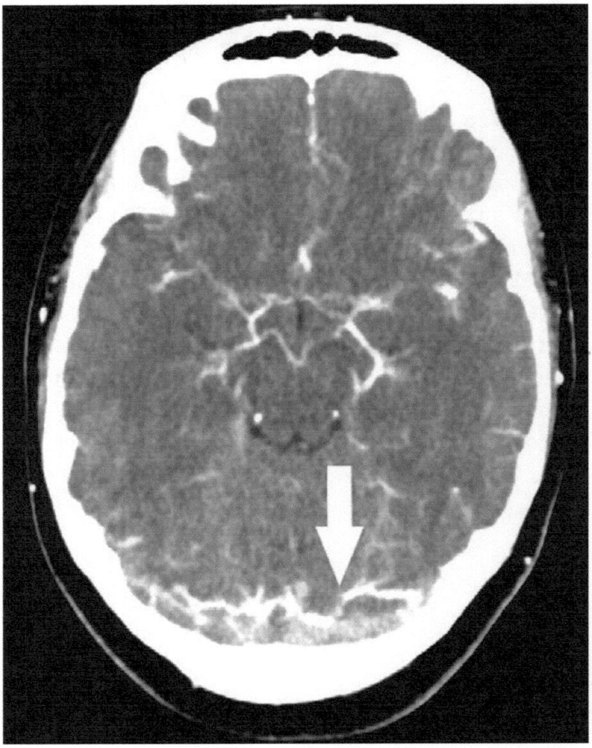

Fig. 12.4 CTV demonstrating reduced contrast opacification in the transverse sinus

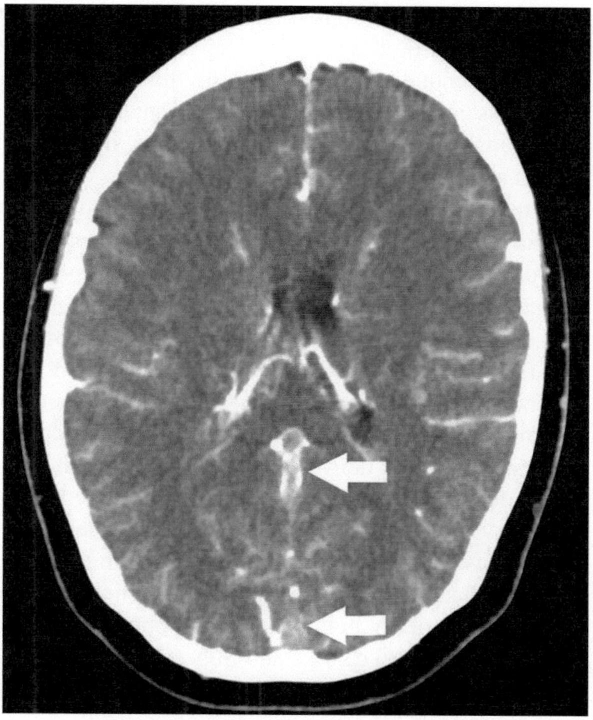

Fig. 12.5 CTV demonstrating reduced contrast opacification in the straight and superior sagittal sinuses

Discussion

Cerebral venous sinus thrombosis (CVT) is an uncommon disorder with an annual incidence of 2–7 cases per million [1] and accounts for 0.5–1% of strokes. It more commonly affects younger patients, with over 75% occurring in those under 50 years of age [2]. With prompt diagnosis and appropriate therapy, the majority of patients make a good recovery, with poor neurological outcome seen in 7–20% of cases largely due to a delay to diagnosis but sometimes due to aggressive clotting dependent on the underlying cause [3].

CVT typically presents with symptoms related to raised intracranial pressure and/ or the more focal effects of venous ischaemia or haemorrhage. Headache is the most common presenting symptom and is typically diffuse and progressively worsens but is occasionally thunderclap. CVT is an important cause of isolated intracranial hypertension ("benign" intracranial hypertension). However, in the context of patients presenting with stroke, the region of brain affected by venous ischaemia or haemorrhage determines the focal clinical manifestations and is influenced by location of the thrombosis, which frequently involves multiple sites. With cortical involvement, as may occur in superior sagittal, transverse sinus or cortical vein thrombosis, there may be seizures, motor deficits, or aphasia. The classical clinical triad of headache, seizures and focal motor deficit should prompt early consideration of the diagnosis. Bilateral signs and gradually deteriorating symptoms are also relatively common features and may help to discriminate venous from arterial ischaemia. With thrombosis of the deep venous system (internal cerebral veins, basal vein of Rosenthal and vein of Galen), the archetypal presentation is depressed consciousness and diencephalic dysfunction; however, partial syndromes with preserved consciousness and focal symptoms, including hemiparesis and visual field defects are well recognised [4].

Although 15–20% of cases are unprovoked, numerous acquired and genetic factors have been shown to predispose to CVT, often a precipitating factor such as dehydration acting simultaneously with a predisposing factor. Prothrombotic states, especially thrombophilia caused by inherited deficiencies of proteins C and S or mutations of the genes encoding factor V Leiden and prothrombin G20210A are all well recognised risk factors, and there is also an association with antiphospholipid antibodies. The incidence of CVT increases during pregnancy due to a transient prothrombotic state that persists for 1–2 months postpartum and may be exacerbated at the time of delivery by dehydration. Oral contraceptives are also a predisposing factor as in this case, with the risk being greater in those women with hereditary prothrombotic conditions. The presence of cancer, particularly myeloproliferative neoplasia, is also associated with increased risk. Less common causes include sinus trauma, parameningeal infections (especially otitis media and mastoiditis), particularly in the paediatric population, and systemic diseases, including inflammatory bowel disease and Behcet's disease [2].

The investigation of suspected CVT should include full blood count and assessment of prothrombin time and activated partial thromboplastin time. D-Dimer levels are usually abnormally high in CVT but false negatives are well recognised, particularly in subacute or chronic presentations, and a normal assay should not discourage further investigation if clinical suspicion is high.

Both CT and MRI are useful non-invasive imaging modalities but routine structural imaging has a limited sensitivity in isolation and should be combined with CT or MR venography when clinical suspicion of CVT is high. The parenchymal changes of venous ischaemia appear as low attenuation regions on plain CT and are frequently haemorrhagic. They may be bilateral, particularly if the superior sagittal sinus or deep venous system is involved. The finding of ischaemia or infarction that does not respect a typical arterial territory is very suggestive of the diagnosis of CVT (Fig. 12.5). Patchy haemorrhage within an infarct suggesting haemorrhagic transformation seen early in the disease course within a few hours of onset on the first CT or MRI is also indicative of venous thrombosis. Another clue may be that the patient does not have as extensive a focal deficit as one would expect from the apparent extent of the abnormality on parenchymal imaging. The secondary parenchymal changes of venous infarction are better demonstrated by MRI than CT. T2* ('gradient echo') and susceptibility weighted imaging (SWI) sequences are very sensitive in detecting associated parenchymal and subarachnoid haemorrhage. The parenchymal appearances on diffusion-weighted imaging are variable and can reflect either vasogenic oedema, cytotoxic oedema or a combination of the two. Lesions with increased diffusion are more likely to resolve without parenchymal sequelae than areas of restricted diffusion, but even the latter may be reversible once the CVT has resolved [5].

The principle role of subsequent venographic imaging is to demonstrate the venous thrombosis itself and any secondary effects on the brain parenchyma. Non-contrast CT is positive in approximately one third of cases [2]. In the early stages, thrombosed dural sinuses or veins appear hyperdense but the intensity on CT reduces as the clot matures and attenuation values decrease. CT venography improves sensitivity by highlighting clot as luminal filling defects or showing isolated enhancement of the dural wall when the sinus is completely occluded. Clot within the superior sagittal sinus, the most common site of CVT, gives rise to the so-called 'delta sign' due its triangular profile on non-contrast CT and the inverse 'empty delta sign' on venography due to enhancement of its dural margins.

Detection of venous thrombus on MRI is complicated by the fact that signal characteristics of clot fluctuate over time and because normal venous structures also have a variable signal due to the effects of flowing blood. The signal intensity of venous thrombus varies according to the interval between formation and imaging, principally reflecting the decomposition of haemoglobin. In the acute stage (0–5 days), deoxyhaemoglobin results in isointense and hypointense signal on T1 and T2-weighted imaging respectively and may mimic normal flow states, making detection of the clot particularly challenging. In the subacute stage (6–15 days), methaemoglobin results in high signal on both T1 and T2-weighted images and is the most straightforward to detect. The signal from chronic thrombus is variable but usually isointense on T1-weighted and isointense or hyperintense on T2-weighted images [1]. Chronic thrombus may also enhance and be difficult to distinguish from the luminal enhancement of a normal patent sinus. Sequences such as T2* and SWI are very sensitive to the presence of paramagnetic blood components and can be used as an adjunct to the standard T1 and T2-weighted sequences. Intense signal loss with a 'blooming' effect often results in thrombosed vessels appearing more expanded than on other sequences and may be particularly useful in identifying cortical or deep vein thrombosis [6]. As with CTV, contrast enhanced MRI can be used to highlight luminal filling defects. MR venography can be used to show lack of flow in the occluded vessels and is particularly important in discriminating acute thrombus from normal flow states.

After confirmed cases of CVT screening for genetic and acquired thrombophilia is required but levels of antithrombin III, protein C and S should only be tested after cessation of anticoagulation. Positive antiphospholipid antibodies require confirmatory repeat assays taken at least 12 weeks apart and specialist haematology assessment is necessitated as false positives due to transiently high titres are relatively common. Investigation for mutations of the JAK2 gene, a specific marker of myeloproliferative neoplasia, should also be considered. Examination and follow up by an ophthalmologist is required for patients with papilloedema or visual symptoms [2]. If vision deteriorates despite medical treatment of CVT, optic nerve decompression may be required.

The mainstay of CVT treatment is low molecular weight heparin followed by oral vitamin K antagonists, although there is some evidence that a direct oral anticoagulant may be a safe alternative for patients without coma, major trauma, central nervous system infections, or active cancer [7]. This has been shown to be safe and probably effective in the adult population [2, 3, 8] and is not contraindicated by venous infarction, parenchymal haemorrhage or subarachnoid haemorrhage [2, 3].

Due to the lack of adequate trial data the optimum duration of oral anticoagulation is not known. However, where a transient risk factor is identified it is reasonable to limit treatment to 3–6 months; if the CVT is unprovoked or there is mild thrombophilia treatment is usually continued for 6–12 months, guided by repeat venography. Indefinite anticoagulation should be considered in severe thrombophilia, malignancy or recurrent thrombosis [2, 3]. Long-term anticoagulation should also be considered if follow up imaging shows persistent stenosis of the affected venous sinus. In the acute phase endovascular clot disruption or thrombolysis may have a role if a patient deteriorates despite anticoagulation but the evidence is limited. Acetazolamide is a reasonable adjunct in patients presenting with intracranial hypertension and interventions such as therapeutic lumbar puncture, CSF shunting and optic nerve sheath fenestration may be considered in those with progressive visual failure [2].

Key Clinical Learning Points

- CVT typically presents with findings related to raised intracranial pressure and/or the more focal effects of venous ischaemia or haemorrhage
- A progressively worsening headache with features of raised intracranial pressure should make the assessor consider CVT
- Bilateral signs, seizures and gradually deteriorating symptoms are common features and may help discriminate from arterial ischaemia
- Deep cerebral venous thrombosis often presents with depressed consciousness and diencephalic dysfunction but the clinical course may be much milder with symptoms such as hemiparesis
- Investigations should include screening for the numerous inherited and acquired thrombophilic states associated with CVT
- Anticoagulation with heparin followed by oral vitamin K antagonist is recommended and is not contraindicated by haemorrhagic venous infarct at the time of presentation

Key Radiological Learning Points

- Imaging is used to detect the venous thrombosis itself, resultant venous ischaemia and complications such as haemorrhage and hydrocephalus
- Non resolving clot with worsening hydrocephalus may be amenable to thrombectomy, serial imaging in the acute phase may be necessary and cases should be discussed with an interventional radiologist
- Plain CT and MR should be supplemented by CT or MR venography when clinical suspicion is high
- The MRI signal of venous thrombus evolves over time and distinguishing from flowing blood may be difficult, particularly in the first few days after clot formation and in the chronic stages
- Venous infarcts are frequently haemorrhagic, bilateral and do not conform to arterial territories

References

1. Leach JL, Fortuna RB, Jones BV, et al. Imaging of cerebral venous thrombosis: current techniques, spectrum of findings, and diagnostic pitfalls. Radiographics. 2006;26(Suppl 1):S19–41.
2. Saposnik G, Barinagarrementeria F, Brown RD Jr, et al. American Heart Association Stroke Council and the Council on Epidemiology and Prevention. Diagnosis and management of cerebral venous thrombosis: a statement for healthcare professionals from the American Heart Association/American Stroke Association. Stroke. 2011;42(4):1158–92.
3. Martinelli I, Passamonti SM, Rossi E, et al. Cerebral sinus-venous thrombosis. Intern Emerg Med. 2012;7(Suppl 3):S221–S5.
4. Van den Bergh WM, van der Schaaf I, van Gijn J. The spectrum of presentations of venous infarction caused by deep cerebral vein thrombosis. Neurology. 2005;65(2):192–6.
5. Mullins ME, Grant PE, Wang B, et al. Parenchymal abnormalities associated with cerebral venous sinus thrombosis, assessment with diffusion weighted MR imaging. AJNR Am J Neuroradiol. 2004;25(10):1666–75.
6. Boukobza M, Crassard I, Bousser MG, et al. MR imaging features of isolated cortical vein thrombosis: diagnosis and follow up. AJNR Am J Neuroradiol. 2009;30(2):344–8.
7. Ferro JM, Coutinho JM, Dentali F, Kobayashi A, Alasheev A, Canhão P, Karpov D, Nagel S, Posthuma L, Roriz JM, Caria J, Frässdorf M, Huisman H, Reilly P, Diener HC, RE-SPECT CVT Study Group. Safety and efficacy of dabigatran etexilate vs dose-adjusted warfarin in patients with cerebral venous thrombosis: a randomized clinical trial. JAMA Neurol. 2019;76(12):1457–65.
8. Coutinho J, de Bruijn SFTM, deVeber G, et al. Anticoagulation for cerebral venous sinus thrombosis. Cochrane Database Syst Rev. 2011;(8):CD002005. https://doi.org/10.1002/14651858.CD002005.pub2.

Chapter 13
An Alternative Solution to a Difficult Problem

Kelvin Kuan Huei Ng

Clinical History

A 64-year-old gentleman was found by his wife slumped to the right side, unable to speak with ongoing epistaxis at about 6 o'clock in the morning. He was last seen well before going to bed just before midnight the previous day. He was accompanied by his wife to the emergency room. She reported he had intermittent epistaxis for the past week and had to stop taking aspirin prescribed for remote post-operative paroxysmal atrial fibrillation. He had a diagnosis of hereditary haemorrhagic telangiectasia and usually required iron supplementation and regular blood transfusion for recurrent epistaxis despite embolization and surgical ligation of his nasal vessels. He had hypertension and a stable type B thoracic aorta dissection and an abdominal aortic aneurysm under routine surveillance. He was not noted to have any other significant vascular malformations elsewhere. He did not smoke or drink alcohol. He had previously had an uncomplicated resection of a left adrenal tumour around 7 years ago.

His medications included pantoprazole, irbesartan, hydrochlorothiazide, atorvastatin and metoprolol. He had been prescribed aspirin 81 mg once daily but took it only intermittently due to his recurrent epistaxis.

K. K. H. Ng (✉)
Medicine (Neurology), McMaster University, Hamilton, ON, Canada

David Braley Cardiac, Vascular and Stroke Research Institute, Hamilton General Hospital, Hamilton, ON, Canada
e-mail: kelvin.ng@phri.ca

S. K. Gill et al. (eds.), *Stroke Medicine*,
https://doi.org/10.1007/978-3-031-58188-5_13

Examination

On arrival to the emergency room, he was alert and cooperative. He had right sided facial weakness sparing the forehead and dense right sided hemiplegia. He had predominantly expressive dysphasia but no neglect. Sensation was intact.

Cardiovascular examination demonstrated a soft ejection systolic murmur loudest over the precordium. Respiratory and abdominal examination were unremarkable apart from a well healed surgical scar.

Investigations and Clinical Progress

Routine blood work on admission was within normal range apart from a normocytic anaemia (haemoglobin of 87 g/L). ECG showed no obvious abnormality and he was in sinus rhythm.

CT Scan of Head on Admission Is Shown (Fig. 13.1)

Carotid Doppler ultrasound showed no evidence of significant stenosis in the extracranial segment of both internal carotid arteries. Extended inpatient telemetry and twenty-four-hour Holter ECG monitor showed sinus rhythm with frequent short runs of atrial tachycardia but no sustained atrial fibrillation.

Both the transthoracic and transoesophageal echocardiogram demonstrated the old type B aortic dissection in the descending aorta distal to the left subclavian artery. There was severe biatrial enlargement but no significant valve disease with preserved left ventricular function and importantly no evidence of right-left shunting with contrast.

After completing the investigations for the underlying aetiology of the stroke, he was diagnosed with likely cardioembolic stroke secondary to paroxysmal atrial fibrillation. His CHA 2 DS 2 -VaSc was 4. He recovered from his initial stroke with minimal residual weakness in his right arm and leg. He continued to have residual mild expressive dysphasia.

Taking into account his propensity to bleed, he was restarted on aspirin but continued to have further nose bleeds requiring inpatient blood transfusions. Ear, nose and throat (ENT) specialists were consulted but the mucocutaneous telangiectasia was not remediable to surgical intervention. As he was intolerant of antithrombotic agents, he was referred to the cardiologists and later the cardiothoracic surgeons for consideration of left atrial excision for stroke prophylaxis. He was deemed to be at low surgical risk of complications. Following a lengthy discussion with the patient and his family, he went on to have an open surgical excision of his left atrial appendage for secondary stroke prevention.

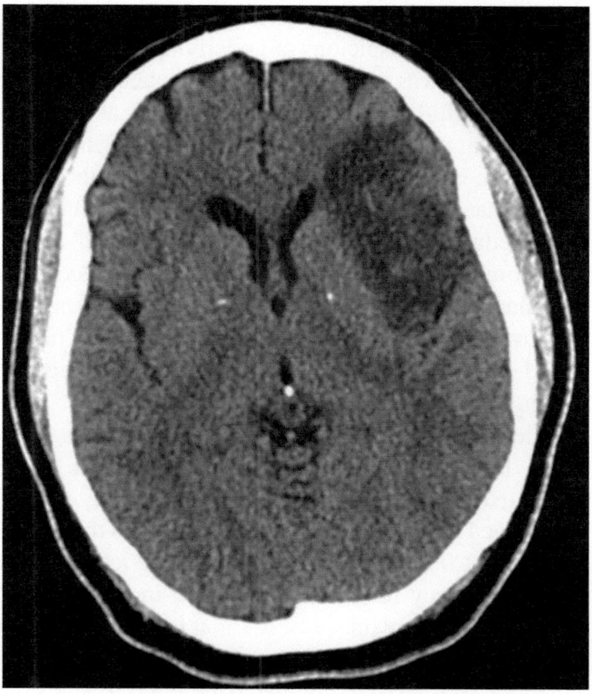

Fig. 13.1 There is significant hypodensity in the left frontal region encompassing most of the insular ribbon and external capsule with mild effacement and mass effect. There is a small amount of petechial haemorrhage within the infarct zone. This cortically based infarct was thought to be due to a proximal embolic source. In the absence of significant cervical carotid artery disease, a cardiogenic embolus from paroxysmal atrial fibrillation was suspected

He had a further period of rehabilitation post-operatively and was eventually discharged home without antiplatelets or anticoagulants.

Discussion

Hereditary haemorrhagic telangiectasia is a rare disorder composed of a triad of mucocutaneous telangiectasia, recurrent epistaxis or gastrointestinal haemorrhage and a family history of the disorder. The condition is inherited in a Mendelian dominant manner. In the central nervous system, vascular anomalies include telangiectasia, arteriovenous malformations, aneurysms and rarely, carotid-cavernous fistulae.

Pulmonary venous fistulae can be responsible for paradoxical embolism resulting in stroke or transient ischaemic attack. Hypoxia due to significant right to left shunting can result in mental obtundation and polycythaemia. Rarely, air embolism or portosystemic encephalopathy can occur. Whilst arteriovenous malformations in hereditary haemorrhagic telangiectasia can be associated with stroke, patients can also have 'classical' risk factors for stroke. Unfortunately, the patients' propensity to bleed may pose therapeutic challenges [1].

In this case, the patient could have been considered to have had an embolic stroke of uncertain source (ESUS) as his history of paroxysmal atrial fibrillation could not be validated. Prior to the results of the NAVIGATE ESUS [2] and RE-SPECT ESUS

[3] trials, there was community equipoise regarding anticoagulation for this patient population. Our suspicions of underlying paroxysmal atrial fibrillation as the cause for his stroke was affirmed following extensive cardiac investigations with no evidence of right-left shunting. Additionally, atrial cardiopathy is recognised as an independent risk factor for strokes outside of atrial fibrillation [4] and the left atrial appendage is well recognised as the source of thromboembolism.

Pharmacological therapy with oral anticoagulants and antithrombotics are effective at reducing the risk of stroke in patients with atrial fibrillation but the benefit of antithrombotics are attenuated with increasing age [5]. The novel selective oral anticoagulants such as dabigatran, rivaroxaban, apixaban and edoxaban are at least as effective as warfarin but appear safer with lower rates of intracranial haemorrhage. Based on the AVERROES trial, the risk of bleeding on apixaban is similar to aspirin [6].

If long-term antiplatelet agents or oral anticoagulation is not tolerated, percutaneous left atrial appendage occlusion can be considered. The WATCHMAN implanted percutaneous device (WATCHMAN; Aritech Inc., Plymouth, Minnesota) is approved by the FDA for this indication. In the combined PROTECT-AF trial and PREVAIL trial [7], the WATCHMAN device is at least as effective as long term warfarin therapy for preventing stroke in selected populations. However, in both trials, patients were on warfarin for at least 45 days after device implantation before going on to dual antiplatelet agents for 6 months and finally aspirin monotherapy thereafter. Neither trials compared the WATCHMAN device against patients deemed unsuitable for long-term warfarin, a population which best describes our patient. In addition, our patient did not tolerate long-term aspirin and was at high risk of further events.

Open surgical left atrial amputation or occlusion can be considered for secondary stroke prevention in the context of atrial fibrillation. The LAAOS III trial comparing left atrial amputation with aspirin against long term anticoagulation for warfarin following open heart surgery demonstrated a significant but attenuated risk reduction in ischemic stroke or systemic embolism [8].

Even though anticoagulation for patients with ESUS is no longer routinely recommended following the results of recent trials in this population [2, 3] and oral anticoagulation for atrial cardiopathy alone is the subject of ongoing study in the ARCADIA trial [4], this patient was thought to have had a stroke secondary to paroxysmal atrial fibrillation. Patients with atrial fibrillation should be offered oral anticoagulation for stroke prophylaxis. Whilst direct-acting oral anticoagulants are safer than warfarin, certain groups of patients may not tolerate any pharmacological anticoagulant or antithrombotic medications. Percutaneous and open surgical options for stroke prophylaxis can be considered but conclusive evidence from randomised controlled trials in this select population is limited.

Key Clinical Learning Points

- Routine anticoagulation for patients with embolic stroke of uncertain source is not recommended.
- Atrial fibrillation is a common and preventable cause for stroke that is managed with direct-acting oral anticoagulation in the majority of patients due to its favourable safety profile.
- Hereditary haemorrhagic telangiectasia is a rare, inherited vascular disorder that may preclude oral anticoagulants and antithrombotics.
- Selected patients may benefit from percutaneous or open surgical left atrial occlusion for stroke prevention if oral anticoagulants or antithrombotics are contraindicated.

References

1. Devlin HL, Hosman AE, Shovlin CL. Antiplatelet and anticoagulant agents in hereditary hemorrhagic telangiectasia. N Engl J Med. 2013;368(9):876–8.
2. Hart RH, Sharma M, Mundi H, et al. Rivaroxaban for stroke prevention after embolic stroke of undetermined source. N Engl J Med. 2018;278:2191–201.
3. Diener HS, Sacco RL, Easton JD, et al. Dabigatran for prevention of stroke after embolic stroke of undetermined source. N Engl J Med. 2019;380:1906–17.
4. Hooman K, Longstreth WT Jr, Tirschwell DL. The AtRial cardiopathy and antithrombotic drugs in prevention after cryptogenic stroke randomized trial: rationale and methods. Int J Stroke. 2019;14(2):207–14.
5. Van Walraven C, Hart RG, Connolly S, et al. Effect of age on stroke prevention therapy in patients with atrial fibrillation: the atrial fibrillation investigators. Stroke. 2009;40(4):1410–6.
6. Connolly SJ, Eikelboom J, Joyner C, et al. Apixaban in patients with atrial fibrillation. NEJM. 2011;364(9):806–17.
7. Reddy VV, Doshi SK, Kar S, et al. 5-year outcomes after left atrial appendate closure: from the PREVAIL and PROTECT AF trials. J Am Coll Cardiol. 2017;70(24):2964–75.
8. Whitlock RP, Belley-Cote EP, Paparella D, et al. Left atrial appendage occlusion during cardiac surgery to prevent stroke. N Engl J Med. 2021;384:2081–91.

Chapter 14
Lower Urinary Tract Dysfunction Following Stroke

Howell T. Jones and Jalesh N. Panicker

Clinical History

A 28-year-old female presented initially 17 years ago with a reduced level of consciousness and was diagnosed with a left frontal intracerebral haemorrhage, which was managed with a left posterior-frontal hemicraniectomy and haematoma evacuation. She had a protracted recovery period during which she had an indwelling urethral catheter for managing incontinence. During her prolonged admission, she was diagnosed with a right below-knee deep vein thrombosis and an inferior vena cava (IVC) filter was inserted. Subsequently, she commenced anticoagulation with Warfarin. She made a partial recovery following a period of rehabilitation, however had residual right hemiparesis with limited movement in the arm and right food drop, expressive dysphasia and higher-level cognitive dysfunction, as well as bladder and bowel symptoms.

Ten years ago, whilst leaning over to pick something up she developed acute lower back pain followed by rapidly progressive left lower limb weakness and numbness which spread to include the saddle area. She presented to the Emergency Department and underwent hyperacute imaging that demonstrated an epidural haematoma at the level of T8/9. The international normalized ratio (INR) was high (4.7). She underwent a T8/9 laminectomy and haematoma evacuation. Following a

H. T. Jones (✉)
Department of Stroke, The National Hospital for Neurology and Neurosurgery, London, UK

MRC Unit for Lifelong Health and Ageing at UCL, London, UK
e-mail: howell.jones@nhs.net

J. N. Panicker
Department of Uro-Neurology, The National Hospital for Neurology and Neurosurgery and UCL Queen Square Institute of Neurology, Faculty of Brain Sciences, UCL, London, UK
e-mail: j.panicker@ucl.ac.uk

S. K. Gill et al. (eds.), *Stroke Medicine*,
https://doi.org/10.1007/978-3-031-58188-5_14

period of rehabilitation, she regained some functions, though was left with new mild weakness in the left leg and persistent sensory loss.

Since the initial Stroke she was experiencing significant overactive bladder symptoms and voiding difficulties. She was incontinent of urine around three times a day, and this was associated with urinary urgency. She would visit the toilet around ten times in the daytime and occasionally overnight. She also reported occasional stress incontinence. She underwent bladder scans and was found to be retaining urine in her bladder consistently, around 300 mL, after voiding. She initially required the insertion of an indwelling urethral catheter (IDC) though this was later removed, and she was started on the anti-muscarinic agent Oxybutynin which she took for nearly 2 years.

Seven years ago, she was reviewed and underwent a urodynamics study that revealed a small capacity bladder of around 195 mL. There was clear evidence for detrusor overactivity and the detrusor pressures rose to a maximum of 122 cm of water, which coincided with a sensation of urinary urgency and was associated with incontinence. Voiding functions could not be adequately assessed because of the incontinence. However, her post-void residual volume after the test was only 30 mL. She was reluctant to pursue the option of intermittent self-catheterisation (ISC) and different options were discussed: oral agents (anti-muscarinic agents, β_3-adrenoceptor agonist), tibial nerve stimulation and botulinum toxin injections into the bladder wall. She opted to trial the anti-muscarinic agent Solifenacin at a low-dose of 5 mg once a day.

On review a year later, Solifenacin was found to be ineffective. The dosage was increased to 10 mg and the β_3-adrenoceptor agonist Mirabegron was also added. The addition of Mirabegron resulted in urinary retention requiring the insertion of an IDC. Urinary retention persisted for some time and she failed several trials without catheters. Eventually the catheter was successfully removed, and her overactive bladder symptoms became apparent once again. She declined botulinum toxin injection into the bladder due to the potential risk of urinary retention necessitating the need to perform ISC. The patient enquired about the use of a long-term urethral IDC; however, it was felt that due to her age and the risk for infection that other options should be explored first. She therefore opted for the insertion of a suprapubic catheter (SPC) and underwent botulinum toxin injection to the bladder wall. In view of the need for repeating botulinum toxin injections periodically, she opted for sacral neuromodulation. After the implant, her lower urinary tract (LUT) symptoms and quality of life improved considerably and she has been able to return to work, live independently and enter a relationship.

Discussion

This case highlights several areas of complexity in regards to LUT dysfunction following a Stroke. We will explore the neural control of the LUT in health, dysfunction following neurological disorders such as Stroke, treatment options and prognosis.

Lower Urinary Tract Dysfunction Post Stroke

Central or peripheral damage to the nervous system can result in LUT dysfunction. Lesions of the suprapontine or spinal pathways affecting the storage phase, resulting in reduced bladder capacity and detrusor overactivity, which is expressed as spontaneous involuntary contractions of the detrusor [1]. Patients may report varying degrees of urinary urgency, frequency, nocturia, and incontinence (collectively known as overactive bladder symptoms) [1]. Incontinence is most commonly caused by detrusor overactivity where the sensation of urinary urgency is experienced as the detrusor begins to contract, and if the pressure rise continues, the patient senses impending micturition [1]. Damage to the suprapontine neural circuitry results in removal of the tonic inhibition of the PMC so that spontaneous involuntary detrusor contractions occur [1].

Therefore, incontinence is not a normal and harmless consequence of Stroke and is frequently overlooked. More than half of all patients will experience urinary incontinence during the acute phase of Stroke with those with multimorbidity or advanced age being at most risk [1, 2]. This number remains high at 1 year, with approximately a quarter of survivors experiencing incontinence [3].

Storage symptoms are more common than voiding symptoms and Sakakibara et al. (1996) noted that nocturia was the most commonly experienced symptom (36%), followed by urge incontinence (29%), voiding difficulty (25%) and urinary retention (6%) [2]. They also observed that on urodynamics that detrusor overactivity was the most common (68%) finding, followed by detrusor-sphincter dyssynergia (14%) [2]. Ischemic Strokes are more commonly associated with detrusor overactivity whilst haemorrhagic Strokes tend to lead to detrusor underactivity, though both can be associated with urinary retention [4].

Patients with large lesions, or those involving the anteromedial frontal lobe, paraventricular white matter, and putamen are more likely to experience incontinence [1]. Detrusor-sphincter dyssynergia has been reported following basal ganglia lesions, whereas retention may occur following lesions involving the cerebellum [1]. Incontinence following Stroke is however multidimensional. Disruptions to the neural pathways controlling the LUT can lead to LUT dysfunction. The pathophysiology of bladder overactivity in Stroke is likely due to reduced suprapontine inhibition leading to detrusor overactivity. A rat cerebral infarction model demonstrated that bladder overactivity was contributed by NMDA receptor mediated glutamatergic and D2 receptor mediated excitatory activity [5, 6]. Alteration in dopaminergic-glutamatergic activity results in up-regulation of excitatory pathways and down-regulation of tonic inhibitory pathways leading to bladder overactivity [5, 6]. However, disabilities arising from Stroke can also contribute to incontinence and other problems with the bladder. For example, immobility, visual inattention and proprioceptive loss lead to difficulties in using a toilet challenging, whereas speech disturbance such as aphasia or dysarthria affect the ability to communicate toilet needs with others [1].

Small-vessel disease of the white matter, or leukoaraiosis, is also associated with LUT dysfunction, particularly urgency incontinence and is now recognised as an important cause of incontinence in functionally independent older people [2, 7–9]. Evidence suggests that white matter changes affecting the anterior thalamic radiation and superior longitudinal fasciculus in particular are most associated with incontinence [7].

Incontinence has been shown to be a poor prognostic marker in the context of acute Stroke with its persistence 7 days after Stroke has been shown to correlate with poor survival, increased severity of neurological disability and increased likelihood to require discharge to a long-term care facility [10]. Continuing to experience incontinence at 1 year post Stroke has been shown to be associated with a four times greater risk for mortality [11].

Neurological Control of Lower Urinary Tract Functions

Prior to considering management of incontinence post-Stroke, one must first understand the neurological control of LUT functions in health. Typically, the coordinated activity of the LUT results in low pressure filling and periodic voluntary emptying controlled by a neural network of parasympathetic, sympathetic, and somatic pathways [1]. The bladder remains in the storage phase for more than 99% of the time, switching to the voiding phase for only a few minutes per day [12, 13]. Voiding is typically initiated by a conscious decision and it is this voluntary control that distinguishes the LUT from other autonomically innervated structures [13].

Storage and voiding both require intact connections between the pons and the sacral spinal cord as well as peripheral innervation that originates from the caudal segments of the cord [1]. The cerebral cortex is involved in the perception of sensations of bladder fullness and timing of micturition, the brainstem for coordination of reflexes, the spinal cord for amplification of these reflexes and the peripheral nerves for relaying signals to the bladder [14]. During bladder filling, sympathetic and pudendal nerves mediate contraction of the internal smooth and external striated muscles of the urethral sphincter, respectively, whereas sympathetic-mediated inhibition of the detrusor prevents contractions and ensures a low pressure, thereby maintaining continence [1, 13]. When voiding is to be initiated, the pontine micturition centre (PMC) or 'Barrington's nucleus' is released from the tonic inhibition of cortical and subcortical centres of the brain, and the reciprocal activation–inhibition of the sphincter–detrusor is reversed [15–18]. Detrusor contraction in response to parasympathetic stimulation, accompanied by relaxation of the pelvic floor and external and internal urethral sphincters, results in effective bladder emptying [1].

Clinical Assessment of Incontinence

We now outline the approach on how to assess incontinence. Assessment of continence requires appreciation of multiple systems and a thorough history and examination.

History

As in the rest of medicine, history taking provides most of the crucial information to make the correct diagnosis. In patients who are able, the use of a bladder diary is recommended as this provides a real-time objective patient-reported measure of symptoms, which might not be obtained through history taking [19]. A bladder diary consists of information charted by time, as to how much fluid a patient drinks, how frequently they micturate and the volume (this can be subjective or objective [19]. It also documents the timing and amount of urinary leakage and urgency symptoms [19].

Initial focus should be on differentiating between storage and voiding dysfunction [20]. Storage symptoms include frequency, urgency, leaking of urine during physical activity and/or nocturia [20]. Voiding symptoms consist of hesitancy, intermittent stream, incomplete bladder emptying, double voiding and post micturition dribbling [20]. Abdominal pain, fever, dysuria, and haematuria should be specifically enquired about to exclude alternative causes such as infection or malignancy [12].

Next, congenital and neurological abnormalities, previous urogenital complications and treatments, and urinary tract, sexual, bowel, obstetric, gynaecological, and neurological function should be explored [20, 21]. Systemic symptoms and those symptoms that could be associated with diseases that predispose a patient to urinary incontinence as well as the presence of co-morbidities should be reviewed [20].

Exploring functional status is crucial as many patients post Stroke report becoming incontinent because of inability to reach the toilet in a timely manner due to their neurological deficits or to poor toilet accessibility, and this is termed functional incontinence [1, 20].

Detailed medication review is essential as many drugs can exacerbate urinary incontinence [20, 21]. Common culprits include opioids use to treat pain following Stroke, α-adrenoceptor agonists, and medications with anticholinergic properties such as antidepressants to treat post Stroke depression, respiratory drugs to manage secretions or antipsychotic drugs [1, 22].

Finally, evaluation of lifestyle factors such as smoking, alcohol, or recreational drugs as well as the impact of symptoms on quality of life important [1].

Physical Examination

Focussed examination consists of examining the abdomen, loins, pelvic and genital organs urogenital sensations and sacral cord mediated reflexes (bulbocavernosus reflex and anal reflex) when appropriate [1].

A general examination should be performed looking for signs of vascular disease, assessment of cognition and consideration of a digital rectal examination to assess anal tone, presence of constipation or rectal masses and in those with a prostate it's the size, symmetry and texture [20].

Investigations

There are several specialist investigations useful when assessing incontinence. Urinalysis and measurement of the postvoid residual form part of the core neuro-urological assessment [1, 21], and we outline the more specialist investigations below:

Urinalysis

In patients presenting with new LUT dysfunction it is prudent to exclude infection [1]. Urinalysis is helpful for excluding infection in younger patients as the cause of new incontinence and though it has a high sensitivity the specificity is limited [23]. In all cases where urinary tract infection is considered possible the gold standard test remains bacterial culture [24].

Most Strokes occur in older people but the accuracy of dipstick testing in adults aged over 65 is poor when compared to younger people [25–28]. In people over 65 years asymptomatic bacteriuria is common but not associated with increased morbidity [27]. Treating asymptomatic bacteriuria unnecessarily with antibiotics is associated with a significant increase in adverse events however with no clinical benefit [27, 29]. Therefore other clinical characteristics should also be considered when diagnosing urinary tract infections in older people such as vital signs and clinical assessment to ensure appropriate management and avoid unnecessary use of antibiotics [27].

Urinalysis is not an effective method for detecting urinary tract infections in patient with an IDC as its sheer presence can induce pyuria, with no relationship between the level of pyuria and the incidence of infection [30–32]. Evidence suggests that as many as 2–7% of patients with an IDC develop bacteriuria each day despite good catheter care [33]. Meanwhile in those who have an IDC long-term almost all patients are bacteriuric often with two or more organisms [34, 35]. To ensure that urinary tract infections are diagnosed accurately and to avoid false positive results, urinalysis should not be performed with focus again being on vital signs, clinical assessment and results of bacterial culture [23, 24, 30–32].

Biochemistry

All patients presenting with new LUT dysfunction should undergo blood tests to assess renal function; urea, creatinine and estimated glomerular filtration rate (eGFR) [21].

In situations such as renal impairment, older people and people with extremes of muscle mass the eGFR result can be inaccurate with the advice to calculate the creatinine clearance (Cockcroft-Gault Formula) to provide a more accurate assessment [36]. This has replaced 24-h urine collection to estimate creatinine excretion as despite it being more accurate it is cumbersome and incomplete collection can result in an underestimation [1, 37]. The GFR is most accurately measured using renal scintigraphy, which is recommended when renal function is poor, in individuals with reduced muscle mass, if function for each renal unit has to be assessed separately and in high-risk patients [21].

Measuring the Post-Void Residual

The postvoid residual (PVR) is the volume of urine remaining in the bladder after micturition or ISC and can be measured either by bedside ultrasound known as a 'bladder scan' or by inserting an IDC to drain the bladder, colloquially known as 'in–out catheterisation' [1, 38, 39]. Measuring the PVR is useful as voiding dysfunction may not always be forthcoming from the history and incomplete bladder emptying is an important cause for urinary storage symptoms as well as predisposing to urinary tract infections [1, 24, 38, 39]. A single reading is useful to assess for significant retention, however if an elevated PVR volume is found this should be repeated ideally at different times and in different circumstances to confirm a pattern [21, 40]. A PVR volume confirms voiding dysfunction, however the cause-whether due to obstructed voiding or poor detrusor contractility- can be established by urodynamics [1].

Ultrasonography

Formal ultrasonography of the kidneys, ureters and bladder is useful to exclude urological pathology such as hydronephrosis, renal or bladder calculi, tumours, prostate size if applicable, or congenital anomalies in those with a relevant history, and to measure the PVR [1, 41–43].

Urodynamics

Urodynamics testing is valuable to understand the nature of LUT dysfunction, assess the risk for developing upper urinary tract damage, provide guidance for appropriate treatment and to monitor response particularly when initial symptom-based therapy has failed [1]. Uroflowmetry non-invasively assesses voiding functions and the finding of abnormally poor flow provides an indicator for voiding dysfunction [1]. However, cystometry, with or without simultaneous fluoroscopic monitoring (video-urodynamics), would be required to assess whether voiding dysfunction is due to detrusor underactivity or bladder outlet obstruction in the pressure-flow study [1]. Filling cystometry provides information about detrusor pressure and compliance [1].

Principles of Management

The purpose of managing LUT dysfunction post Stroke is to maintain independence and quality of life, preserve renal function and prevent infection [21]. Specific management is dependent on whether the problem is related to storage or voiding dysfunction.

Management of Storage Dysfunction

The management of storage dysfunction ranges from conservative to invasive which will be outlined below.

Physical Treatments

Behavioural interventions are an important part of managing storage symptoms [1]. Behavioural interventions are useful post Stroke using strategies such as personalised toileting scheduled with timed voiding based around a person's natural voiding pattern [1]. These techniques however have a limited evidence base and often require not only patient engagement but also that of caregivers or care professionals to be successful [44–46]. Pelvic floor muscle training can enhance the inhibitory effect of pelvic floor contraction on the detrusor with evidence that this results in an improvement in urinary frequency and the number of daily incontinence episodes, whilst also increasing the mean cystometric capacity [47].

Antimuscarinic Agents

Antimuscarinic agents competitively antagonise muscarinic acetylcholine receptor of which the M2 receptor is the most relevant subtype in the bladder, whilst it is the M3 receptor that is found in the detrusor, urothelium, and suburothelium [1]. Blocking of these receptors results in detrusor relaxation, lower intravesical pressures and reduced storage symptoms [1]. Oxybutynin has been available for several years, and several new agents are now available such as Solifenacin, Darifenacin and Tolterodine [48–52].

Antimuscarinic agents have a range of adverse effects due to their non-specific anticholinergic action such as dry mouth, blurred vision and constipation [1]. Antimuscarinic drugs have also been found to have a significant effect on cognition and a study in healthy volunteers demonstrated that using Oxybutynin resulted in a significant decline in alpha activity on electroencephalography (EEG) [53]. The effect is magnified in older people, with evidence that the degree in memory deterioration is comparable to 10 years of brain ageing [54]. The effects of antimuscarinic medications are cumulative so reviewing the total acetylcholine burden of a patient's medications is essential prior to commencing treatment for overactive bladder [55]. This can be done using the anticholinergic burden (ACB) scale [56, 57]. If it is felt the benefit outweighs the risk then choosing a medication that does not cross the blood–brain barrier (such as trospium chloride) or has a relatively high affinity for the muscarinic receptors of the bladder (such as darifenacin) is preferable as theoretically they have less effect on cognition, though patients should still be counselled on the potential impact on cognition [58–61].

Measurement of the PVR volume should be performed prior to commencing antimuscarinic medications and this should be repeated to exclude incomplete bladder emptying if the patient's symptoms fail to improve or paradoxically deteriorate, or if the patient begins to experience urinary tract infections [40]. In many circumstances the combination of antimuscarinic medication with ISC provides the most effective management of LUT symptoms [1].

Desmopressin

Desmopressin is a synthetic analogue of arginine vasopressin that temporarily reduces urine production and volume-determined detrusor overactivity, by promoting water reabsorption at the distal and collecting tubules of the kidney [1, 62]. It is most useful in managing nocturnal polyuria, however should be avoided in older adults, or those with heart failure due to the risk of hyponatremia and fluid overload [1].

β_3-Adrenoceptor Agonists

The oral β_3-adrenoceptor agonist Mirabegron is licensed for overactive bladder [21]. A study has reported a significant subjective improvement in overactive bladder symptoms in neuro-urological patients using Mirabegron without any negative effects on voiding function [63]. However, other studies have not demonstrated any substantial effect on detrusor pressure or cystometric capacity, despite reported improvement in symptoms [64, 65]. Mirabegron is not associated with the side effects of antimuscarinic drugs, however instead affecting the cardiovascular system and may be associated with side effects such as palpitations, raised blood pressure and rarely atrial fibrillation [66].

Botulinum Toxin

Botulinum toxin injections were first injected into the detrusor muscle in 2000, and has been used for the management of neurogenic detrusor overactivity and shown to be highly effective, safe, and well tolerated [67–72]. There are seven subtypes but it is type A that is used in the context of urological disorders, with onabotulinumtoxinA being the only formulation licensed for treatment of detrusor overactivity [73, 74]. The procedure can be performed under local anaesthesia through either rigid or flexible cystoscopy with thirty injections made into the bladder wall. Evidence suggests that injections are efficacious with results lasting from 9 to 13 months, as well as being cost-effective when compared to best supportive care [21, 75–78]. There is however a risk of developing detrusor underactivity necessitating the need for ISC in up to 42% of patients so pre-procedural counselling is vital [73, 74].

Neuromodulation

Electrical stimulation of peripheral nerves such as the sacral nerve roots, tibial nerve, pudendal nerve, and dorsal genital nerves has been shown to improve symptoms of overactive bladder [79].

Percutaneous tibial nerve stimulation (PTNS) has been shown to improve overactive bladder symptoms and urodynamic parameters and is a safe and effective treatment for urgency incontinence caused by detrusor overactivity [80–82]. A typical course consists of once weekly 30-min treatments over 8 to 12 weeks where the tibial nerve is stimulated via a fine gauge needle using a fixed electrical signal [1]. Transcutaneous tibial nerve stimulation (TTNS) is an effective alternative that can be performed at home [83, 84]. Both are minimally invasive with few adverse effects, and is a treatment for the overactive bladder than does not cause an increase in PVR volume. However the results can be short lived [85].

Sacral neuromodulation (SNM) is an effective treatment for both LUT and bowel dysfunction and unlike botulinum toxin, does not increase the PVR volume [86–88]. SNM involves modulation of spinal cord reflexes and brain networks by peripheral afferents rather than direct stimulation of the motor response of the detrusor or urethral sphincter (or anal sphincter) and presumably mediates an inhibitory effect [89–94]. Patients post Stroke can be good candidates for SNM as they have had a discrete neurological event as opposed to a progressive neurological disorder, however it is important to note insertion of a SNM system involves the insertion of metallic implants potentially complicating future investigations such as magnetic resonance imaging (MRI) [1, 87, 88].

Management of Voiding Dysfunction

The decision to commence treatment for voiding dysfunction is based on the PVR volume and risk for developing renal damage [1]. Patients with neurogenic LUT dysfunction often have reduced bladder capacity and so a PVR volume of more than 100 mL in a symptomatic patient is often considered an indication for treatment [40].

Intermittent Self-Catheterisation

Intermittent self-catheterisation (ISC) is often used as an adjunct to other treatment options as incomplete bladder emptying can exacerbate overactive bladder symptoms and render treatments such as antimuscarinic drugs or botulinum toxin less effective [1]. ISC can be challenging for patients following a Stroke if lesions have resulted in poor manual dexterity, weakness, spasticity, impaired visual acuity or cognitive impairment [95]. Patients should be referred to a local continence service to facilitate ongoing education and support [1]. Current recommendations are to perform ISC between four and six times a day for individuals with complete retention and one and three times for those with incomplete bladder emptying [1]. Individual strategies will be based upon bladder volume, fluid intake, PVR volume and results from urodynamics [1]. The risk for developing urinary tract infections is generally low if performed regularly [40].

Other Treatments

The use ofα-Adrenoceptor blockers to relax the internal urethral sphincter in men could be considered if there is concomitant bladder outlet obstruction caused by a nonrelaxing bladder neck or benign prostate enlargement [40].

Surgical Treatment

Surgical interventions can be considered in cases where conservative measures have been unsuccessful and include external sphincter/bladder neck incision, transurethral resection of prostate or continent/incontinent urinary diversion [1]. These are less likely to be pursued post Stroke due to the increasing availability of non-invasive options and the fact that post Stroke, patients may not be suitable surgical candidates [1].

Conclusion

LUT dysfunction is common post Stroke and has a poor prognosis. When reviewing Stroke patients, a regular review of continence should be performed. The availability of multiple non-invasive treatments means that patients do not need to experience these symptoms long-term and should be referred to a multi-speciality service including Stroke Physicians or Neurologists, Urologists, specialist continence nurses and if relevant Uro-Gynaecologists for assessment and formulation of an individualised care plan.

Key Clinical Learning Points

- Ischemic Strokes are more associated with detrusor overactivity whilst haemorrhagic Strokes tend to lead to detrusor underactivity.
- Initial bladder assessment can be performed by any healthcare professional adopting a systematic approach that includes history taking and examination.
- Bladder diaries are a useful tool providing a real-time assessment of symptoms.
- Assessment of LUT symptoms include urinalysis, measurement of the post-void residual, serum urea and creatinine measurement, ultrasonography of the kidneys and urinary bladder and possibly urodynamics.
- Antimuscarinic agents are the first line treatment for managing overactive bladder symptoms.

References

1. Panicker JN, Fowler CJ, Kessler TM. Lower urinary tract dysfunction in the neurological patient: clinical assessment and management. Lancet Neurol. 2015;14(7):720–32.
2. Sakakibara R, Hattori T, Yasuda K, Yamanishi T. Micturitional disturbance after acute hemispheric stroke: analysis of the lesion site by CT and MRI. J Neurol Sci. 1996;137(1):47–56.

3. Kolominsky-Rabas PL, Hilz MJ, Neundoerfer B, Heuschmann PU. Impact of urinary incontinence after stroke: results from a prospective population-based stroke register. Neurourol Urodyn. 2003;22(4):322–7.
4. Han KS, Heo SH, Lee SJ, Jeon SH, Yoo KH. Comparison of urodynamics between ischemic and hemorrhagic stroke patients; can we uggest the category of urinary dysfunction in patients with cerebrovascular accident according to type of stroke? Neurourol Urodyn. 2010;29(3):387–90.
5. Yokoyama O, Komatsu K, Ishiura Y, Akino H, Kodama K, Yotsuyanagi S, et al. Overactive bladder—experimental aspects. Scand J Urol Nephrol Suppl. 2002;210:59–64.
6. Yoshimura Y, Ohmura T, Komatsu Y. Two forms of synaptic plasticity with distinct dependence on age, experience, and NMDA receptor subtype in rat visual cortex. J Neurosci. 2003;23(16):6557–66.
7. Tadic SD, Griffiths D, Murrin A, Schaefer W, Aizenstein HJ, Resnick NM. Brain activity during bladder filling is related to white matter structural changes in older women with urinary incontinence. Neuro Image. 2010;51(4):1294–302.
8. Sakakibara R, Hattori T, Uchiyama T, Yamanishi T. Urinary function in elderly people with and without leukoaraiosis: relation to cognitive and gait function. J Neurol Neurosurg Psychiatry. 1999;67(5):658–60.
9. Kuchel GA, Moscufo N, Guttmann CR, Zeevi N, Wakefield D, Schmidt J, et al. Localization of brain white matter hyperintensities and urinary incontinence in community-dwelling older adults. J Gerontol A Biol Sci Med Sci. 2009;64(8):902–9.
10. Wade DT, Hewer RL. Outlook after an acute stroke: urinary incontinence and loss of consciousness compared in 532 patients. QJM. 1985;56(3–4):601–8.
11. Anderson CS, Jamrozik KD, Broadhurst RJ, Stewart-Wynne EG. Predicting survival for 1 year among different subtypes of stroke. Results from the Perth Community Stroke Study. Stroke. 1994;25(10):1935–44.
12. Fowler CJ. Integrated control of lower urinary tract—clinical perspective. Br J Pharmacol. 2006;147(SUPPL 2):S14–24.
13. Fowler CJ, Griffiths D, De Groat WC. The neural control of micturition. Nat Rev Neurosci. 2008;9(6):453–66.
14. de Groat WC, Kawatani M, Hisamitsu T, Cheng CL, Ma CP, Thor K, et al. Mechanisms underlying the recovery of urinary bladder function following spinal cord injury. JANS. 1990;30:S71–S7.
15. Griffiths DJ. The pontine micturition centres. Scand J Urol Nephrol Suppl. 2002;36(210):21–6.
16. Michels L, Blok BFM, Gregorini F, Kurz M, Schurch B, Kessler TM, et al. Supraspinal control of urine storage and micturition in men-an fMRI study. Cereb Cortex. 2015;25(10):3369–80.
17. Griffiths D, Holstege G, Dalm E, Wall HD. Control and coordination of bladder and urethral function in the brainstem of the cat. Neurourol Urodyn. 1990;9:63–82.
18. Blok BF, Willemsen AT, Holstege G. A PET study on brain control of micturition in humans. Brain. 1997;120(Pt 1):111–21.
19. Kessler TM. Diagnosis of urinary incontinence. JAMA. 2008;300(3):283.
20. British Geriatrics Society. CGA in primary care settings: patients presenting with urinary incontinence. In: Comprehensive geriatric assessment toolkit for primary care practitioners. London: British Geriatrics Society; 2019. p. 42–4.
21. European Association of Urology. EAU Guidelines. In: Edn. presented at the EAU Annual Congress Amsterdam 2020. Arnhem: EAU Guidelines Office; 2020.
22. Panicker JN, Game X, Khan S, Kessler TM, Gonzales G, Elneil S, et al. The possible role of opiates in women with chronic urinary retention: observations from a prospective clinical study. J Urol. 2012;188(2):480–4.
23. Simerville JA, Maxted WC, Pahira JJ. Urinalysis: a comprehensive review. Am Fam Physician. 2005;71(6):1153–62.
24. Schmiemann G, Kniehl E, Gebhardt K, Matejczyk MM, Hummers-Pradier E. The diagnosis of urinary tract infection: a systematic review. Dtsch Arztebl Int. 2010;107(21):361–7.

25. Roy-O'Reilly M, McCullough LD. Age and sex are critical factors in ischemic stroke pathology. Endocrinol. 2018;159(8):3120–31.
26. Kelly-Hayes M. Influence of age and health behaviors on Stroke risk: lessons from longitudinal studies. JAGS. 2010;58(Suppl 2):S325–S8.
27. Nicolle LE, Mayhew WJ, Bryan L. Prospective randomized comparison of therapy and no therapy for asymptomatic bacteriuria in institutionalized elderly women. Am J Med. 1987;83(1):27–33.
28. Abrutyn E, Berlin J, Mossey J, Pitsakis P, Levison M, Kaye D. Does treatment of asymptomatic bacteriuria in older ambulatory women reduce subsequent symptoms of urinary tract infection? J Am Geriatr Soc. 1996;44(3):293–5.
29. Harding GK, Zhanel GG, Nicolle LE, Cheang M. Antimicrobial treatment in diabetic women with asymptomatic bacteriuria. N Engl J Med. 2002;347(20):1576–83.
30. Tambyah PA, Maki DG. The relationship between pyuria and infection in patients with indwelling urinary catheters: a prospective study of 761 patients. Arch Intern Med. 2000;160(5):673–7.
31. Steward DK, Wood GL, Cohen RL, Smith JW, Mackowiak PA. Failure of the urinalysis and quantitative urine culture in diagnosing symptomatic urinary tract infections in patients with long-term urinary catheters. Am J Infect Control. 1985;13(4):154–60.
32. Mimoz O, Bouchet E, Edouard A, Costa Y, Samii K. Limited usefulness of urinary dipsticks to screen out catheter-associated bacteriuria in ICU patients. Anaesth Intensive Care. 1995;23(6):706–7.
33. Pratt RJ, Pellowe C, Loveday HP, Robinson N, Smith GW, Barrett S, et al. The epic project: developing national evidence-based guidelines for preventing healthcare associated infections. Phase I: guidelines for preventing hospital-acquired infections. Department of Health (England). J Hosp Infect. 2001;47:S3–82.
34. Warren JW, Anthony WC, Hoopes JM, Muncie HL Jr. Cephalexin for susceptible bacteriuria in afebrile, long-term catheterized patients. JAMA. 1982;248(4):454–8.
35. Breitenbucher RB. Bacterial changes in the urine samples of patients with long-term indwelling catheters. Arch Intern Med. 1984;144(8):1585–8.
36. Helou R. Should we continue to use the Cockcroft-Gault formula? Nephron Clin Pract. 2010;116(3):c172–c86.
37. Kalantari K, Bolton WK. A good reason to measure 24-hour urine creatinine excretion, but not to assess kidney function. Clin J Am Soc Nephrol. 2013;8(11):1847–9.
38. Haylen BT, Lee J. The accuracy of post-void residual measurement in women. Int Urogynecol J Pelvic Floor Dysfunct. 2008;19(5):603–6.
39. Venkatesan M, Nasto L, Tsegaye M, Grevitt M. Bladder scans and postvoid residual volume measurement improve diagnostic accuracy of cauda equina syndrome. Spine. 2019;44(18):1303–8.
40. Fowler CJ, Panicker JN, Drake M, Harris C, Harrison SC, Kirby M, et al. A UK consensus on the management of the bladder in multiple sclerosis. J Neurol Neurosurgery Psych. 2009;80(5):470–7.
41. Jiménez Cidre MA, López-Fando Lavalle L, Quicios Dorado C, de Castro GC, Fraile Poblador A, Mayayo DT. Ultrasound for the diagnosis of female urinary incontinence. Arch Esp Urol. 2006;59(4):431–9.
42. O'Neill WC. Renal relevant radiology: use of ultrasound in kidney disease and nephrology procedures. Clin J Am Soc Nephrol. 2014;9(2):373–81.
43. Mitterberger M, Horninger W, Aigner F, Pinggera GM, Steppan I, Rehder P, et al. Ultrasound of the prostate. Cancer Imaging. 2010;10(1):40–8.
44. Wallace SA, Roe B, Williams K, Palmer M. Bladder training for urinary incontinence in adults. Cochrane Database Sys Rev (Online). 2004;1:CD001308.
45. Eustice S, Roe B, Paterson J. Prompted voiding for the management of urinary incontinence in adults. Cochrane Database Sys Rev (Online). 2000;2:CD002113.
46. Ostaszkiewicz J, Johnston L, Roe B. Timed voiding for the management of urinary incontinence in adults. Cochrane Database Sys Rev (Online). 2004;1:CD002802.

47. De Ridder D, Vermeulen C, Ketelaer P, Van Poppel H, Baert L. Pelvic floor rehabilitation in multiple sclerosis. Acta Neurol Belg. 1999;99(1):61–4.
48. Gajewski JB, Awad SA. Oxybutynin versus propantheline in patients with multiple sclerosis and detrusor hyperreflexia. J Urol. 1986;135(5):966–8.
49. Stöhrer M, Mürtz G, Kramer G, Schnabel F, Arnold EP, Wyndaele JJ. Propiverine compared to oxybutynin in neurogenic detrusor overactivity-results of a randomized, double-blind, multicenter clinical study. Eur Urol. 2007;51(1):235–42.
50. van Rey F, Heesakkers J. Solifenacin in multiple sclerosis patients with overactive bladder: a prospective study. Adv Urol. 2011;2011:834753.
51. Ethans KD, Nance PW, Bard RJ, Casey AR, Schryvers OI. Efficacy and safety of tolterodine in people with neurogenic detrusor overactivity. J Spinal Cord Med. 2004;27(3):214–8.
52. Mazo EB, Babanina GA. Trospium chloride (spasmex) in the treatment of lower urinary tract symptoms in patients with neurogenic hyperactive urinary bladder caused by vertebrogenic lesions. Urologii. 1999;2007(3):15–9.
53. Todorova A, Vonderheid-Guth B, Dimpfel W. Effects of tolterodine, trospium chloride, and oxybutynin on the central nervous system. J Clin Pharm. 2001;41(6):636–44.
54. Kay G, Crook T, Rekeda L, Lima R, Ebinger U, Arguinzoniz M, et al. Differential effects of the antimuscarinic agents darifenacin and oxybutynin ER on memory in older subjects. Eur Urol. 2006;50(2):317–26.
55. Gray SL, Anderson ML, Dublin S, Hanlon JT, Hubbard R, Walker R, et al. Cumulative use of strong anticholinergics and incident dementia: a prospective cohort study. JAMA Intern Med. 2015;175(3):401–7.
56. Boustani M, Campbell N, Munger S, Maidment I, Fox C. Impact of anticholinergics on the aging brain: a review and practical application. Aging Health. 2008;4(3):311–20.
57. Campbell N, Boustani M, Limbil T, Ott C, Fox C, Maidment I, et al. The cognitive impact of anticholinergics: a clinical review. Clin Interv Aging. 2009;4:225–33.
58. Davis TP, Sanchez-Covarubias L, Tome ME. P-glycoprotein trafficking as a therapeutic target to optimize CNS drug delivery. Adv Pharmacol. 2014;71:25–44.
59. Chancellor MB, Staskin DR, Kay GG, Sandage BW, Oefelein MG, Tsao JW. Blood-brain barrier permeation and efflux exclusion of anticholinergics used in the treatment of overactive bladder. Drugs Aging. 2012;29(4):259–73.
60. Wagg A, Verdejo C, Molander U. Review of cognitive impairment with antimuscarinic agents in elderly patients with overactive bladder. Int J Clin Pract. 2010;64(9):1279–86.
61. Isik AT, Celik T, Bozoglu E, Doruk H. Trospium and cognition in patients with late onset Alzheimer disease. J Nutr Health Aging. 2009;13(8):672–6.
62. Bosma R, Wynia K, Havlíková E, De Keyser J, Middel B. Efficacy of desmopressin in patients with multiple sclerosis suffering from bladder dysfunction: a meta-analysis. Acta Neurologica Scand. 2005;112(1):1–5.
63. Chen SF, Kuo HC. Therapeutic efficacy of low-dose (25 mg) mirabegron therapy for patients with mild to moderate overactive bladder symptoms due to central nervous system diseases. Low Urin Tract Symptoms. 2019;11(2):O53–o8.
64. Krhut J, Borovička V, Bílková K, Sýkora R, Míka D, Mokriš J, et al. Efficacy and safety of mirabegron for the treatment of neurogenic detrusor overactivity-prospective, randomized, double-blind, placebo-controlled study. Neurourol Urodyn. 2018;37(7):2226–33.
65. Welk B, Hickling D, McKibbon M, Radomski S, Ethans K. A pilot randomized-controlled trial of the urodynamic efficacy of mirabegron for patients with neurogenic lower urinary tract dysfunction. Neurourol Urodyn. 2018;37(8):2810–7.
66. Chapple CR, Cardozo L, Nitti VW, Siddiqui E, Michel MC. Mirabegron in overactive bladder: a review of efficacy, safety, and tolerability. Neurourol Urodyn. 2014;33(1):17–30.
67. Schurch B, Stöhrer M, Kramer G, Schmid DM, Gaul G, Hauri D. Botulinum-A toxin for treating detrusor hyperreflexia in spinal cord injured patients: a new alternative to anticholinergic drugs? Preliminary results. J Urol. 2000;164(3 Pt 1):692–7.

68. Schurch B, Schmid DM, Stöhrer M. Treatment of neurogenic incontinence with botulinum toxin A. N Engl J Med. 2000;342(9):665.
69. Mangera A, Apostolidis A, Andersson KE, Dasgupta P, Giannantoni A, Roehrborn C, et al. An updated systematic review and statistical comparison of standardised mean outcomes for the use of botulinum toxin in the management of lower urinary tract disorders. Eur Urol. 2014;65(5):981–90.
70. Sussman D, Patel V, Del Popolo G, Lam W, Globe D, Pommerville P. Treatment satisfaction and improvement in health-related quality of life with onabotulinumtoxinA in patients with urinary incontinence due to neurogenic detrusor overactivity. Neurourol Urodyn. 2013;32(3):242–9.
71. Chancellor MB, Patel V, Leng WW, Shenot PJ, Lam W, Globe DR, et al. OnabotulinumtoxinA improves quality of life in patients with neurogenic detrusor overactivity. Neurology. 2013;81(9):841–8.
72. Rovner E, Dmochowski R, Chapple C, Thompson C, Lam W, Haag-Molkenteller C. OnabotulinumtoxinA improves urodynamic outcomes in patients with neurogenic detrusor overactivity. Neurourol Urodyn. 2013;32(8):1109–15.
73. Cruz F, Herschorn S, Aliotta P, Brin M, Thompson C, Lam W, et al. Efficacy and safety of onabotulinumtoxinA in patients with urinary incontinence due to neurogenic detrusor overactivity: a randomised, double-blind, placebo-controlled trial. Eur Urol. 2011;60(4):742–50.
74. Ginsberg D, Gousse A, Keppenne V, Sievert KD, Thompson C, Lam W, et al. Phase 3 efficacy and tolerability study of onabotulinumtoxinA for urinary incontinence from neurogenic detrusor overactivity. J Urol. 2012;187(6):2131–9.
75. Giannantoni A, Mearini E, Del Zingaro M, Porena M. Six-year follow-up of botulinum toxin A intradetrusorial injections in patients with refractory neurogenic detrusor overactivity: clinical and urodynamic results. Eur Urol. 2009;55(3):705–11.
76. Kennelly M, Dmochowski R, Ethans K, Karsenty G, Schulte-Baukloh H, Jenkins B, et al. Long-term efficacy and safety of onabotulinumtoxinA in patients with urinary incontinence due to neurogenic detrusor overactivity: an interim analysis. Urology. 2013;81(3):491–7.
77. Carlson JJ, Hansen RN, Dmochowski RR, Globe DR, Colayco DC, Sullivan SD. Estimating the cost-effectiveness of onabotulinumtoxinA for neurogenic detrusor overactivity in the United States. Clin Ther. 2013;35(4):414–24.
78. Wöllner J, Kessler TM. Botulinum toxin injections into the detrusor. BJU Int. 2011;108(9):1528–37.
79. Bartley J, Gilleran J, Peters K. Neuromodulation for overactive bladder. Nat Rev Urol. 2013;10(9):513–21.
80. Peters KM, Carrico DJ, Perez-Marrero RA, Khan AU, Wooldridge LS, Davis GL, et al. Randomized trial of percutaneous tibial nerve stimulation versus sham efficacy in the treatment of overactive bladder syndrome: results from the SUmiT trial. J Urol. 2010;183(4):1438–43.
81. Kabay SC, Kabay S, Yucel M, Ozden H. Acute urodynamic effects of percutaneous posterior tibial nerve stimulation on neurogenic detrusor overactivity in patients with Parkinson's disease. Neurourol Urodyn. 2009;28(1):62–7.
82. Kabay S, Kabay SC, Yucel M, Ozden H, Yilmaz Z, Aras O, et al. The clinical and urodynamic results of a 3-month percutaneous posterior tibial nerve stimulation treatment in patients with multiple sclerosis-related neurogenic bladder dysfunction. Neurourol Urodyn. 2009;28(8):964–8.
83. De Sèze M, Raibaut P, Gallien P, Even-Schneider A, Denys P, Bonniaud V, et al. Transcutaneous posterior tibial nerve stimulation for treatment of the overactive bladder syndrome in multiple sclerosis: results of a multicenter prospective study. Neurourol Urodyn. 2011;30(3):306–11.
84. Monteiro ÉS, De Carvalho LBC, Fukujima MM, Lora MI, Do Prado GF. Electrical stimulation of the posterior tibialis nerve improves symptoms of post Stroke neurogenic overactive bladder in men: a randomized controlled trial. Urology. 2014;84(3):509–14.
85. Gobbi C, Digesu GA, Khullar V, El Neil S, Caccia G, Zecca C. Percutaneous posterior tibial nerve stimulation as an effective treatment of refractory lower urinary tract symptoms in

patients with multiple sclerosis: preliminary data from a multicentre, prospective, open label trial. Multiple Sclerosis J. 2011;17(12):1514–9.
86. Wöllner J, Hampel C, Kessler TM. Surgery illustrated—surgical atlas sacral neuromodulation. BJU Int. 2012;110(1):146–59.
87. Knüpfer SC, Liechti MD, Mordasini L, Abt D, Engeler DS, Wöllner J, et al. Protocol for a randomized, placebo-controlled, double-blind clinical trial investigating sacral neuromodulation for neurogenic lower urinary tract dysfunction. BMC Urol. 2014;14(1):65.
88. Kessler TM, La Framboise D, Trelle S, Fowler CJ, Kiss G, Pannek J, et al. Sacral neuromodulation for neurogenic lower urinary tract dysfunction: systematic review and meta-analysis. Eur Urol. 2010;58(6):865–74.
89. Amend B, Matzel KE, Abrams P, De Groat WC, Sievert KD. How does neuromodulation work. Neurourol Urodyn. 2011;30(5):762–5.
90. Wyndaele JJ, Michielsen D, Van Dromme S. Influence of sacral neuromodulation on electrosensation of the lower urinary tract. J Urol. 2000;163(1):221–4.
91. Braun PM, Baezner H, Seif C, Boehler G, Bross S, Eschenfelder CC, et al. Alterations of cortical electrical activity in patients with sacral neuromodulator. Eur Urol. 2002;41(5):562–7.
92. Malaguti S, Spinelli M, Giardiello G, Lazzeri M, Van Den Hombergh U. Neurophysiological evidence may predict the outcome of sacral neuromodulation. J Urol. 2003;170(6 I):2323–6.
93. Fowler CJ, Swinn MJ, Goodwin RJ, Oliver S, Craggs M. Studies of the latency of pelvic floor contraction during peripheral nerve evaluation show that the muscle response is reflexly mediated. J Urol. 2000;163(3):881–3.
94. Schurch B, Reilly I, Reitz A, Curt A. Electrophysiological recordings during the peripheral nerve evaluation (PNE) test in complete spinal cord injury patients. World J Urol. 2003;20(6):319–22.
95. Seth JH, Haslam C, Panicker JN. Ensuring patient adherence to clean intermittent self-catheterization. Patient Prefer Adherence. 2014;8:191–8.

Chapter 15
Stroke Presenting as Hemiballismus

Heather Angus-Leppan

Clinical History

A 73-year-old man with a past history of diabetes Type II and hypertension awoke with sudden flinging movements of his right arm, involving the whole arm, which were irregular, high velocity and large amplitude. During the movements, his arm hit objects, and he sustained extensive bruising. Occasionally he had irregular, large amplitude leg movements. His face was unaffected. He had no control of these movements which were continuous while awake, and interfered with attempts at purposeful movements. He felt otherwise well, but alarmed by the uncontrolled movements.

His medications were metformin, atorvostatin and amlodipine. He was a non-smoker, drunk no alcohol and was usually independent in all his activities.

The patient continued to have spontaneous movements for 3 days which gradually reduced and then disappeared. Acute treatment with haloperidol 0.5 mg twice daily was given, and weaned after 3 days. Aspirin 300 mg stat was given and continued daily at 75 mg, and amlodipine and atorvastatin increased. At 3 and 12 months, the patient remained well with no further spontaneous movements and no residual weakness or impairment in daily functions.

H. Angus-Leppan (✉)
Department of Clinical and Movement Neurosciences, UCL Queen Square Institute of Neurology London, London, UK

Royal Free London NHS Foundation Trust, London, UK
e-mail: heather.angus-leppan@nhs.net

S. K. Gill et al. (eds.), *Stroke Medicine*,
https://doi.org/10.1007/978-3-031-58188-5_15

Examination

On arrival in the emergency department, he was alert with a Glasgow coma scale of 15/15, orientated in time place and person and his speech was normal in terms of comprehension and expression. Vital signs were normal apart from blood pressure of 154/93, reducing to 145/86 over the next 4 h. He had a mild right sided drift of his outstretched arm, and purposeful arm movements were disrupted by the involuntary movements. Attempted ambulation was disrupted by spontaneous involuntary movements which pushed him off balance, and he required assistance to walk. Cranial nerve examination was normal, upper limb examination revealed mild weakness of extensors (4+/5), lower limb examination was normal for tone, power, reflexes were present and symmetrical apart from reduced ankle jerks, and plantar responses were flexor, sensation was normal apart from absent vibration at both toes.

Investigations

Baseline blood tests revealed an elevated HbA1c of 48mmol/mol, blood glucose level was 6.3 mmol/L, creatinine was 123 μmol/L, reminder of blood tests unremarkable including normal full blood count, normal electrolytes with a sodium of 140 mmol/L, normal liver function tests and cholesterol was 4.3 mmol/L. Electrocardiogram showed sinus rhythm, and no acute changes.

Acute CT head scan showed age-related changes, acute MRI on day 1 was degraded by movement and did not show any acute lesions. MRI scan at 1 week was reported as showing mild-moderate involutional changes. Carotid Dopplers did not reveal any significant stenosis.

Discussion

Involuntary movement disorders are a rare presentation of stroke, occurring in <4% of patients in the largest series of 1500 consecutive patients with immediate, or delayed onset [1]. Chorea was the most commonly described, sometimes associated with hemiballismus; followed by tremor, dystonia and parkinsonism. Movement disorders were more commonly associated with deeper lesions, either ischaemic or haemorrhagic.

Hemiballismus is a rare movement disorder characterised by unilateral, irregular, involuntary large amplitude violent flinging movement of the limbs, estimated to occur in 1/500,000 people [2], and comprising <1% of all movement disorders in a large tertiary centre series [3]. It involves proximal arm, and/or leg; and in 50% of cases there may be facial involvement [4]. Movements occur, or are worsened with attempted activity, reduce with rest and disappear with sleep (as for most movement disorders with the exceptions of sleep related parasomnias and myoclonus). Hemiballismus must be differentiated from chorea (Fig. 15.1), which is proximal. Some authors describe combinations of chorea-hemiballismus [1, 4]. Tics may also be a mimic, clearly differentiated by age of onset, nature and setting. Other movement disorders such as tremor, dystonia and parkinsonism are readily distinguished from hemiballismus by clinical features [3].

Stroke is the most commonly reported aetiology for hemiballismus, but it can also occur with structural lesions (neoplastic or infective), metabolic derangement (especially non-ketotic hyperglycaemia), demyelination or connective tissue disease (systemic vasculitis, systemic lupus erythematosis) and complications of HIV such as toxoplasmosis [4, 5] (Fig. 15.2).

Early reports postulated the pathophysiology of hemiballismus as a lesion in the contralateral subthalamic nucleus causing excitation on the internal segment of the globus pallidus. One suggestion is that damage to the contralateral subthalamic nucleus reduces the inhibitory g-aminobutyric acid (GABA) input to the external globus pallidus, resulting in increased activity. Through feedback loops, this in turn reduces globus pallidus interna inhibition of the motor thalamus and a release phenomenon on motor activity [6]. Given the complexity of this circuitry, it is

	Hemiballismus	Chorea	Tic
Age of onset	Usually elderly	Variable	Childhood
Duration	Usually self-limited, days to weeks	Variable, determined by aetiology	Usually disappear or reduces in adulthood
Aetiology	Stroke most common (see Figure 3)	Multiple Genetic, post infectious	Usually unknown May be post-infectious
Muscles involved	Proximal limb muscles	Distal limb muscles	Any
Site	Unilateral	bilateral	Any, often changing
Nature	Hyperkinetic Irregular, high amplitude	Hyperkinetic Irregular, dance-like	Hyperkinetic Explosive, variable
Vocal utterances	Nil	Nil	Frequent
Suppressible	No	No, may be converted to apparently purposeful movement	Yes

Fig. 15.1 Differentiating hemiballismus from chorea and tic

Aetiology	Subtypes	Clinical features
Stroke	Ischaemic Haemorrhagic	Most common cause May occur in isolation Mild associated pyramidal weakness in some Various sites reported
Structural	Vascular malformations Neoplasia	Deep lesions
Metabolic / toxic	Nonketotic hyperglycemia Hypoglycaemia/ anoxia Drug toxicity eg phenytoin	Gradual worsening over hours or days May be associated with encephalopathy
Neuroinflammatory	Demyelination Systemic lupus erythematosis	Young age of onset Associated clinical features of the cause will be present
Degenerative / destructive	Amyotrophic lateral sclerosis Traumatic brain injury	Clinical features of the aetiology will establish diagnosis
Infection	Tuberculomas HIV infection – eg toxoplasmosis	Can be due to structural effect of infection, toxic or diffuse effect

Fig. 15.2 Aetiology of hemiballismus

unsurprising that there may be a number of sites, or multiple sites, of disruption, both through GABA and dopaminergic imbalance [4, 5].

Although some reported cases involve strokes in the subthalamic nucleus, pure subthalamic strokes are rare, occurring in only 1/25 in a series of patients with hemiballismus [5]. Simultaneous lesions of the subthalamic nucleus and other parts of the basal ganglia, pons, or midbrain are more common. There are also reports of hemiballismus after strokes in the parietal lobe and bilateral frontal cortex [5, 7], but cortical lesions are a much rarer cause than deep basal ganglia lesions [1]. Other stroke localisations found in of hemiballismus include the thalamus, pons, posterior limb of the internal capsule, external capsule and corona radiata [4]. In two-thirds of patients developing hemiballismus due to stroke, the pathophysiology is small vessel disease with lacunar infarction. This is the likely mechanism in our patient. Haemorrhage, and large and vessel atherothrombosis (or cardioembolism), account for the remainder, with a case report also of middle cerebral artery dissection in a young woman [8]. The most common vascular territories affected are the middle cerebral artery (M1, M2, and lateral lenticulostriate arteries), posterior cerebral artery (thalamogeniculate, thalamoperforating, and choroidal arteries), and occasionally the anterior cerebral artery (recurrent artery of Huebner and leptomeningeal arteries) [5, 7]. Most importantly, in more than 25% of cases, the exact site of the stroke is unclear, as in this case [5]. The likely reasons for this are that small perforating vessel events may be below resolution of MRI scanning, there is commonly background microvascular disease, making it difficult to pick out new lacunar lesions, and because initial scanning may be obscured by movement artefacts, even with sedation [6].

Most strokes affecting the basal ganglia do not produce hemiballismus, and predisposing factors for this are uncertain. It seems likely that risk factors for small vessel disease are important, particularly diabetes, suggesting unique predisposing factors for this rare clinical phenotype.

Management of hemiballismus involves establishment a definitive diagnosis and excluding infection, structural lesions, toxins and metabolic or inflammatory causes. Imaging should be acute, and will often require sedation with a small dose of benzodiazepine, where this can be done safely. Prevention of injury is paramount as the movements are distressing and can cause injury. Counselling of the patient of this is a treatable and usually temporary phenomena with a good prognosis [9] in almost all cases is important. The usual stroke work-up is essential, and treatment as per stroke guidelines should be followed.

Stroke-associated hemiballismus may not require specific treatment because the disorder may be rapidly self-limited [6, 9]. Early reports of the prognosis of hemiballismus suggested a poor outlook, but more recent series suggest a good immediate outcome, usually with resolution of stroke related hemiballismus [1, 5]. The patient's overall prognosis will depend on their specific vascular risk factor profile, and previous vascular events, particularly cardiovascular events.

If pharmacological treatment is necessary, antidopaminergic drugs (antipsychotics such as haloperidol, or dopamine blockade with tetrabenazine) may be used, although evidence is based on small case reports and series [5, 10, 11]. Our patient was treated with haloperidol, and hemiballismus settled within 3 days, and did not recur on weaning the haloperidol. It is very possible that the patient would have improved without this treatment. Other treatments that have been used include benzodiazepines, anticonvulsants (most recently reported is topiramate) [10]. In rare refractory cases, botulinum toxin, intrathecal baclofen, and occasionally functional neurosurgery have been used [11]. Invasive treatments will almost never be required for stroke-related hemiballismus.

There is no evidence about whether thrombolytic therapy should be used for treatment of hemiballismus, with a few case reports of good outcome with use [6]. As this is a rare stroke presentation, it may present late, meaning that often the decision does not come into play, as the window of potential therapy with thrombolysis is past before Neurology or Stroke services are alerted. Given the usually good outcome of stroke-related hemiballismus, it is difficult to evaluate whether thrombolysis is helpful, or necessary.

Key Clinical Learning Points

- Hemiballismus is a unilateral hyperkinetic movement disorder presenting as explosive proximal movements of the arm or leg
- Hemiballismus is a rare stroke presentation, occurring in <4% of strokes
- Movements may cause injury and it is important to protect the patient
- Many patients will require only symptomatic treatment, but dopamine blockers (antipsychotics or tetrabenazine) are reported in case studies and small series to be effective
- The prognosis for the hemiballismus is good, and the patient's overall prognosis will depend on their vascular risk factors and previous events

Key Radiological Learning Points

- The contralateral subthalamic nucleus is the first described site of pathophysiology but multiple other stroke sites have been described
- Most commonly the lesion will be subcortical, lacunar, and involving the basal ganglia
- Rarely cortical or brainstem strokes may cause hemiballismus
- The stroke is usually ischaemic (2/3), but may be haemorrhagic
- In 25% of cases there will be no acute lesion, usually in the setting of small vessel disease

References

1. Alarcón F, Zijlmans JC, Dueñas G, Cevallos N. Post-stroke movement disorders: report of 56 patients. J Neurol Neurosurg Psychiatry. 2004;75:1568–74.
2. Ballismus MR. In: Vinken PJ, Bruun GW, editors. Handbook of clinical neurology, vol. 6. Amsterdam: Elsevier Press; 1968. p. 476–90.
3. Dewey RB, Jankovic J. Hemiballism-hemichorea: clinical and pharmacologic findings in 21 patients. Arch Neurol. 1989;46:862–7.
4. Postuma RB, Lang AE. Hemiballism: revisiting a classic disorder. Lancet Neurol. 2003;2:661–8.
5. Vidaković A, Dragasević N, Kostić VS. Hemiballism: report of 25 cases. J Neurol Neurosurg Psychiatry. 1994;57(8):945–9. https://doi.org/10.1136/jnnp.57.8.945.
6. McCollum D, Silvers S, Dawson SB, Barrett KM. Resolution of acute onset hemichorea-hemiballismus after treatment with intravenous tissue plasminogen activator. Neurohospitalist. 2013;3:131–4.
7. Wu MC, Yen RF, Lin CH, Wu RM. Hemiballism in a patient with parietal lobe infarction. Neurology. 2013;80:e22.
8. Chen H, Xu Z. Hemichorea-hemiballismus as the initial manifestation of symptomatic middle cerebral artery dissection: a case report. Medicine (Baltimore). 2020;99(36):e22116. https://doi.org/10.1097/MD.0000000000022116.

9. Klawans HL, Moses H, Nausieda PA, et al. Treatment and prognosis of hemiballisms. N Engl J Med. 1976;295:1348–50.
10. Driver-Dunckley E, Evidente VG. Hemichorea-hemiballismus may respond to topiramate. Clin Neuropharmacol. 2005;28(3):142–4.
11. Hawley JS, Weiner WJ. Hemiballismus: current concepts and review. Parkinsonism Relat Disord. 2012;18(2):125–9. https://doi.org/10.1016/j.parkreldis.2011.08.015. Epub 17 Sep 2011. PMID: 21930415.

Chapter 16
Balloon to Brain Bubbles

Rawan Matar, Mamoun Saeed, Soma Banerjee, Zoe Brown, and Joseph Kwan

Introduction

Ischemic stroke during air travel is rare with a reported incidence of one stroke per 35,000 flights in a prospective study, none of which attributed to cerebral air embolism [1]. Notably, pulmonary bulla causing air embolism during air travel affecting other body parts have been reported including that to the skin, manifesting as livedo reticularis of the upper limbs and thorax [2]. However, pulmonary bulla causing cerebral air embolism during air travel is extremely rare with the first reported case dating to 1985 [3]. We report a case of a pulmonary bulla causing cerebral air embolism during air travel, where a bronchogenic connection to the systemic circulation was radiologically established.

Case

A 67-year-old right-handed Caucasian lady was touring in the United Kingdom with her partner. She was at her normal state of health upon departure from Newark International Airport to London. However, during her return flight from London to the United States, she became acutely unwell 1 h into the flight. It was presumed to

R. Matar (✉) · M. Saeed · S. Banerjee · Z. Brown
Imperial College NHS Trust, London, UK
e-mail: rawan.matar@nhs.net; mamoun.saeed@nhs.net; zoe.brown14@nhs.net

J. Kwan
Imperial College NHS Trust, London, UK

Imperial College London, London, UK
e-mail: joseph.kwan@nhs.net

S. K. Gill et al. (eds.), *Stroke Medicine*,
https://doi.org/10.1007/978-3-031-58188-5_16

be symptoms of hypoglycemia due to her history of diabetes. However, this was immediately followed by a short period of loss of consciousness which resulted in an emergency landing in Ireland. On arrival to the nearest local hospital, she fully regained consciousness and the examination was unremarkable. Blood work-up and electrocardiogram were normal. She was discharged the following day with a diagnosis of "possible syncope" and was deemed fit to fly back to the United States through London.

One day after discharge, she boarded a flight from Ireland to London and again became acutely unwell 20 min after take-off. She lost consciousness and had urinary incontinence, resulting in an emergency landing in London. Upon arrival to London, she was taken to our hospital where she remained unconscious, hence intubated, ventilated, and admitted to the intensive care unit (ICU).

Her medical background includes diet-controlled diabetes and a gastric bypass surgery in 2005, which was complicated by an incidental left lung bulla on imaging. She was advised against air ballooning and scuba diving, but she continued air travel without any incidents for more than 17 years.

Admission non-contrast computed tomography (CT) of the brain showed multiple air locules in both cerebral hemispheres, in keeping with cerebral air embolism (Fig. 16.1a, b). Magnetic Resonance Imaging (MRI) of the brain performed on day four into her admission revealed bilateral multiple small subacute embolic infarcts across multiple supratentorial territories on the diffusion-weighted images, as well as diffuse white matter T2 hyperintensity (Fig. 16.1c, d). No hemorrhage was demonstrated. Chest x-ray showed a pulmonary bulla occupying the left lower lobe (Fig. 16.2a). CT of the thorax confirmed an 88 mm air-containing bulla in the left lung with large pulmonary vessels leading directly to the edge of the bulla, indicative of a direct communication between the bulla and the pulmonary circulation. (Fig. 16.2b).

When she was extubated on day six, she was found to be dysphagic, dysarthric and quadriplegic. Neurologic examination revealed left UMN facial weakness, flickering movements with an MRC grading of 1/5 of the left thumb, right hip flexion and toe movements bilaterally. She was then stepped down from ICU to the Hyperacute Stroke Unit where she received ongoing acute stroke management and neurorehabilitation. After extensive discussions with respiratory and cardiothoracic surgery teams, the consensus decision was to continue conservative management without surgery until she was repatriated back to the United States.

During the first 4 weeks, she remained quadriplegic with a man-in-a-barrel pattern of weakness consistent with bilateral watershed infarcts. Her bulbar function continued to improve. This was evident by regaining swallowing function. After 6 weeks, she fully regained her muscle power in the upper and lower extremities as well as truncal strength. The aim of the neurorehabilitation was to help her become medically fit to travel back to the United States by a cruise ferry. 10 weeks later, she arrived back to New York.

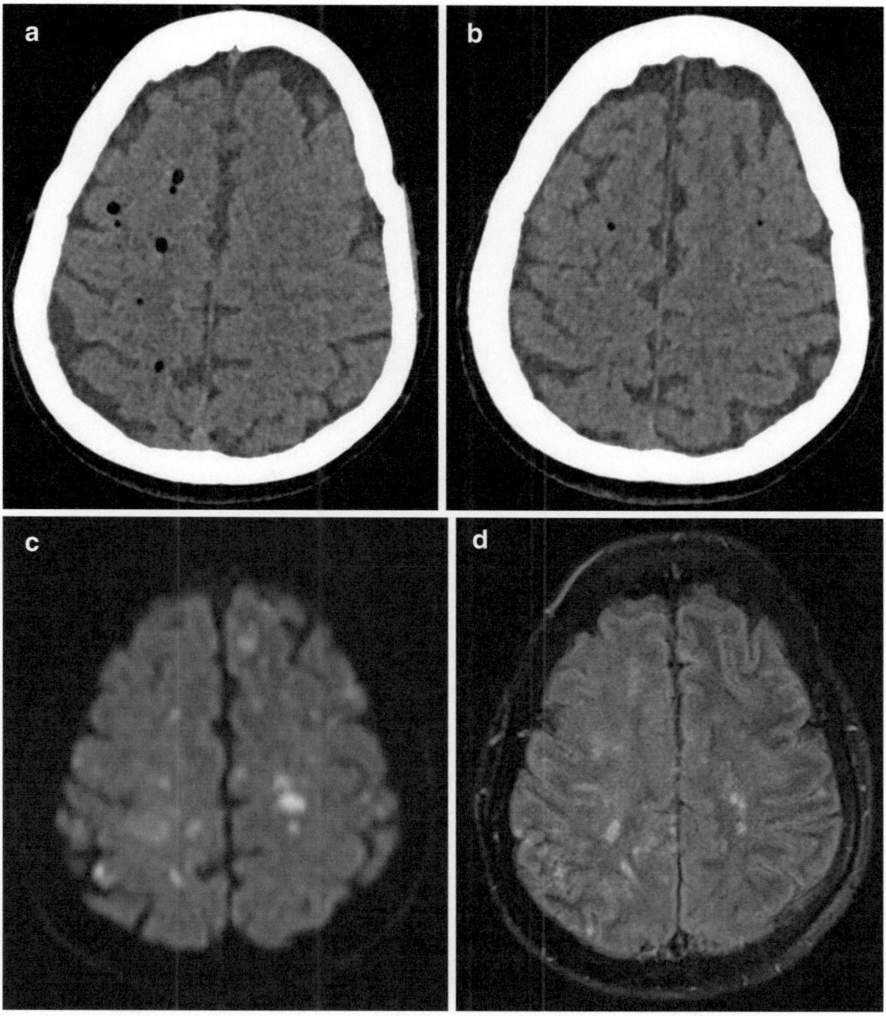

Fig. 16.1 (**a** and **b**) Brain CT non contrast Axial imaging showing multiple small gas locules involving the subcortical white matter of the right frontal and parietal lobes. (**c**) Brain MRI diffusion weighted images revealing multiple area of acute infarction of bilateral cerebral hemispheres. (**d**) Brain MRI FLAIR images demonstrating bilateral white matter signal abnormality most conspicuous in the juxtacortical and subcortical white matter of the MCA border zones

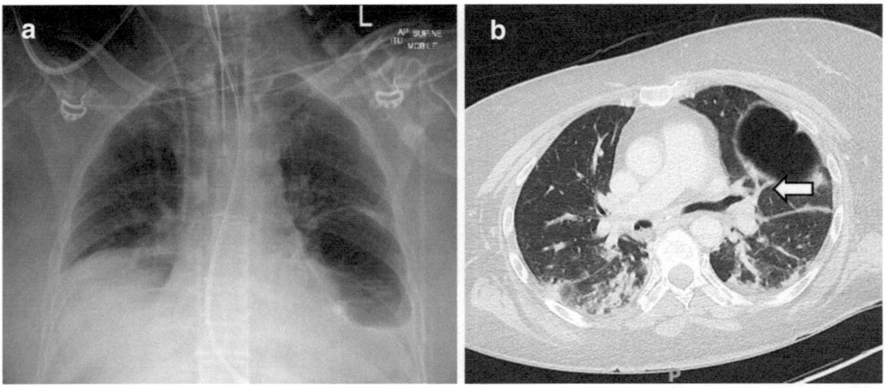

Fig. 16.2 (**a**) CXR demonstrates a large bulla projected over the left lower lung zone. (**b**) CT Thorax enhanced images demonstrating a bulla measuring 88 mm within the left lingula with a number of large pulmonary vessels (arrow) running to the edge of the cavity

Discussion

Pulmonary bulla causing cerebral air embolism is extremely rare. It presents clinically with a variable presentation ranging from minor motor weakness, headache, seizures, loss of consciousness and coma [4, 5]. Cerebral air embolism manifesting with loss of consciousness shortly after take-off, as in our patient, has previously been reported [2–4, 6–14]. The loss of consciousness in most could be attributed to the massive cerebral oedema, bi-hemispheric infarcts, thalamic or brainstem involvement, for which most suffered a fatal outcome [2–4, 7–11, 13, 14]. Despite presenting unconscious, our patient made a surprisingly good outcome which could possibly be explained by the absence of cerebral oedema, thalamic and brainstem involvement [6, 14]. CT/MR mismatch in our patient can be explained by the time interval between the two imaging and the dynamic nature of the air embolism itself. These together would result in discrepancy between the two modalities.

Cerebral air embolism in individuals with a pre-existing lung pathology is likely related to decompression during ascent [11]. The pathophysiology of arterial gas embolism in relation to a pulmonary bulla during air travel is poorly understood and is presumed to be secondary to the bulla expansion due to changes in atmospheric pressure encountered on plane ascent [2–16]. Identification of the bronchial connection is always challenging, and determination of its anatomical location is usually not possible [2]. None of the previous reported cases demonstrated a communication between the bulla and the pulmonary circulation [2–15]. In our case, CT of the thorax enabled us to identify a connection between the bulla and the pulmonary vein as a mechanistic explanation of air embolization to the systemic circulation hence the brain.

Optimal treatment of cerebral air embolism remains to be elucidated, as there is no high-quality research evidence available. However, hyperbaric oxygen therapy is currently considered a first line treatment of cerebral air embolism by limiting cerebral oedema and reducing the size of air bubbles by depleting intravascular nitrogen [17]. Ultimately, the risk of further air embolism by air travel can be eliminated by surgical resection of the pulmonary bulla prior to air travel [5].

References

1. Álvarez-Velasco R, Masjuan J, de Felipe A, Corral I, Estévez-Fraga C, Crespo L, et al. Stroke in commercial flights. Stroke. 2016;47:1117–9. https://doi.org/10.1161/STROKEAHA.115.012637.
2. Zaugg M, Kaplan V, Widmer U, Baumann PC, Russi EW. Fatal air embolism in an airplane passenger with a giant intrapulmonary bronchogenic cyst. Am J Respir Crit Care Med. 1998;157(5 Pt 1):1686–9.
3. Neidhart P, Suter PM. Pulmonary bulla and sudden death in a young aeroplane passenger. Intensive Care Med. 1985;11:45–7.
4. Farshchi Zarabi S, Parotto M, Katznelson R, Downar J. Massive ischemic stroke due to pulmonary barotrauma and cerebral artery air embolism during commercial air travel. Am J Case Rep. 2017;18:660–4. https://doi.org/10.12659/AJCR.903354.
5. Gudmundsdottir JF, Geirsson A, Hannesson P, Gudbjartsson T. Major ischaemic stroke caused by an air embolism from a ruptured giant pulmonary bulla. BMJ Case Rep. 2015;2015:bcr2014208159. https://doi.org/10.1136/bcr-2014.
6. Closon M, et al. Air embolism during an aircraft flight in a passenger with a pulmonary cyst: a favorable outcome with hyperbaric therapy. Anesthesiology. 2004;101:539–42.
7. Almeida FA, DeSouza BX, Meyer T, Gregory S, Greenspon L. Intrapulmonary bronchogenic cyst and cerebral gas embolism in an aircraft flight passenger. Chest. 2006;130:575–7. https://doi.org/10.1378/chest.130.2.575.
8. Edwardson M, Wurth D, Lacy JM, Fink J, Becker K. Cerebral air embolism resulting in fatal stroke in an airplane passenger with a pulmonary bronchogenic cyst. Neurocrit Care. 2009;10:218–21. https://doi.org/10.1007/s12028-008-9126-3.
9. Salameh J. A 62-year-old woman with cerebral artery air embolism during commercial air travel. Neurologist. 2010;16:136–7. https://doi.org/10.1097/NRL.0b013e3181cf8695.
10. Arnaiz J, Marco De Lucas E, Piedra T, Elena M, Garcia A, Patel AD, et al. In-flight seizures and fatal air embolism the importance of a chest radiograph. Arch Neurol. 2011;68:661–4.
11. Yeung JTH, Ma JKF, Mak YF, Lam VSC. Fatal cerebral air embolism related to an air flight. Hong Kong Med J. 2013;19:352–3. https://doi.org/10.12809/hkmj133898.
12. Desgranges FP, Cour M, Hernu R, Delafosse B, Argaud L. Cerebral air embolism during an aircraft flight in a passenger with an air-filled lung cavity associated with remote lung surgery. J Thorac Cardiovasc Surg. 2013;146:e20. https://doi.org/10.1016/j.jtcvs.2013.05.008.
13. Saliou G, Leblanc PE, Cauquil C, Theaudin M, Ract C, Ducreux D. Sudden loss of consciousness during a flight. Cerebrovasc Dis. 2014;37:470–1. https://doi.org/10.1159/000363370.
14. Oyanguren B. Cerebral air embolism in commercial flights: a potentially fatal complication of intrathoracic lesions. Int J Crit Care Emer Med. 2017;3:3. https://doi.org/10.23937/2474-3674/1510022.
15. Machicado JD, Davogustto G, Burgeois S, Kaldis P, Jani PP, Gidwani R. Fatal air embolism: a rare complication of bronchogenic cysts in an airplane passenger. Am J Respir Crit Care Med. 2013;188:249–50. https://doi.org/10.1164/rccm.201210-1956IM.
16. Ramadas P, Chakravarty R, Krishnan P, Nadkarni A. Dangers of flying high and diving low! An unusual case of dyspnea. Respir Med Case Rep. 2017;20:1–3. https://doi.org/10.1016/j.rmcr.2016.10.015.
17. Laus C, Uth MM, Hank RSS. Gas embolism. New Engl J Med. n.d.;

Chapter 17
Ischaemic Stroke Presenting with Isolated Dysarthria

Talal Al-Mayhani

A 51-year-old right-handed man, with background of hypertension, Type II Diabetes Mellitus, bipolar disorder and active cigarette smoking, presented to the Emergency Stroke Unit (ESU). He had a 1-day history of left sided neck pain, 2-h history of ache around the left eye and left temple, followed by sudden onset slurred speech that persisted while the pain resolved. There was no history of trauma, cough or sneezing, alcohol consumption or substance abuse.

Examination and Localization

He was brought by the ambulance services and walked into ESU with no need for assistance. He was alert, fully oriented and engaged. There was severe dysarthria, with no evidence of expressive or receptive aphasia. He had a longstanding anisocoria with the left pupil smaller than the right. The remaining cranial nerves were normal. The vital signs on admission were within normal range.

Investigations and Management

The routine blood tests were unremarkable. The 12 L ECG showed sinus rhythm. The plain CT head was normal, and the CT angiogram of head and neck excluded large vessel occlusion. MRI head, however, showed evidence of acute stroke in the crus cerebri in left side of the midbrain (Fig. 17.1).

T. Al-Mayhani (✉)
National Hospital for Neurology and Neurosurgery, London, UK
e-mail: talal.al-mayhani@nhs.net

S. K. Gill et al. (eds.), *Stroke Medicine*,
https://doi.org/10.1007/978-3-031-58188-5_17

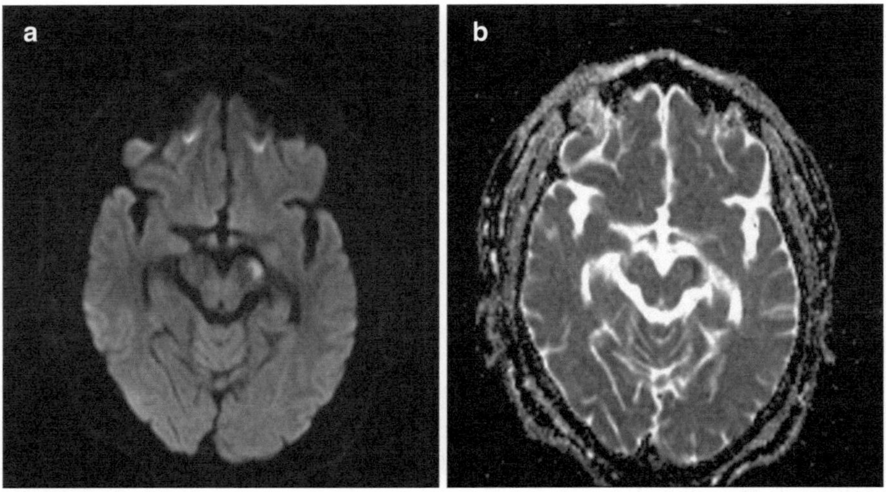

Fig. 17.1 (**a** and **b**) axial MRI head DWI and ADC sequences showing a small area of restricted diffusion in the left crus cerebri in the midbrain, indicating acute ischaemic lesion

Further blood tests for young stroke screen were normal or negative. Although inpatient investigations did not reveal evidence of dysrhythmia or structural or valvular heart disease, the normal angiogram studies, and the relatively young age, raised the unconfirmed possibility of cardioembolic etiology. The patient was treated initially with dual antiplatelets (Aspirin and Clopidogrel) for 3 weeks, then with lifelong Clopidogrel.

Discussion

Defined as a disorder of articulation, dysarthria is a symptom and/or sign of poor localizing value [1]. It may result from structural neurological lesions in the central or peripheral nervous system, along with array of non-neurological pathologies. Dysarthria should be distinguished from dysphasia, a disorder of language, and can overlap with dysphonia, a disorder of vocalization.

Classically, dysarthria is classified into different types depending on the disturbance of speech quality, and the presumed site of lesion, as follows:

- Ataxic dysarthria: the speech is slow, scanning and/or explosive and has a staccato quality, with discoordination between the speech and breathing. It is part of the cerebellar syndrome with wide range of underlying vascular, demyelination and structural pathologies.
- Flaccid dysarthria: the speech has a nasal quality, and fasciculation and wasting may develop in the tongue. It is usually due to lesion in the lower motor neuron (progressive bulbar palsy), nerves (facial diplegia in Guillain-Barré syndrome) or neuromuscular junction disorders (myasthenia gravis).

- Spastic dysarthria: the speech is effortful and slow, and can be associated with prominent jaw reflex, and emotional lability (pseudobulbar affect). Since the lower cranial nerves receive inputs from both hemispheres, this type of dysarthria results usually from bilateral lesions in the corticobulbar tracts disrupting the upper motor neuron projections.
- More profound and persistent forms of spastic dysarthria can be encountered in pseudobulbar palsy or amyotrophic lateral sclerosis forms of the motor neuron disease, or in bilateral vascular damage in the classical anterior opercular syndrome of Foix-Chavany-Marie. Notably, patients with left hemiparesis due to right subcortical stroke tend to present with particularly severe dysarthria, although it tends to improve with time [2].
- Hypokinetic dysarthria: the speech is expressed rapidly and can usually be hypophonic and monotonous. It can be seen in extrapyramidal lesions resulting in parkinsonism syndrome.
- Hyperkinetic: the speech is usually loud with inappropriate stresses, pauses, and intonation. There can be associated involuntary hyperkinetic movements of the underlying disorder. This type of dysarthria can be seen in from extrapyramidal lesions resulting in dystonia, tremor, myoclonus or chorea.

Most cases of acute dysarthria can be attributed to systemic conditions with transient impact on neurological function such as alcohol intoxication, delirium, medications side effects and encephalopathic states. Careful history taking usually helps in clarifying the clinical picture. Similarly, chronic neurological conditions or mature stroke, known to be associated in the past with dysarthria, may present with acute decompensation or recrudescence in context of acute systemic upset.

As mentioned in spastic dysarthria above, acute presentation of dysarthria is also known to accompany acute stroke [3], however, it is usually part of a wider clinical syndrome due to lesions in the corticospinal or corticobulbar tracts.

Very rarely, isolated dysarthria, with no other focal neurological deficits, can be the only feature of acute stroke [4], as demonstrated in this case report. Again, the clinical history is a key, as careful questioning helps in elucidating the sudden onset of the presentation, exploring the cardiovascular risk factors and excluding other possibilities, for instance, alcohol intoxication, medications (narcotics, antiepileptics and neuroleptics), of masked old stroke, stress and fatigue (as the motor system is affect sensitive).

The author came across two additional cases in a 64-year-old man and a 73-year-old man, both with similar presentation of sudden onset, isolated and persistent dysarthria. The work up did show ischaemic stroke in the left corona radiata of undetermined etiology in one patient (Fig. 17.2a, b), while in the other patient there was a small ischaemic lesion in the right side of basis pontis, likely due to small vessel disease (Fig. 17.2c, d).

A few case series studied the presentation of dysarthria in stroke patients. In one report, isolated dysarthria was found only in 2.9% of patients presenting with dysarthria due to stroke, and the vast majority of cases dysarthria was associated with other symptoms such as lingual paresis, facial paresis, clumsy hand syndrome, pure motor hemiparesis or hemi-ataxia [5].

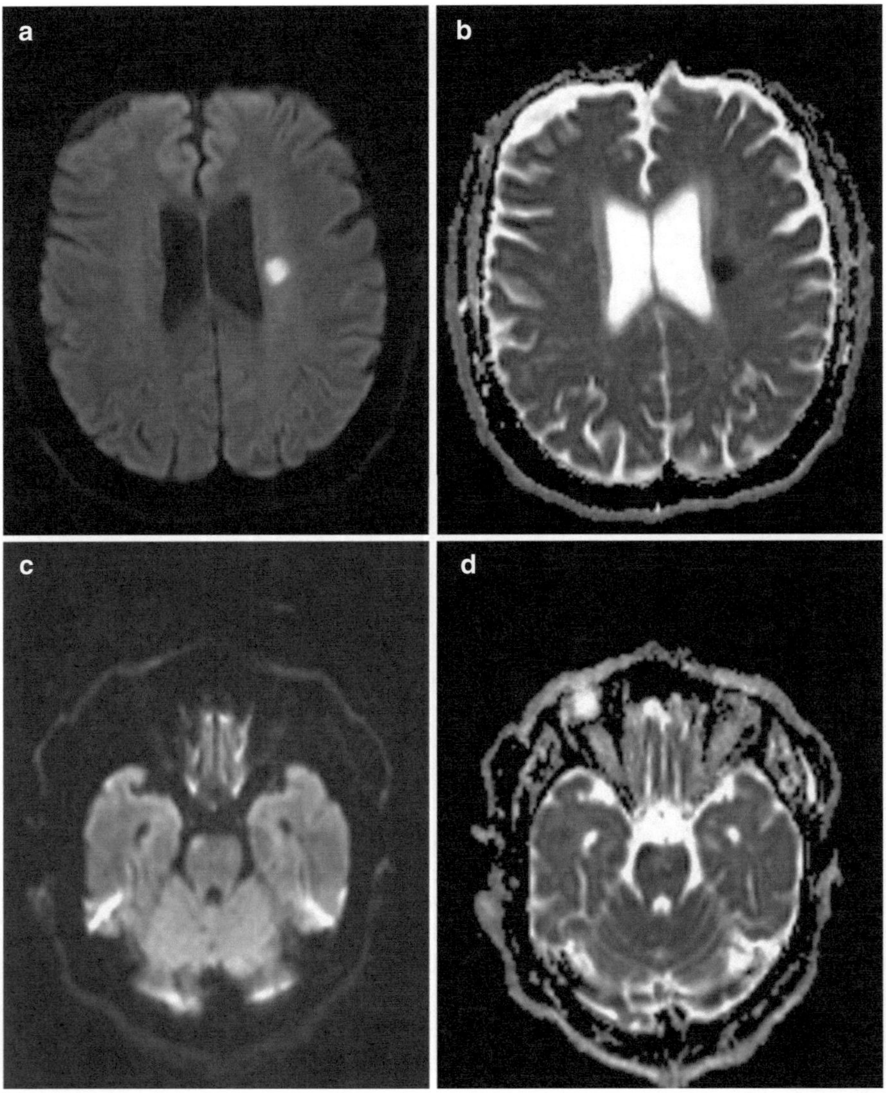

Fig. 17.2 (**a** and **b**): axial MRI head DWI and ADC sequences showing a small area of restricted diffusion in the left corona radiata, indicating acute ischaemic lesion. (**c** and **d**): axial MRI head DWI and ADC sequences showing a small area of restricted diffusion in the right anterior basis pontis, indicating acute ischaemic lesion

Such unusual presentation with isolated dysarthria can easily be missed, and high index of suspicion in patients with clear history, and relevant cardiovascular risk factors, should warrant stroke work up to guide optimum management and secondary prevention, and to reduce the risk of future stroke that may result in more profound disability. It is unclear, however, whether the stroke presenting with such isolated dysarthria indicates a successful compensating mechanism in a brain of good functional reserve, or whether it is a harbinger of impeding and evolving more severe events. Further questions about the long-term prognosis of such isolated presentation, and the risk of future strokes, remain to be elucidated.

Key Clinical Learning Points

- Isolated dysarthria may be a presenting feature of stroke or occur as a part of stroke syndrome for example dysarthria -clumsy hand syndrome (one of five lacunar syndromes)
- Clinical history is key: a sudden onset dysarthria which occurs in the context of vascular risk factors warrants further investigation with brain imaging
- Causes of dysarthria associated with systemic disease should be excluded e.g. encephalopathy, delirium, medications

Key Radiological Learning Points

- Isolated dysarthria should prompt a search on imaging for an ischaemic lesion in the pons, internal capsule or as in this case the midbrain
- MRI with diffusion weighted imaging can clarify smaller lesions in the brainstem which may not be evident of CT head

References

1. Alpert J. The neurological diagnosis. A practical bedside approach. Springer; 2019.
2. Ropper AH. Severe dysarthria with right hemisphere stroke. Neurology. 1987;37(6):1061–3.
3. Fisher CM. A Lacunar Stroke. The dysarthria-clumsy hand syndrome. Neurology. 1967;17(6):614–7.
4. Urban PP, et al. Isolated dysarthria due to extracerebellar lacunar stroke: a central monoparesis of the tongue. J Neurol Neurosurg Psychiatry. 1999;66(4):495–501.
5. Urban PP, et al. Dysarthria in acute ischemic stroke: lesion topography, clinicoradiologic correlation and etiology. Neurology. 2001;56(8):1021–7.

Chapter 18
Hole in One: Golf-Associated Dissection

Oishik Raha and Paul Bentley

Clinical History

A 46 year-old right-handed man, AB, was brought to the local Emergency Department by his wife after he collapsed at home. There was a witnessed transient loss of consciousness followed by inability to speak, and left hemiparesis. He had been playing golf several hours earlier. There were no other triggering activities identified; and he had been feeling well according to the family. Past medical history consisted of: hypertension treated with perindopril, type 1 diabetes mellitus and asthma. He was compliant with medications, and blood pressure had been controlled.

Examination

AB was drowsy and unable to verbalise or sit up, but able to communicate non-verbally with simple gestures of the right-hand. Left arm and left leg were both graded as no better than 3/5 power throughout; and all limbs were ataxic. He was

O. Raha
Department of Stroke and Neuroscience, Charing Cross Hospital, Imperial College London NHS Healthcare Trust, London, UK
e-mail: oishik.raha@nhs.net

P. Bentley (✉)
Department of Stroke and Neuroscience, Charing Cross Hospital, Imperial College London NHS Healthcare Trust, London, UK

Imperial College London, London, UK
e-mail: paul.bentley2@nhs.net

S. K. Gill et al. (eds.), *Stroke Medicine*,
https://doi.org/10.1007/978-3-031-58188-5_18

Table 18.1 National Institute for Health Stroke Score (NIHSS)

Domain	Score
1a—Level of consciousness	1
1b—Orientation	0
1c—Commands	0
2—Gaze paresis	0
3—Visual field defect	0
4—Facial paresis	0
5a—Left arm motor	2
5b—Right arm motor	0
6a—Left leg motor	2
6b—Right leg motor	0
7—Limb ataxia	2
8—Sensation	0
9—Language	3
10—Dysarthria	2
11—Extinction/inattention	0
Total:	12

drooling, and had pooled secretions in the oropharynx requiring suctioning. Palatal elevation and gag reflex were impaired. A nasopharyngeal airway was inserted. The following were recorded as intact: visual acuity; visual fields; eye movements; facial power; sensation. There was no visuo-spatial neglect or sensory inattention. Admission NIHSS was 12 (breakdown shown in Table 18.1):

Investigations

An urgent non-contrast CT (NCCT) (Fig. 18.1) showed hyperdensity in the mid basilar artery indicating acute thrombosis, although brain parenchyma was normal. Tissue plasminogen activator was administered as onset time was ~4 h.

A CT angiogram (CTA) of intracranial and aortic arch regions confirmed occlusion of the basilar artery and the right dominant vertebral artery shortly after the ostium (Fig. 18.2).

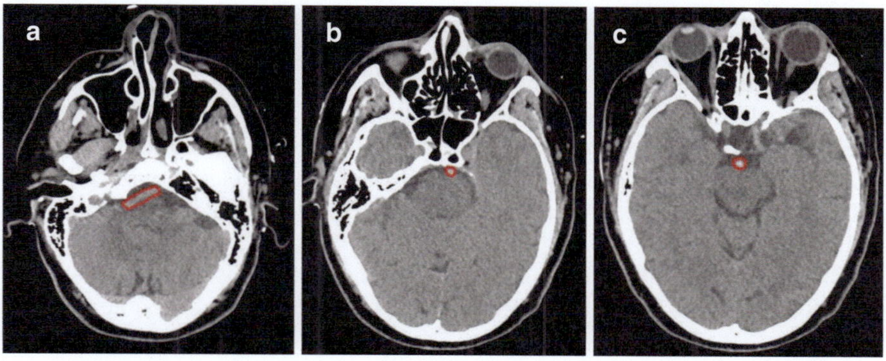

Fig. 18.1 Posterior circulation vessels highlighted with red outline in a series of slices in this NCCT. (**a**) demonstrates the dominant right vertebral artery with density equivalent to surrounding brain parenchyma. (**b**) demonstrates the proximal basilar artery with density equivalent to surrounding brain parenchyma. (**c**) demonstrates the middle to distal basilar artery with hyperdensity concerning for basilar artery occlusion

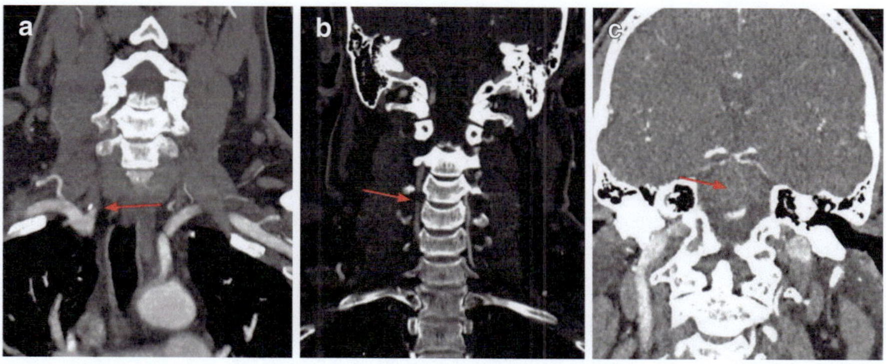

Fig. 18.2 CT angiogram imaging performed at PSC. (**a**) Abrupt cessation of contrast flow distal to vertebral artery ostium. (**b**) In comparison to the contralateral vertebral artery, the right vertebral demonstrates patchy flow. (**c**) Intracranially, there is contrast in the right vertebral and bilateral posterior cerebral artery and superior cerebellar arteries but no flow in where the basilar artery runs indicative of basilar artery occlusion

Treatment & Course

The patient was intubated, because of drowsiness, poor swallowing, vomiting, oxygen desaturation, and for transfer to a tertiary centre for thrombectomy. Intravenous antibiotics were started for suspected aspiration pneumonitis. At thrombectomy, a vertebral artery occlusion was identified within the intraforaminal (V2) segment, with evidence of a dissection and associated free floating thrombus (FFT). This was crossed to gain access to the intracranial circulation where the middle and distal basilar artery was occluded with soft thrombus. Using a thromboaspiration technique the basilar artery was recanalised after two passes. The FFT in the vertebral artery was also aspirated as it increased the risk of basilar artery re-occlusion. The dissection was not actively treated during the endovascular procedure. The post-procedure TICI score (Thrombolysis in Cerebral Infarction) was 3 indicating complete recanalisation of the target vessel and its distal branches (Fig. 18.3). A residual 70% stenosis of the vertebral artery remained at the dissection. To mitigate for the risk of basilar artery re-occlusion, high dose single antiplatelet regime of Aspirin 300 mg was administered. A flat detector CT scan excluded haemorrhagic transformation (Fig. 18.4a).

The day after thrombectomy, an MRI scan revealed extensive infarction of the posterior circulation (Fig. 18.4b). In the next 24 h, an episode of asystole occurred

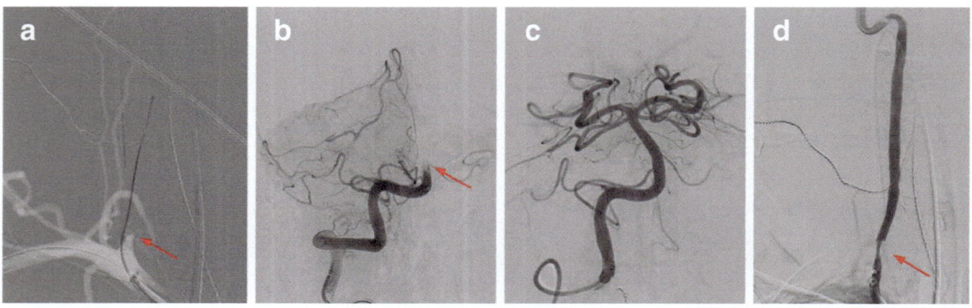

Fig. 18.3 (**a**) Abrupt cessation of contrast flow distal to vertebral artery ostium. The angiographic run demonstrates crossing the occlusion with a microwire and microcatheter. (**b**) Intracranial angiographic run demonstrates basilar artery occlusion with no distal run-off = TICI 0. (**c**) After thromboaspiration, the basilar artery and its distal branches are fully recanalised = TICI 3. (**d**) Residual 70% stenosis at the point of vertebral artery dissection

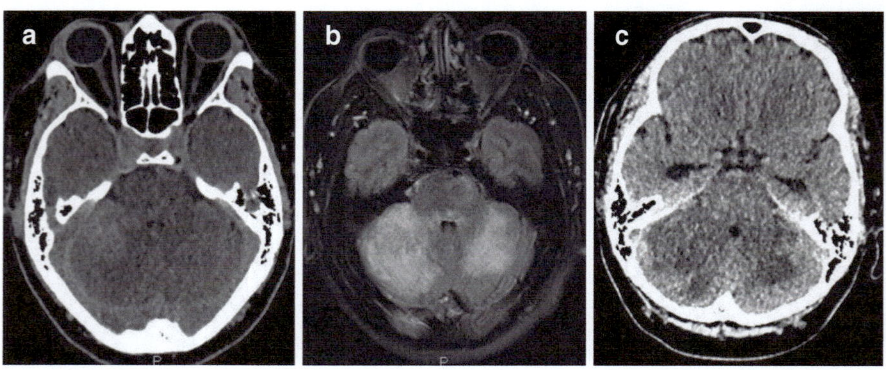

Fig. 18.4 (**a**) Post-thrombectomy NCCT demonstrates no evidence of haemorrhagic transformation in the posterior fossa. The slight hyperdense area in the right cerebellum is an area of "luxury perfusion". Following recanalisation, blood flow to the area is in excess of the local metabolic demands of the infarcted brain tissue. (**b**) T2 FLAIR sequences from an MRI head scan shows extensive hyperintense areas of both cerebellar hemispheres with effacement of the fourth ventricle. (**c**) NCCT demonstrates extensive cerebellar infarction with effacement of the fourth ventricle and early dilatation of the temporal horns of the lateral ventricles, a sign of early hydrocephalus and malignant cerebellar syndrome

and a repeat NCCT scan confirmed the presence of malignant cerebellar syndrome (Fig. 18.4c). A multi-disciplinary team meeting was conducted involving the neurosurgical, intensive care and stroke teams. Due to the extent of brainstem infarction with an associated poor prognosis for recovery, a decision was made in conjunction with the family to not perform a suboccipital decompressive craniectomy and to opt for palliation. There was no neurological recovery once anaesthetic and sedative drugs were held. Ventilation was withdrawn and he died shortly afterwards.

Discussion

The case highlights, firstly, challenges in the management of acute ischaemic stroke secondary to Basilar Artery Occlusion (BAO); and secondly, how vertebral artery dissection can be triggered by seemingly innocuous activities such as golf playing.

The posterior circulation is affected in only one-fifth of acute ischaemic strokes, but its associated morbidity and mortality is proportionately higher than anterior circulation strokes. After BAO, one-third are left with severe disability (modified Rankin Score of 4 or 5), and a further one-third die [1]. Posterior circulation strokes present ~1 h later than anterior circulation strokes [2], resulting in less effective treatment. This delay arises partly because posterior circulation ischaemia often present with non-specific symptoms such as nausea, vomiting, headache, dizziness, vertigo, fainting, or imbalance. The standard stroke disability metric NIHSS (National Institute of Health Stroke Scale), under-represents disability due to posterior circulation stroke, which risks undertreatment [3]. To correct for this, a posterior-circulation disability correction can be applied (Posterior—NIHSS) [3]. Additional points are attributed for gait or truncal ataxia, dysphagia and an abnormal cough—all of which were present in our case. In addition to triggering the need for mechanical thrombectomy, the POST-NIHSS prompts early assessment of airway function. Early endotracheal intubation can prevent complications of aspiration pneumonitis, including hypoxia, septicaemia, and hypotension, that may exacerbate brainstem ischaemia.

The radiological assessment of posterior circulation strokes also differs from anterior circulation strokes. The presence of hyperdense basilar sign (Fig. 18.1) is a key early ischaemic finding. Artefact from the bony skull base in NCCT makes identification of early ischaemic change in the posterior fossa challenging. Appropriate windowing of CT angiogram source imaging can provide adequate assessment of the posterior fossa using either the posterior-circulation Acute Stroke Prognosis Early CT Score (pc-ASPECTS, Fig. 18.5) or the Pons-Midbrain Index [4]. Whilst pc-ASPECTS helps to prognosticate for severity, the Pons-Midbrain Index has been shown to predict mortality outcomes in comatose patients with basilar stroke [5].

The BAOCHE and ATTENTION randomised clinical trials provide Level 1 evidence in support of endovascular therapy for BAO [6, 7]. A meta-analysis of four basilar RCTs demonstrated a positive treatment effect with endovascular therapy

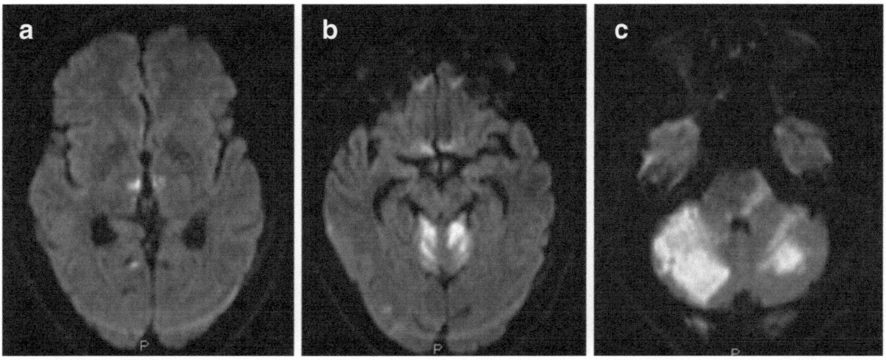

Fig. 18.5 pc-ASPECTS score assigns points to each of the territories of the posterior circulation (1 for each cerebellar hemisphere, 1 for each occipital lobe, 1 for each thalamus, 2 for pons and 2 for midbrain). Evidence of infarction in each territory subtracts points from a total score of 10. In our case (**a**–**c**) demonstrates slices from diffusion-weighted imaging on MRI head with a pc-ASPECTS score of 3 (pontine, bilateral cerebellar, bilateral thalamic, right occipital involvement).

compared to best medical therapy. There were improved rates of good functional outcome as defined by modified Rankin Scale score of 0–3 (Relative Risk 1.54) with significant lower mortality rates in the intervention arm (Relative Risk 0.76) [8].

In the current case, the BAO occurred in conjunction with a separate vertebral artery occlusion (so called "tandem" lesion). In general, it is preferable to treat the BAO first, either by entering the unaffected vertebral artery (if wide enough); or, as in this case, passing a wire through the vertebral occlusion first. Subsequently the vertebral occlusion is removed, and if narrowing is still present then balloon dilatation or stent may be deployed [9]. Registry data from carotid tandem occlusion favours targeting the intracranial occlusion first, to achieve quicker flow restoration and better functional outcomes [10]. Active intervention of the vertebral tandem lesion is demonstrably safe [11], but it is unknown if mechanical treatment of vessel dissection, and/or high-intensity anti-platelet or anticoagulation therapy, post-thrombectomy, leads to improved outcomes.

Basilar artery occlusions arise from three main mechanisms: (a) embolism without vertebral artery steno-occlusive disease; (b) embolism secondary to vertebral artery steno-occlusive disease; (c) in-situ atherosclerotic thrombosis [11]. In our case, an embolism originated from a likely acute vertebral artery dissection, with accompanying free floating thrombus. The cause of the dissection cannot be known with absolute certainty, but the close temporal association of clinical presentation with participation in a game of golf; absence of other reported triggers; and a recognised association of golf with vertebral artery dissection [12–14], make this a likely cause in the current case.

Dissection refers to the abrupt tearing of the inner layer (intima) of an arterial wall. The resultant blood pooling in the false lumen, with secondary stenosis and turbulence within the true lumen, combined with an intimal tear, create the conditions for thrombosis formation. Cervical arterial dissection is associated with prior manoeuvres that exert mechanical shear forces across the vessel wall. One observational case-control study of ~1000 cervical artery dissections recorded that prior minor cervical trauma (e.g. extreme neck movements or heavy lifting) was identified in ~40% of cases, including 6% that were sports associated [15]. By comparison, minor cervical trauma was recorded in only 10–20% of non-dissection stroke, or matched healthy subjects, over an equivalent time window. However, in this study, the delay between traumatic event and dissection presentation was as long as 1 month. This long delay range, together with the risk of recall bias makes it plausible that many reported neck injuries are coincidental rather than causal. On the other hand, if only a trivial mechanical trigger is required to inflict a dissection, then many such events may go unrecognised by patients.

Alternative non-traumatic triggers for arterial dissection include sympathetic overactivity [16], blood pressure surges [17]; or reflexes such as sneezing, coughing or Valsalva manoeuvres [18]. Whilst an external or internal, mechanical shearing force may be necessary to trigger arterial dissection, it is unlikely to be sufficient, given the far higher number of incidences of people playing golf etc. who do not incur dissection. Thus affected subjects are likely to be predisposed to dissection, for example due to defects in vascular collagen, elastin or extracellular matrix. This may be caused by a combination of genetic mutation (e.g. Marfan's or Ehlers Danlos syndromes; hyperhomocystinaemia [19, 20]; and comorbidities, such as migraine [21], hypertension (also present in our patient) [22]; and, curiously low cholesterol, and low body weight [23].

In the case of vertebral artery dissection, the commonest sites are V2 (intraforaminal segments of C2-C7 vertebrae) or V3 (axial-occipital, C2-dura, loop), accounting for ~35% cases each. In healthy subjects, active neck rotation is coupled to lateral spinal flexion in the direction of rotation, stretching the contralateral vertebral artery, and reducing its blood flow (which if extreme can cause so-called "bow-hunter's stroke"). In certain healthy subjects, dynamic occlusion of the vertebral artery within C2 foramen occurs during contralateral rotation due to anatomical variation: namely, a small arterial loop or excessive C1-C2 rotation [24]. Transient occlusion may redirect arterial pulsatility into adjacent parts of the vertebral artery wall, causing stretching, and ultimately a tear [25].

Key Clinical Learning Points

1. Posterior circulation stroke can present with non-specific symptoms, and worsen progressively or fluctuate. Such atypical stroke presentations result in delayed presentation and reduced treatment effectiveness.
2. Basilar artery occlusions result in a significantly higher disability and mortality than other types of ischaemic stroke.
3. A focused history can help to identify minor mechanical triggers, including sports, that may be associated preferentially with either carotid or vertebral arterial dissections.
4. The Posterior-NIHSS appropriately weights disability due to posterior circulation stroke; and highlights the need to assess airway compromise.
5. Mechanical thrombectomy is a highly effective treatment for basilar artery occlusions.

Key Radiological Learning Points

1. A hyperdense basilar artery is often the only finding in early basilar artery occlusion stroke, on non-contrast CT.
2. CT angiography confirms basilar artery occlusion; while the angiography source images can enable semi-quantitative estimation of posterior circulation ischaemia; using scoring systems such as pc-ASPECTS and PMI.
3. Tandem vertebral-basilar artery occlusions require a sequential approach to thrombectomy, usually starting with the basilar occlusion.

References

1. Schonewille WJ, Wijman CAC, Michel P, Rueckert C, Weimar C, Mattle H, et al. Treatment and outcomes of acute basilar artery occlusion in the Basilar Artery International Cooperation Study (BASICS): a prospective registry study. Lancet Neurol [Internet]. 2009;8(8):724–30. Available from: https://pubmed.ncbi.nlm.nih.gov/19577962/. Cited 16 Dec 2022.
2. Sommer P, Seyfang L, Posekany A, Ferrari J, Lang W, Fertl E, Serles W, Töll T, Kiechl S, Greisenegger S. Prehospital and intra-hospital time delays in posterior circulation stroke: results from the Austrian Stroke Unit Registry. J Neurol. 2017;264(1):131–8.
3. Alemseged F, Rocco A, Arba F, Schwabova JP, Wu T, Cavicchia L, et al. Posterior National Institutes of Health Stroke Scale improves prognostic accuracy in posterior circulation stroke. Stroke [Internet]. 2022;53(4):1247–55. Available from: https://www.ahajournals.org/doi/abs/10.1161/STROKEAHA.120.034019. Cited 16 Dec 2022.
4. Schaefer PW, Yoo AJ, Bell D, Barak ER, Romero JM, Nogueira RG, et al. CT angiography-source image hypoattenuation predicts clinical outcome in posterior circulation strokes treated with intra-arterial therapy. Stroke [Internet]. 2008;39(11):3107–9. Available from: https://www.ahajournals.org/doi/abs/10.1161/STROKEAHA.108.517680. Cited 16 Dec 2022.
5. Pallesen LP, Khomenko A, Dzialowski I, Barlinn J, Barlinn K, Zerna C, et al. CT-angiography source images indicate less fatal outcome despite coma of patients in the Basilar Artery International Cooperation Study. Int J Stroke [Internet]. 2017;12(2):145–51. Available from: https://pubmed.ncbi.nlm.nih.gov/27698280/. Cited 16 Dec 2022.
6. Jovin TG, Li C, Wu L, Wu C, Chen J, Jiang C, et al. Trial of thrombectomy 6 to 24 hours after stroke due to basilar-artery occlusion. New England J Med [Internet]. 2022;387(15):1373–84. Available from: https://www.nejm.org/doi/full/10.1056/NEJMoa2207576. Cited 16 Dec 2022.
7. Tao C, Qureshi AI, Yin Y, Li J, Li R, Xu P, et al. Endovascular treatment versus best medical management in acute basilar artery occlusion strokes: results from the ATTENTION Multicenter Registry. Circulation [Internet]. 2022;146(1):6–17. Available from: https://www.ahajournals.org/doi/abs/10.1161/CIRCULATIONAHA.121.058544. Cited 16 Dec 2022.
8. Malik A, Drumm B, D'Anna L, Brooks I, Low B, Raha O, et al. Mechanical thrombectomy in acute basilar artery stroke: a systematic review and Meta-analysis of randomized controlled trials. BMC Neurol [Internet]. 2022;22(1):1–8. Available from: https://bmcneurol.biomedcentral.com/articles/10.1186/s12883-022-02953-2. Cited 16 Dec 2022.
9. Baik SH, Jung C, Kim BM, Kim DJ. Mechanical thrombectomy for tandem vertebrobasilar stroke: characteristics and treatment outcome. Stroke [Internet]. 2020;51:1883–5. Available from: https://www.ahajournals.org/doi/abs/10.1161/STROKEAHA.120.029503. Cited 16 Dec 2022.
10. Feil K, Herzberg M, Dorn F, Tiedt S, Küpper C, Thunstedt DC, et al. Tandem lesions in anterior circulation stroke: analysis of the German Stroke Registry-endovascular treatment. Stroke [Internet]. 2021;52(4):1265–75. Available from: https://pubmed.ncbi.nlm.nih.gov/33588589/. Cited 16 Dec 2022.

11. Baik SH, Park HJ, Kim JH, Jang CK, Kim BM, Kim DJ. Mechanical thrombectomy in subtypes of basilar artery occlusion: Relationship to recanalization rate and clinical outcome. Radiology [Internet]. 2019;291(3):730–7. Available from: https://pubs.rsna.org/doi/10.1148/radiol.2019181924. Cited 16 Dec 2022.
12. Schlemm L, Nolte CH, Engelter ST, Endres M, Ebinger M. Cervical artery dissection after sports—an analytical evaluation of 190 published cases. Eur Stroke J. 2017;2(4):335–45. https://doi.org/10.1177/2396987317720544.2. Available from: https://www.karger.com/Article/FullText/94530.
13. Engelter ST, Traenka C, Grond-Ginsbach C, Brandt T, Hakimi M, Worrall BB, et al. Cervical artery dissection and sports. Front Neurol [Internet]. 2021;12:663830. Available from: /pmc/articles/PMC8200565/. Cited 16 Dec 2022.
14. Saw AE, McIntosh AS, Kountouris A, Newman P, Gaida JE. Vertebral artery dissection in sport: a systematic review. Sports Med [Internet]. 2019;49(4):553–64. Available from: https://link.springer.com/article/10.1007/s40279-019-01066-0. Cited 16 Dec 2022.
15. Engelter ST, Grond-Ginsbach C, Metso TM, et al. Cervical artery dissection: trauma and other potential mechanical trigger events. Neurology. 2013;80:1950–7.
16. Mawet J, Debette S, Bousser MG, Ducros A. The link between migraine, reversible cerebral vasoconstriction syndrome and cervical artery dissection. Headache. 2016;56(4):645–56.
17. Shanmugalingam R, Reza Pour N, Chuah SC, Vo TM, Beran R, Hennessy A, Makris A. Vertebral artery dissection in hypertensive disorders of pregnancy: a case series and literature review. BMC Pregnancy Childbirth. 2016;16(1):164.
18. Nomura M, Kannuki S, Kuwayama K, Kohyama Y, Hayashi Y, Yamamoto E, Kaji T, Uehara K, Nishikado A, Ito S, Nakaya Y, Nagahiro S. A patient with Wallenberg's syndrome induced by severe cough. J Clin Neurosci. 2004;11(2):179–82.
19. Giossi A, Ritelli M, Costa P, et al. Connective tissue anomalies in patients with spontaneous cervical artery dissection. Neurology. 2014;83:2032–7.
20. Wang K, Zhao S, Zhang Q, Yuan J, Liu J, Ding X, Song X, Lin J, Du R, Zhou Y, Sugimoto M, Chen W, Yuan B, Liu J, Yan Z, Liu B, Zhang Y, Li X, Niu Y, Long B, Shen Y, Zhang S, Abe K, Su J, Wu Z, Wu N, Liu P, Yang X, Deciphering Disorders Involving Scoliosis & Comorbidities (DISCO) study. Whole-exome sequencing reveals known and novel variants in a cohort of intracranial vertebral-basilar artery dissection (IVAD). J Hum Genet. 2018;63(11):1119–28. https://doi.org/10.1038/s10038-018-0496-x. Epub 16 Aug 2018. PMID: 30115950.
21. Rist PM, Diener HC, Kurth T, Schürks M. Migraine, migraine aura, and cervical artery dissection: a systematic review and meta-analysis. Cephalalgia. 2011;31(8):886–96.
22. Pezzini A, Caso V, Zanferrari C, Del Zotto E, Paciaroni M, Bertolino C, Grassi M, Agnelli G, Padovani A. Arterial hypertension as risk factor for spontaneous cervical artery dissection. A case-control study. J Neurol Neurosurg Psychiatry. 2006;77(1):95–7.
23. Debette S, Metso T, Pezzini A, Abboud S, Metso A, Leys D, Bersano A, Louillet F, Caso V, Lamy C, Medeiros E, Samson Y, Grond-Ginsbach C, Engelter ST, Thijs V, Beretta S, Béjot Y, Sessa M, Lorenza Muiesan M, Amouyel P, Castellano M, Arveiler D, Tatlisumak T, Dallongeville J, Cervical Artery Dissection and Ischemic Stroke Patients (CADISP) Group. Association of vascular risk factors with cervical artery dissection and ischemic stroke in young adults. Circulation. 2011;123(14):1537–44.
24. Dumas JL, Salama J, Dreyfus P, Thoreux P, Goldlust D, Chevrel JP. Magnetic resonance angiographic analysis of atlanto-axial rotation: anatomic bases of compression of the vertebral arteries. Surg Radiol Anat. 1996;18(4):303–13. https://doi.org/10.1007/BF01627609. PMID: 8983110.
25. Haynes MJ, Cala LA, Melsom A, Mastaglia FL, Milne N, McGeachie JK. Vertebral arteries and cervical rotation: modeling and magnetic resonance angiography studies. J Manip Physiol Ther. 2002;25(6):370–83. https://doi.org/10.1067/mmt.2002.126130. PMID: 12183695.

Chapter 19
Chemotherapy Emboli as an Iatrogenic Cause of Ischaemic Stroke Arising from a Misplaced Central Venous Access Line

Natalie Marzouqa, Geoffrey Chow, and Daryll M. Baker

Introduction

Central venous catheters are widely used in chronically ill patients in need of long-term treatments. Oncology patients in particular benefit from the ease such lines offer for chemotherapy delivery and long-term administration of fluids, blood products, medications, parenteral nutrition and regular blood sampling [1, 2]. We present a case of recurrent ischemic strokes caused by emboli from a "Port-A-Cath" central venous access line incorrectly positioned in the ascending aorta occurring during chemotherapy.

Clinical History

A 73-year-old male was admitted to the oncology department to receive chemotherapy via a "port-a-cath" central venous catheter for gastro-oesophageal junction adenocarcinoma (HER2 negative) with lung nodules and mediastinal lymph nodes, and metastatic bowel cancer in the mediastinum (normal MMR gene, RAS/RAF wild type). He was not in atrial fibrillation and did not have a history of cardiac disease. There was no history of a previous stroke or other neurological problem. There was no history of thromboembolic disease.

N. Marzouqa · G. Chow · D. M. Baker (✉)
National Hospital for Neurology and Neurosurgery, London, UK

University College London Hospitals NHS Foundation Trust, London, UK
e-mail: natalie.marzouqa@nhs.net; geoffrey.chow@nhs.net; daryll.baker@nhs.net

S. K. Gill et al. (eds.), *Stroke Medicine*,
https://doi.org/10.1007/978-3-031-58188-5_19

The day following his first chemotherapy, he experienced an episode of unresponsiveness with lip smacking movements for two minutes, confusion and expressive dysphasia. He had two further episodes during the same day, with persistent expressive dysphasia. MRI demonstrated acute infarcts in the left posterior insula, supramarginal gyrus and deep white matter (Fig. 19.1). It was thought that the infarcts could be secondary to viral vasculitis/encephalitis and he was commenced on IV acyclovir, as well as IV methylprednisolone given his background of vasculitis. EEG did not show any evidence of epileptiform activity.

Around 3 weeks after this event, the patient developed aphasia, a right arm drift with reduced power in his right upper and lower limbs. CT head demonstrated a new hyperdensity within the distal M1/proximal M2 segments of the left Middle cerebral artery suggestive of an acute thrombus, which was subsequently confirmed on CT angiogram. Additionally, when compared with previous studies, imaging showed multiple bilateral infarcts of varying ages, with overall appearances suggesting an embolic source (Figs. 19.2 and 19.3). IV thrombolysis (alteplase) was administered and the patient was transferred to the Hyperacute Stroke Unit at UCLH. He was started on antiplatelet therapy.

The stroke physicians conducted multiple investigations in an attempt to identify a possible embolic source. Carotid artery Doppler ultrasound was normal, identifying no carotid artery stenosis. An echocardiogram showed no evidence of intracardiac thrombus, with a normal left ventricle. The aortic valve was calcified (sclerotic), but there was no significant stenosis. Repeated ECGs were normal and identified no cardiac arrhythmias. Testing for a hypercoagulable state, abnormal lipid profile, metabolic abnormalities (lactate, pyruvate, urine organic acids, serum amino acids), inflammatory conditions (erythrocyte sedimentation rate, antinuclear antibody) were either not altered.

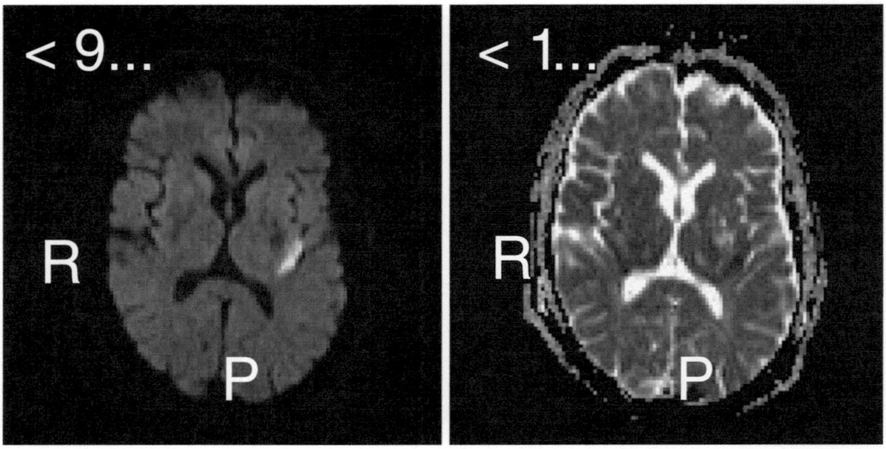

Fig. 19.1 MRI brain Diffusion weighted images and ADC images demonstrating left insular and deep white matter infarcts soon after the patient had clinically suffered a stroke following miss insertion of a venous access catheter

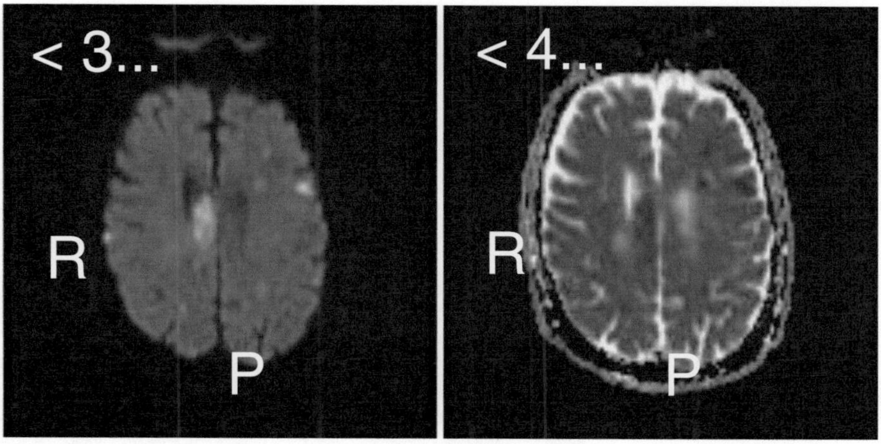

Fig. 19.2 Follow up MRI brain showing diffusion weighted images and ADC images demonstrating further infarcts right cingulum after the patient had clinically suffered further strokes following further chemotherapy through a miss-inserted central venous access catheter

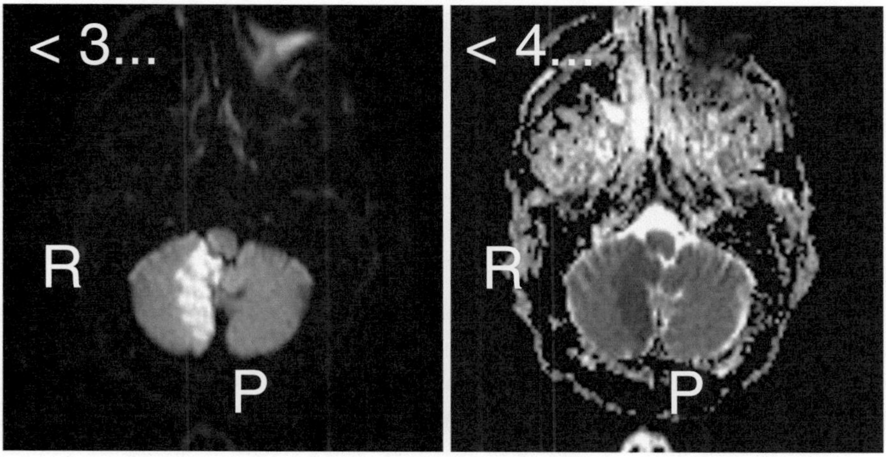

Fig. 19.3 Follow up MRI brain showing diffusion weighted images and ADC images demonstrating further infarcts this time in the right cerebellum after the patient had clinically suffered further strokes following further chemotherapy through a miss-inserted central venous access catheter

The “Embolic Stroke of Undetermined Source” was assumed due to hypercoagulability related to the underlying tumours and their treatment and anticoagulation was considered. However, a PET scan to assess disease status during chemotherapy showed the port-a-catheter tip in the ascending aorta (Fig. 19.4). The Port-A-Cath appeared to traverse the right internal jugular vein before entering the right common carotid artery thus identifying the embolic source.

The “port-a-cath” was removed and a covered stent placed across the arterial puncture site.

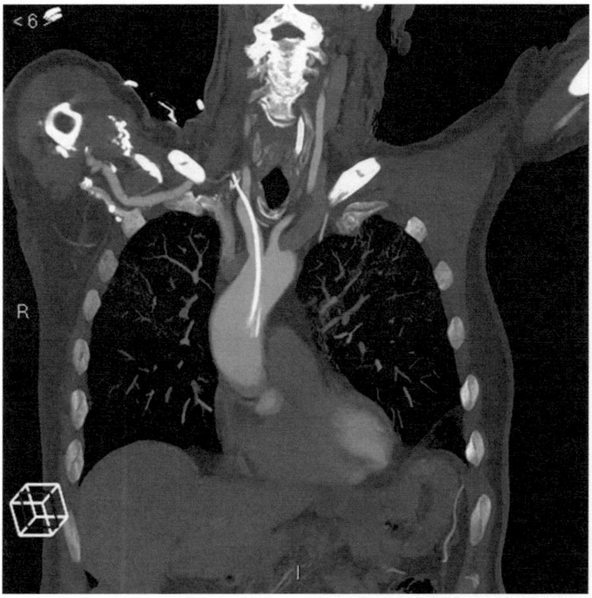

Fig. 19.4 CTC+ CorMIP (contrast enhanced aortogram version)—highlighting the position of the central venous in the right common carotid, brachiocephalic and ultimately the aorta

The patient had no further ischaemic episodes, however, following his prolonged 3 month hospital admission, he was globally deconditioned and required assistance of one to mobilise around his room.

Discussion

This case reports the inadvertent insertion of a central venous catheter into the aortic arch that was not immediately identified. Recurrent ischaemic embolic strokes developed as a result of intra-arterial chemotherapy medication delivery. No new stokes developed once the line was removed.

Direct arterial injury complicates less than one percent of attempted central venous cannulation. This is usually identified straight away during insertion as a high flow arterial blood pulses from the catheter [3–7]. There are a few similar cases in the literature reporting stroke following inadvertent intra-arterial central venous line insertion (Table 19.1). In most cases the stroke occurred very soon after line insertion and occasionally after its use. In over 50% of cases the subclavian artery was punctured inadvertently and in 30% the carotid artery was punctured. In 60% the consequence of this was either death or a residual neurological deficit.

This present case report demonstrates the difficulty sometimes experienced in identifying the embolic source of an ischaemic stroke. Embolic Stroke of Undetermined Source (ESUS) involves approximately 17% of all ischemic stroke patients and has an annual rate of stroke recurrence of 4–5% [15]. As such all efforts to determine the embolic source need to be undertaken so recurrent stroke

Table 19.1 Literature review of cases of arterially inserted miss placed central venous catheter lines resulting in stroke

	Line Indication	Artery puncture	Brain lesion	Timing of stroke	Vessel Repair	Outcome	Ref
1	Cancer Chemotherapy	Right Subclavian artery	Multi-territory stroke	At line insertion	Endovascular/open repair	Full recovery	[8]
2	TPN	Right Common carotid artery	Right MCA stroke (right frontal cortex)	6 hours after TPN infusion	?	Residual Deficit	[9]
3	Cardiogenic shock	Right Common carotid artery	Right MCA stoke (right frontal cortex)	2 days after line insertion	Endovascular	Full recovery	[3]
4	Cancer Chemotherapy	?	Right MCA Stroke (parietal)	Soon after TPN infusion started	Open repair	Died	[10]
5	Sepsis	Right subclavian artery	no changes on brain imaging	During antibiotic infusion	Open repair	Full recovery	[10]
6	Sepsis	Right subclavian artery	?	During antibiotic infusion	Open repair	Residual deficit	[10]
7	Cancer Chemotherpay	Right Subclavian artery	Multiteretory stroke	During chemotherapy infusion	Endovascular repair	Residual deficit	This case
8	TPN	Right Subclavian artery	Right MCA stroke & right eye symptoms	Fourth day of chemotherapy	Removed bedside	Full recovery	[11]
9	Antibiotics post surgery	Right brachial artery into Common Carotid Artery	single ischemic lesion involving the right genu of the internal capsule, and right basal ganglia	2 weeks of treatment	Removed bedside	Full recovery	[12]
10	Pre Cardiac bypass surgery	Right internal carotid artery	Right MCA stroke	At line insertion	open	Died	[13]
11	Emergency Diabetic ketoacidosis	Right Subclavian artery	Right MCA stroke	3 days after line insertion	Thrombectomy and endovascualar	Residual deficit	[14]
12	TPN	Left common carotid artery	Left MCA stroke	At line insertion	Removed bedside	Died	[7]
13	TPN	Right Subclavian artery	Multi territory stoke (Lt thalamu, right cerebella)	At line insertion	Removed bedside	Died	[7]

preventative treatment can be targeted. Usually, a battery of tests are performed to identify the most common causes of embolic stroke. These include cardiac echo, ECG and 72 h heart monitor, carotid duplex scan, CT angiogram and MRI, as well as blood samples to exclude infective, inflammatory or thrombogenic causes. If these tests do not initially reveal the embolic source, the stroke(s) are usually eventually found, or assumed, to be due to a cardiac origin (atrial cardiopathy, covert atrial fibrillation, left ventricular disease, cardiac valvular disease or patent foramen ovale). Other aetiologies are assumed to be atherosclerotic plaque rupture or cancer induced thrombogenesis [15]. An iatrogenic cause, as occurred in this case, is rare. Depending on the assumed aetiology (altered blood flow or atherosclerotic plaque rupture) patients are usually either formally anticoagulated with a DOAC or managed with an antiplatelet medication. Neither would have been successful in this particular case.

This case, although an unusual cause for ischaemic stroke, emphasises that there are many aetiologies and in complex cases a careful history, examination and review of ALL the imaging is needed to determine the embolic source of the ischaemic stroke.

Key Clinical Learning Points

- Recurrent embolic strokes have a poor prognosis.
- If after initial review no cause is found, rarer causes of stroke need to be considered so that appropriate treatment can be implemented.
- Always order chest as well as neck and brain CT angiograms for stroke patients. This will help identify more unusual sources of emboli.

Key Radiological Learning Points

- On central venous line insertion always check and re-check that the line tip is within the planned vein. Any concerns consider line pressure wave form analysis.

References

1. D'Souza PC, Kumar S, Kakaria A, Al-Sukaiti R, Zahid KF, Furrukh M, Burney IA, Al-Moundhri MS. Use of port-a-cath in cancer patients: a single-center experience. J Infect Dev Ctries. 2014;8(11):1476–82.
2. Machat S, Eisenhuber E, Pfarl G, Stubler J, Koelblinger C, Zacheri J, Schima W. Complications of central venous port systems: a pictorial review. Insights Imaging. 2019;10:86.
3. Katyal N, Korzep A, Newey C. Inadvertent central arterial catheterization: an unusual cause of ischemic stroke. J Neurosci Rural Pract. 2018;9(1):155–8.
4. Bowdle A. Vascular complications of central venous catheter placement: evidence-based methods for prevention and treatment. J Cardiothorac Vasc Anesth. 2014;28:358–68.

5. Vats HS. Complications of catheters: tunneled and nontunneled. Adv Chronic Kidney Dis. 2012;19:188–94.
6. Kornbau C, Lee KC, Hughes GD, Firstenberg MS. Central line complications. Int J Crit Illn Inj Sci. 2015;5:170–8.
7. Hurwitz BJ, Posner JB. Cerebral infarction complicating subclavian vein catheterization. Ann Neurol. 1977;1:253–4.
8. Jahromi BS, Tummala RP, Levy EI. Inadvertent subclavian artery catheter placement complicated by stroke: endovascular management and review. Catheter Cardiovasc Interv. 2009;73:706–11.
9. Bohlega S, McLean DR. Case report Hemiplegia caused by inadvertent intra-carotid infusion of total parenteral nutrition. Clin Neurol Neurosurg. 1997;99(3):217–9.
10. Shah PM, Leong B, Babu SC, Goyal AM, Mateo RB. Cerebrovascular events associated with infusion through arterially malpositioned triple-lumen catheter report of three cases and review of literature. Cardiol Rev. 2005;13(6):304–8.
11. Wang RC, Katz SE, Lubow M. Visual loss and central venous catheterization: cortical blindness and hemianopsia after inadvertent subclavian artery entry. JNO. 2000;20:32–4.
12. Parikh S, Narayanan V. Misplaced peripherally inserted central catheter: an unusual cause of stroke. Pediatr Neurol. 2004;30:210–2.
13. Marie-Christine Guilbert MC, Elkouri BD, Corriveau MM, Beaudoin N, Dubois MJ, Bruneau L, Blair JF. Arterial trauma during central venous catheter insertion: case series, review and proposed algorithm. J Vasc Surg. 2008;48(4):918–25.
14. Rilling WS. Central line misplacement leading to stroke. Moderator Endovascular Today. 2019;18(8)
15. Ntaios G. Embolic stroke of undetermined source. JACC review topic of the week. J Am Coll Cardiol. 2020;75:333–40.

Chapter 20
Recurrent Thunderclap Headache

Nicholas F. Brown

History

A 22-year-old female right-handed investment banker presented with a three-week history of recurrent thunderclap occipital headaches. Headaches were initially frontal and left sided, then right sided, and then became occipital. She described the headaches as "being hit from behind by a bat" and subsequently "pounding" with associated photophobia and hyperacusis. Each headache was precipitated by physical exertion at the gym. The headaches initially lasted approximately thirty minutes but in the week before presentation were lasting nine to ten hours. There were no relieving factors.

She had no past medical history and was not on any regular medications. There was no family history of note. She did not smoke or drink alcohol, and denied recreational drug use. She had recently started taking diphenhydramine sleeping tablets and unnamed Chinese herbal supplements.

Examination

She was alert and oriented. Blood pressure was 110/68. Cardiac, respiratory, and abdominal examination was unremarkable. Neurological examination of her cranial nerves, upper limbs, and lower limbs was normal. Dilated fundoscopy was normal. There were no visible rashes or arthralgia.

N. F. Brown (✉)
University College London Hospitals, London, UK

S. K. Gill et al. (eds.), *Stroke Medicine*,
https://doi.org/10.1007/978-3-031-58188-5_20

Investigations

Routine blood tests including CRP and ESR were normal. 12 lead ECG displayed sinus rhythm.

MRI Brain revealed normal brain parenchyma. MR Angiogram of the intracranial arteries (Fig. 20.1) demonstrated irregular calibre with beading of multiple arterial segments of the circle of Willis bilaterally consistent with a severe vasculopathic process. These findings were confirmed on a four-vessel catheter angiogram (Fig. 20.1). CT Abdomen with contrast revealed normal extra-cranial blood vessels.

Vasculitis and thrombophilia screens were negative. Cerebrospinal fluid (CSF) opening pressure at lumbar puncture was 14 cm water. CSF was acellular with protein count of 0.5. CSF culture and viral serology was negative.

She was diagnosed with cerebral vasoconstriction syndrome and commenced on oral nimodipine. She was discharged home and her headaches gradually subsided. Repeat MR Angiogram (Fig. 20.2) of the intracranial vessels five months post presentation revealed normal intracranial vessels, confirming the diagnosis of reversible cerebral vasoconstriction syndrome (RCVS). Nimodipine was gradually withdrawn, and she remains headache free.

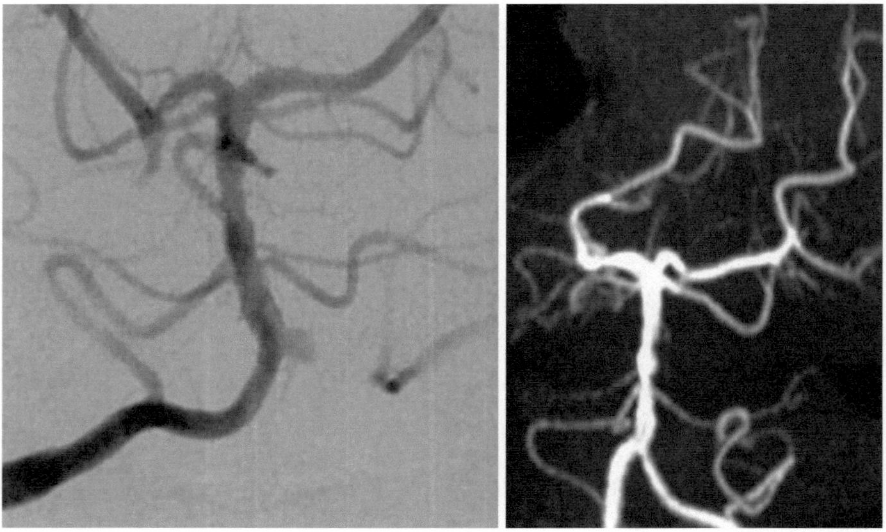

Fig. 20.1 Four-vessel catheter cerebral angiogram and MR Angiogram. Irregularity of the basilar artery and bilateral irregular calibre with 'beading' of multiple arterial segments at the circle of Willis

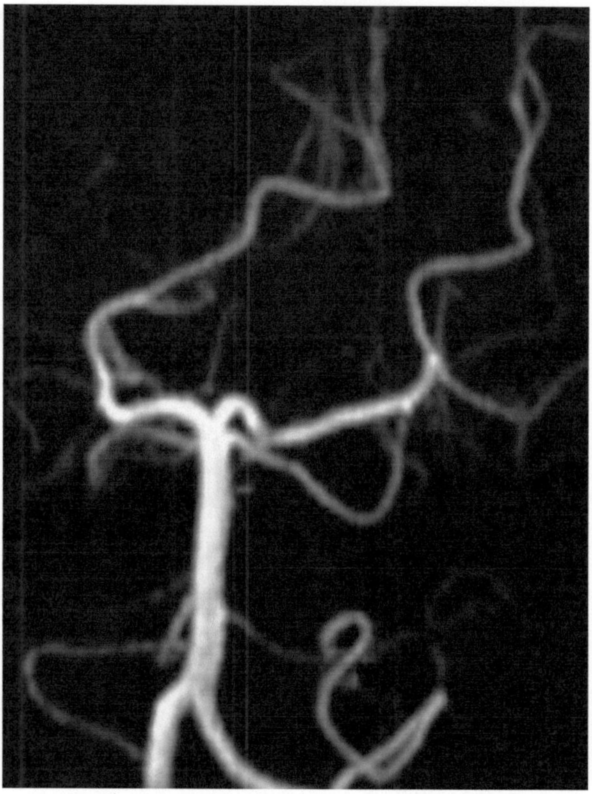

Fig. 20.2 Interval MR Angiogram five months post presentation. Normal intracranial vessels

Discussion

Reversible cerebral vasoconstriction syndrome (RCVS) is characterised by transient dysregulation of cerebral vascular tone leading to prolonged but reversible constriction of intracranial arteries, with resolution within three months. Peak incidence is between 20 and 50 years of age, with a female predominance [1–10]. Accurate incidence is difficult to define as it is underdiagnosed, particularly in pure cephalgic cases.

The most common clinical presentation is with severe acute headache (typically thunderclap), with or without additional neurological symptoms including focal neurology (9–64%) and seizures (0–21%) [4–6]. The acute headache is typically bilateral, with posterior onset and associated nausea, vomiting, and photophobia. In contrast to aneurysm-rupture, the severe headache of RCVS is short lived. Most patients (>90%) will present with recurrent thunderclap headaches, recurring on average seven days apart, with a milder background headache between attacks [2, 3, 6, 7].

The pathophysiology of RCVS is not fully understood. Brain biopsies have not revealed abnormalities, and have not demonstrated vascular inflammation [8]. The prevailing hypothesis is that it is secondary to transient and reversible disturbance in the control of cerebral vascular tone, with subsequent multifocal and segmental arterial constriction and dilatation [5, 9]. Since intracranial vascular tone and calibre is dependent on both vascular receptor activity and sensitivity, a central vascular discharge (either spontaneous or evoked) with a multifactorial trigger may determine the relapsing and reversible nature of RCVS [4]. The temporal clinical progression suggests that the underlying disturbance first involves small distal arteries, potentially causing haemorrhage or a clinical syndrome identical to the posterior reversible encephalopathy syndrome (PRES), and then progresses to involve medium and large calibre vessels, with subsequent ischaemia and potential infarction [2].

The syndrome may be spontaneous (idiopathic), or may occur secondary to a precipitant (25–60%) [5]. Precipitants have been implicated due to a temporal relationship with RCVS which may occur several months after precipitant use [4, 5]. Reported precipitants include vasoactive substances, pregnancy/puer-partum, catecholamine-secreting tumours, and immunosuppressants or blood products (Fig. 20.3). The most commonly reported precipitants are serotonin selective re-uptake inhibitors, cannabis, and over-the-counter nasal decongestants [2]. A trigger immediately prior to the onset of headache is recounted by 80% of patients, including sexual intercourse, straining, physical exertion, urination, high emotional state, showering, and head movements [5].

Complications of RCVS include seizures, PRES, subarachnoid haemorrhage (SAH), and intracerebral haemorrhage during the first seven days after headache-onset when small calibre vessels are affected, followed by ischaemic infarcts during the second week when medium and larger calibre arteries are affected [5]. Subarachnoid haemorrhage is of small volume and tends to be localised, overlying the cortical surface with limited spread over one to three sulci [1, 5, 6]. Infarction is due to ischaemia distal to affected vessels, typically within arterial "watershed" regions, and occurs in 7–50% of cases [1, 4–6].

CT/MR Brain imaging at presentation is frequently normal. Angiography, either transfemoral or indirect (MRA/CTA) shows multifocal segmental narrowing and dilatation, in a "string of beads" pattern. Transcranial doppler can be used both for diagnosis and serial monitoring of vasoconstriction [10, 11]. Typically the anterior

Pregnancy & Puerperum
Vasoactive substances: *Cocaine, Cannabis, Amphetamines, SSRIs, Nasal decongestants, ergotamine, methergine, bromocriptine, triptans, nicotine patches, ginseng*
Catecholamine secreting tumours
Immunosuppressants or blood products: *tacrolimus, cyclophosphamide, interferon-alpha, erythropoietin, intravenous immunoglobulin, packed red cells*
Head trauma

Fig. 20.3 Precipitants attributed to RCVS. (Adapted from [5])

and posterior cerebral circulations are bilaterally and diffusely affected, with potential involvement of the carotid artery and basilar siphon [5]. If performed in the first few days after presentation, angiography may appear normal, due to the poor sensitivity of angiography to small vessel involvement. Follow-up cerebral imaging is abnormal in three quarters of cases, including infarcts (39%), subarachnoid haemorrhage (34%), intracerebral haemorrhage (20%), and oedema (20%) [6]. Serial angiography has found peak involvement of arterial segments 16 days after headache onset, with unsynchronised progression and regression of vasoconstricted arterial segments [1]. Complete reversal of angiographic abnormalities is apparent between one and three months after presentation, and is required to confirm the diagnosis of RCVS [3].

Cerebrospinal fluid at presentation is frequently abnormal, and may show mild elevation in protein and white cell count [5]. Serum inflammatory markers may show a modest elevation [5].

The differential diagnosis for a single thunderclap headache includes aneurysmal subarachnoid haemorrhage, intracranial haemorrhage, cervical or intracranial dissection, hypertensive encephalopathy, post-partum vasculopathy, venous thrombosis, giant cell arteritis, and pituitary apoplexy. Recurrent thunderclap headaches are much more likely to be RCVS. Appropriate imaging and serum inflammatory markers should differentiate the above presentations. RCVS-SAH with vasospasm is distinguished from aneurysmal-SAH on imaging with typical appearances of a small volume bleed overlying the superior or lateral cortical surface, with multifocal vessel abnormalities remote from the site of bleeding, and no evidence of aneurysm rupture [5, 6, 12]. The differential diagnosis for the imaging appearances of RCVS is primary CNS angiitis but the clinical presentation of the two syndromes is very different. CNS angiitis rarely presents with thunderclap headache, progresses over more than 4 weeks, and has marked cerebrospinal fluid and serum abnormalities [8]. In patients found to have intracranial arteriopathy, the $RCVS_2$ score (Fig. 20.4) combines clinical and radiographic features to differentiate RCVS from other causes, with a sensitivity of 94% and specificity of 86% in those with a score ≥ 5 [13].

Criterion	*Value*
Sex	
Female	1
Male	0
Thunderclap headache	
Present	5
Absent	0
Vasoconstrictive trigger	
Present	3
Absent	0
Subarachnoid haemorrhage	
Present	1
Absent	0
Intracranial carotid artery narrowing	
Affected	–2
Not affected	0

Fig. 20.4 The $RCVS_2$ score to distinguish RCVS from other intracranial arteriopathies [13]

The following diagnostic criteria for RCVS have been proposed [4]:

1. Acute severe headache with or without neurological signs or symptoms
2. Multifocal segmental vasoconstriction of cerebral arteries demonstrated by angiography
3. No evidence for aneurysmal subarachnoid haemorrhage
4. Normal or near-normal cerebrospinal fluid analysis (protein <1 g/l, white cells <15 mm^3, glucose normal)
5. Reversibility of angiographic abnormalities within 12 weeks after onset

Initial management includes cessation of potential precipitants, analgesia, blood pressure control, and medical management of seizures. There have been no clinical trials evaluating pharmacotherapy in RCVS and open studies have not identified any significant clinical benefit with calcium channel blockers or glucocorticoids. Patients with RCVS are often given glucocorticoids at presentation due to diagnostic uncertainty of primary CNS angiitis and evidence of benefit in aneurysmal subarachnoid haemorrhage in animal studies [8]. However, there is no clear clinical indication for glucocorticoids in RCVS, and their use has demonstrated a trend towards poor outcomes [6]. Calcium channel blockers (particularly nimodipine) are frequently used as vasodilators, but care must be taken to avoid hypotension and subsequent watershed infarction in areas perfused by the constricted artery [4, 6]. The optimum treatment duration is unclear, but they are generally stopped after resolution of symptoms and angiographic abnormalities. Hypertension should be managed as per acute stroke guidelines, but with caution given the increased the risk watershed infarction with hypotension [3]. Simple analgesics are usually sufficient for headache, with triptans and ergot derivatives contraindicated due to their vasoactivity. Intra-arterial administration of vasodilators and balloon angioplasty have a controversial role in RCVS, with variable success and a risk of reperfusion injury [3, 14–16].

The prognosis in RCVS in favourable, with excellent recovery in uncomplicated cases. One series reported modified Rankin of 0 to 1 in 78% of patients, 2–3 in 11%, and 4–5 in 9% [6]. Cerebral infarction (but not haemorrhage) is associated with a poor outcome [6]. Deaths have rarely been reported. Relapse is very uncommon.

Key Learning Points

- RCVS is a transient disturbance in cerebral vascular tone with subsequent multifocal segmental intracerebral arterial constriction and dilatation.
- RCVS should be considered in all presentations with cryptogenic strokes or thunderclap headache, particularly if recurrent.
- Differentiation from primary CNS angiitis can be made clinically, and from aneurysmal subarachnoid haemorrhage radiologically.
- Management includes enquiring about and discontinuing potential precipitants. Calcium channel blocker initiation may be beneficial.
- Prognosis is favourable, but dependent on the extent of cerebral infarction.

Key Radiology Learning Points

- All patients with recurrent thunderclap headaches with or without cerebral haemorrhage should have intracranial angiography.
- Multifocal segmental narrowing and dilatation with a "string of beads" pattern on angiography (transfemoral or indirect), with normalisation within three months is diagnostic of RCVS.
- Angiography at presentation may be normal, and repeat angiography may be required to demonstrate vascular abnormalities.

References

1. Chen SP, Fuh JL, Wang SJ, Chang FC, Lirng JF, Fang YC, et al. Magnetic resonance angiography in reversible cerebral vasoconstriction syndromes. Ann Neurol. 2010;67(5):648–56.
2. Ducros A, Boukobza M, Porcher R, Sarov M, Valade D, Bousser MG. The clinical and radiological spectrum of reversible cerebral vasoconstriction syndrome. A prospective series of 67 patients. Brain. 2007;130(Pt 12):3091–101.
3. Ducros A. Reversible cerebral vasoconstriction syndrome. Lancet Neurol. 2012;11(10):906–17.
4. Calabrese LH, Dodick DW, Schwedt TJ, Singhal AB. Narrative review: reversible cerebral vasoconstriction syndromes. Ann Intern Med. 2007;146(1):34–44.
5. Ducros A, Bousser MG. Reversible cerebral vasoconstriction syndrome. Pract Neurol. 2009;9(5):256–67.
6. Singhal AB, Hajj-Ali RA, Topcuoglu MA, Fok J, Bena J, Yang D, et al. Reversible cerebral vasoconstriction syndromes: analysis of 139 cases. Arch Neurol. 2011;68(8):1005–12.
7. Chen SP, Fuh JL, Lirng JF, Chang FC, Wang SJ. Recurrent primary thunderclap headache and benign CNS angiopathy: spectra of the same disorder? Neurology. 2006;67(12):2164–9.
8. Sattar A, Manousakis G, Jensen MB. Systematic review of reversible cerebral vasoconstriction syndrome. Expert Rev Cardiovasc Ther. 2010;8(10):1417–21.
9. Schwedt TJ, Matharu MS, Dodick DW. Thunderclap headache. Lancet Neurol. 2006;5(7):621–31.
10. Chen SP, Fuh JL, Chang FC, Lirng JF, Shia BC, Wang SJ. Transcranial color doppler study for reversible cerebral vasoconstriction syndromes. Ann Neurol. 2008;63(6):751–7.
11. Marsh EB, Ziai WC, Llinas RH. The need for a rational approach to vasoconstrictive syndromes: transcranial doppler and calcium channel blockade in reversible cerebral vasoconstriction syndrome. Case Rep Neurol. 2016;8(2):161–71.
12. Hsiao J-R, Chang Y, Chen Y-L, Hsieh S-H, Hsu K-F, Wang C-F, et al. Cyclic αvβ 6-targeting peptide selected from biopanning with clinical potential for head and neck squamous cell carcinoma. Head Neck. 2010;32(2):160–72.
13. Rocha EA, Topcuoglu MA, Silva GS, Singhal AB. $RCVS_2$ score and diagnostic approach for reversible cerebral vasoconstriction syndrome. Neurology. 2019;92(7):e639–e47.
14. Ioannidis I, Nasis N, Agianniotaki A, Katsouda E, Andreou A. Reversible cerebral vasoconstriction syndrome: treatment with multiple sessions of intra-arterial nimodipine and angioplasty. Interv Neuroradiol. 2012;18(3):297–302.
15. Elstner M, Linn J, Müller-Schunk S, Straube A. Reversible cerebral vasoconstriction syndrome: a complicated clinical course treated with intra-arterial application of nimodipine. Cephalalgia. 2009;29(6):677–82.
16. Singhal AB, Kimberly WT, Schaefer PW, Hedley-Whyte ET. Case records of the Massachusetts General Hospital. Case 8-2009. A 36-year-old woman with headache, hypertension, and seizure 2 weeks post partum. N Engl J Med. 2009;360(11):1126–37.

Chapter 21
Cerebral Venous Thrombosis Due to Vaccine-Induced Thrombotic Thrombocytopenia

Talal Al-Mayhani and Richard Perry

A 22-year-old right-handed man, previously fit and well, was brought by his family to a local hospital, before being transferred to our institute for further investigation and management. Twelve days prior, he had received the first dose of ChAdOx1-nCoV-19 (Oxford-AstraZeneca) vaccine. For 4 days before admission, he complained of gradual onset but progressive headache with no nausea, vomiting or other migrainous features. For 1 day before his admission, he became confused and developed right arm weakness.

Examination and Localization

On arrival in hospital, he was initially awake, but disorientated and unable to provide history or follow commands with GCS 13/15 (E4, V3, M6). There was bilateral disc swelling on fundoscopy, weakness of 2/5 and 3/5 in the right upper and lower limbs respectively, and brisk reflexes throughout. The focal neurological findings in the right hemibody localized to the left cortical/subcortical hemisphere, but the presence of disc swelling and encephalopathy raised also the likelihood of diffuse or multifocal intracranial pathological process.

T. Al-Mayhani (✉) · R. Perry
National Hospital for Neurology and Neurosurgery, London, UK
e-mail: tala.al-mayhani@nhs.net; richard.perry2@nhs.net

S. K. Gill et al. (eds.), *Stroke Medicine*,
https://doi.org/10.1007/978-3-031-58188-5_21

Investigations and Management

The vital signs were within normal range. The blood tests showed haemoglobin 109 g/dL, platelets 24×10^9/L, monocytes elevated, potassium 3.2 mmol/L, calcium 2.15 mmol/L, folate <2 ng/mL, C-reactive protein 36.7 mg/L, extractable nuclear antigen positive (with equivocal anti-Ro), hepatitis A antibody (positive), hepatitis B anti-surface AB (positive), hepatitis E antibody (positive), D-dimer 25580 (H), heparin-induced platelet factor 4 (PF4) antibodies positive (optical density 1.823, Asserachrom HPIA IgG assay).

CT/CT venogram and MRI head revealed extensive dural venous sinus thrombosis with venous infarctions and haemorrhage (Fig. 21.1), and systemic imaging detected segmental pulmonary embolism, and right portal vein thrombosis.

He was diagnosed with vaccine-induced immune thrombotic thrombocytopenia and he underwent daily plasma exchange for total of four sessions, and received steroids (methylprednisolone IV, then prednisolone PO) and intravenous

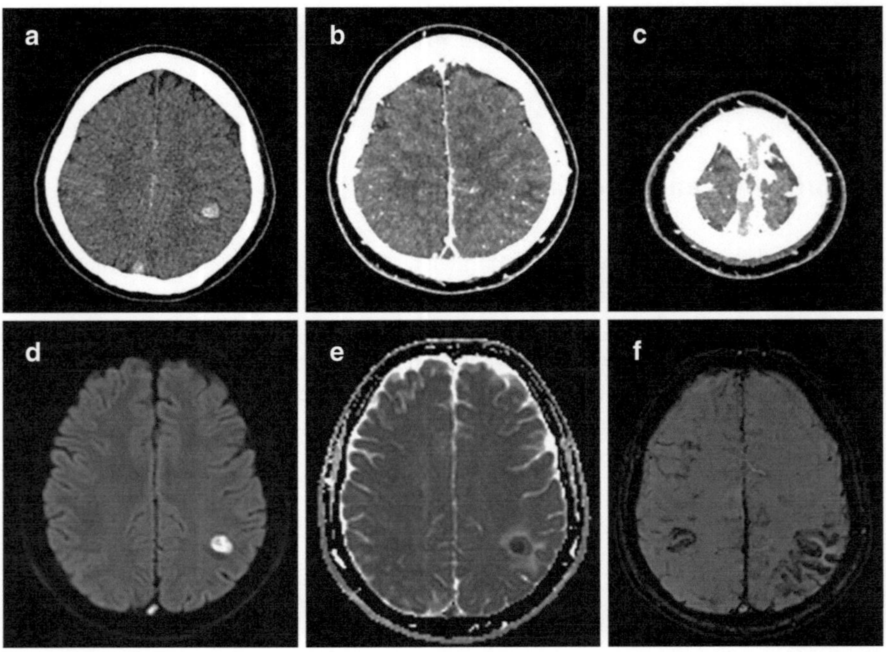

Fig. 21.1 (**a**): axial CT head with no contrast showing global cerebral oedema, parenchymal hyperdensity in the left hemisphere and hyperdense area in the superior sagittal sinus. (**b** and **c**): axial CT venogram showing filling defects in the superior sagittal sinus with delta sign in demonstrated **b**, indicating CVT. (**d** and **e**): axial MRI head DWI and ADC sequences showing areas of restricted diffusion in the left hemisphere, indicating venous infarct, and inside the superior sagittal sinus, indicating acute thrombus. (**f**): axial MRI head SWI image showing bilateral blooming, indicating haemorrhagic lesions associated with CVT

immunoglobulin (IVIG, a total of 2 g/kg over 4 days). He was also commenced on argatroban which was subsequently changed to fondaparinux.

His admission was complicated by seizures resulting in low Glasgow coma scale and respiratory compromise that required short intensive care unit (ICU) admission. Levetiracetam was introduced to control the seizures. While in ICU he developed hospital-acquired pneumonia for which he received the appropriate course of antibiotics.

He was extubated on day 8, stepped down to ward on day 10 and discharged home on day 14 of admission.

On follow up he subjectively reported being back to his baseline, and the examination revealed objective improvement, residual papilloedema and no other focal deficits.

Final Diagnosis

ChAdOx1-nCoV-19 vaccine-induced thrombotic thrombocytopenia (VITT) with cerebral and multisystem venous thrombosis.

Discussion

This case demonstrated some of the classical features of extensive cerebral dural venous sinus thrombosis, in addition to systemic thrombosis, in context of VITT, a rare complication of ChAdOx1-nCoV-19 vaccine.

The cerebral venous system consists of three interconnected components; dural venous sinuses, cortical veins and deep cerebral veins. They drain into the internal jugular veins, and to less extent into the external jugular veins and vertebral venous plexus. However, as demonstrated in 1972 by Browder and Kaplan [1], there is also extensive, complex and highly variable tuberculation, arachnoid granulation and villi, venous anastomotic plexi and lacuna and emissary veins that connect intracranial, diploical and extracranial venous structures whose neuro-anatomical details are beyond the scope of this chapter [2].

Pathologically, cerebral venous thrombosis (CVT) can result in various combinations of venous congestion, oedema, infarctions and haemorrhage.

The location of CVT produces differing clinical syndromes and are important to highlight so they can be recognised in clinical practice:

- cerebral dural venous sinus thrombosis constitutes most CVT presentations, with 70% involving the superior sagittal sinus and/or the transverse sinus [3]. The typical clinical syndrome presents with headache, vomiting, papilloedema and seizures, and the focal neurological deficits can be absent or subtle as back-pressure builds in the venous system. Cavernous sinus thrombosis forms 5% of

total cases of CVT, and results in distinct clinical syndrome that variably present with painful ophthalmoplegia, with or without chemosis and proptosis.
- Occlusion of a cortical vein, especially the superior anastomotic vein (of Trolard) or the inferior anastomotic vein (of Labbé), tend to present with seizures or focal neurological deficits and can be complicated locally by subarachnoid haemorrhage. While the classical description of the thrombosis of vein of Trolard includes proximal weakness of the contralesional arm and leg, that of vein of Labbé includes weakness of contralesional face and arm, with speech disturbance. Anatomical variations make the symptomatology highly inconsistent in clinical practice [4].
- The deep cerebral veins form a complex drainage system from the deep brain structures (mainly the basal ganglia and thalami) and the choroid plexi of the ventricles. A pair of internal cerebral veins joins the two basal veins of Rosenthal to form the great vein of Galen, which in turn joins the inferior sagittal sinus to form the straight sinus. Thrombosis of deep cerebral veins can be encountered in up to 10% of CVT cases [5], tending to present with change in mentation leading to coma, that heralds generally worse prognosis.

It is estimated that CVT forms less than 1–2% of total stroke cases [3]; the exact incidence remains largely unknown. Similarly, autopsy studies provided conflicting data regarding the CVT prevalence with various figures between 1% and 9%, raising the concept of latent and clinically silent venous sinus thrombosis [6]. The true incidence is likely to be higher, given the protean symptoms of CVT presentation, and the possibility of under-diagnosis.

The prospective International Study on Cerebral Vein and Dural Venous Thrombosis (ISCVT) followed 684 patients across 21 countries, and provided valuable insight on this condition [7]. CVT has a 3:1 female preponderance, and average age of 37 years [8]. About 50% of the cases are due to hypercoagulable states of hormonal factors or haematological pathologies. The hormonal factors include pregnancy, peri-partum period and puerperium. Combined oral contraceptives use is a factor in 10% of CVT cases, although 35% of these cases were found to have underlying thrombophilia [8]. The haematological pathologies include the genetic prothrombotic disorders (thrombophilia) such as factor V Leiden mutation, or the acquired disorders such as polycythaemia, thrombocytosis, severe anaemia and nephrotic syndrome. Infectious causes have become less common in developed countries, but facial and dental infections, sinusitis, otitis, mastoiditis and meningitis should always be considered. Neoplasia can result in CVT, either by direct compression or infiltration by metastatic or primary lesions or, more commonly, by malignancy-associated prothrombotic state.

The management of CVT focuses, in the acute stage, on dissipating the thrombus. The priority is to commence the patient on anticoagulation (low molecular weight heparin, LMWH and then warfarin) even in presence of haemorrhagic lesions [9]. In selected cases, endovascular thrombectomy can be offered, especially in patients with expanding thrombus or declining consciousness in spite of anticoagulation, although the only randomized-controlled trial of this intervention did not show benefit [10]. Decompressive hemicraniectomy, a lifesaving procedure, should be considered in certain cases complicated by severe mass effect from swollen venous infarction. The management should also address the predisposing factors and the potential complications e.g. systemic vasculitis or neoplasia, seizures.

In the era of the COVID-19 pandemic, the prothrombotic state and endotheliopathy associated with SARS-CoV-2 infection have resulted in an increase in the thrombotic events in the venous system [11]. Similarly, there have been reports of cases of CVT after receiving COVID-19 vaccines, as illustrated in this case of VITT. This recently described condition shares many features of heparin-induced thrombocytopenia (HIT) [12], a complication of heparin use which has been recognized since the last 1950s.

In HIT, antibodies are formed against the platelet factor-4 (anti-PF4 antibodies) usually within 2 weeks of commencing the treatment in heparin-naïve patients, with an estimated incidence of 0.2–3% of patients started on heparin [13]. Use of unfractionated heparin, especially of bovine source, appears to confer a higher risk than LMWH.

VITT has an estimated incidence of approximately 1 per 100,000 of individuals receiving their first dose of ChAdOx1-nCoV-19 vaccination [14]. The diagnosis can be made by history of recent vaccine, the distinct biochemical profile (significant thrombocytopenia, raised D-dimer and positive anti-PF4 antibodies) and the clinical presentation including venous thrombosis as in this case or, more rarely, arterial stroke [15]. The D-dimer tends to be extremely high in VITT, although a normal D-dimer value does not exclude the diagnosis. In all types of CVT (including VITT), an MRI head with MR venogram is the preferred imaging modality, as MRI has a higher sensitivity for picking up parenchymal lesions than CT. In practice, though, in an emergency setting the first imaging is often done using CT.

By contrast with the conventional management of CVT without VITT, heparins (including LMWH) are currently considered to be contraindicated in VITT, and the mainstay of includes non-heparin anticoagulants, such as fondaparinux, along with steroids, plasma exchange and/or IVIG [16].

Data regarding the long-term prognosis of CVT in general are limited and vary depending on the complications such as disability due to infarcts and bleedings, seizures, intracranial hypertension and dural venous fistulas. The International Study on Cerebral Vein and Dural Sinus Thrombosis (ISCVT) [7] reported mortality rate of 3.4% within 30 days of onset, recurrence rate at around 2% and thrombotic events in other organs in 4% of cases. CVT in the context of VITT appears to have a much worse outcome, with an in-hospital mortality rate of 30–40% [16, 17], although patients who survive hospital admission appear to do well at subsequent follow-up [17].

Key Clinical Learning Points

- CVT can present insidiously with patients presenting several times to healthcare professionals with headaches, seizures and focal neurological deficits
- VITT is associated with an elevated D-dimer and the diagnosis is confirmed by the presence of anti-PF4 antibodies in most cases
- Patients with VITT and CVT will require treatment with ivIG and non-heparin anticoagulation

Key Radiological Learning Points

- Venous infarcts do not map arterial vascular territories and are prone to haemorrhagic transformation
- MRI/MR venogram is preferred to CT/CT venogram in the assessment of CVT as MRI is more sensitive to the detection of parenchymal lesions

References

1. Browder J, Browder A, Kaplan HA. The venous sinuses of the cerebral dura mater: I. Anatomical structures within the superior sagittal sinus. Arch Neurol. 1972;26(2):175–80.
2. Chandra A, Li WA, Stone CR, Geng X, Ding Y. The cerebral circulation and cerebrovascular disease I: anatomy. Brain Circ. 2017;3(2):45–56.
3. Allroggen H, Abbott RJ. Cerebral venous sinus thrombosis. Postgrad Med J. 2000;76:12–5.
4. Murumkar V, Goyal S. Isolated thrombosis of cortical veins–clinical and radiological correlation. J Clin Neurosci. 2021;91:369–77.
5. Kumar P, Sasmal G, Mahto SK, Gupta S, Gupta H. Deep cerebral vein thrombosis: a clinical masquerader. J Clin Diagn Res. 2017;11(4):OD16–8.
6. Bienfait HP, van Duinen S, Tans JT. Latent cerebral venous and sinus thrombosis. J Neurol. 2003;250(4):436–9.
7. Ferro JM, Canhão P, Stam J, Bousser MG, Barinagarrementeria F, ISCVT Investigators. Prognosis of cerebral vein and dural sinus thrombosis: results of the International Study on Cerebral Vein and dural Sinus Thrombosis (ISCVT). Stroke. 2004;35(3):664–70.
8. Martinelli I, Saachi E. High risk of cerebral-vein thrombosis in carriers of a prothrombin-gene mutation and in users of oral contraceptives. N Engl J Med. 1998;338:1793–7.
9. Saposnik G, Barinagarrementeria F, American Heart Association Stroke Council and the Council on Epidemiology and Prevention, et al. Diagnosis and management of cerebral venous thrombosis: a statement for healthcare professionals from the American Heart Association/American Stroke Association. Stroke. 2011;42(4):1158–92.
10. Coutinho JM, Zuurbier SM, et al. Effect of endovascular treatment with medical management vs standard care on severe cerebral venous thrombosis: the TO-ACT randomized clinical trial. JAMA Neurol. 2020;77(8):966–73.
11. Taquet M, et al. Cerebral venous thrombosis and portal vein thrombosis: a retrospective cohort study of 537,913 COVID-19 cases. EClinicalMedicine. 2021;39:101061.

12. Scully M, Singh D, et al. Pathologic antibodies to platelet factor 4 after ChAdOx1 nCoV-19 vaccination. N Engl J Med. 2021;384:2202–11.
13. Arepally GM, Ortel TL. Heparin-induced thrombocytopenia. Annu Rev Med. 2010;61:77–90.
14. Pai M. Epidemiology of VITT. Semin Hematol. 2022;59(2):72–5.
15. Al-Mayhani T, Saber S, et al. Ischaemic stroke as a presenting feature of ChAdOx1 nCoV-19 vaccine-induced immune thrombotic thrombocytopenia. J Neurol Neurosurg Psychiatry. 2021;92(11):1247–8.
16. Perry RJ, Tamborska A, et al. Cerebral venous thrombosis after vaccination against COVID-19 in the UK: a multicentre cohort study. Lancet. 2021;398(10306):1147–56.
17. van de Munckhof A, Lundgren E, et al. Outcomes of cerebral venous thrombosis due to vaccine-induced immune thrombotic thrombocytopenia after the acute phase. Stroke. 2022;53:3206–10.

Chapter 22
Between a Clot and a Hard Place: Ischaemic Stroke and COVID-19

R. Beyrouti, A. Chandratheva, and D. J. Werring

A 65-year-old right-handed gentleman presented on the 28th of March 2020 with a 10-day history of fever, cough, shortness of breath, myalgia and anorexia. On examination, he was dyspnoeic with bilateral basal crackles on chest auscultation and his oxygen saturation was 94% on 10 L O2. His chest x-ray showed bilateral pulmonary infiltrates and his laboratory tests showed lymphopenia at 0.50 × 10^9/L with raised inflammatory markers as follow CRP 287 mg/L, ferritin 4927 μg/L, LDH 654 μg/L, fibrinogen 9.5 μg/L and D-dimer 2390 μg/L. He tested positive for Severe Acute Respiratory Syndrome Coronavirus 2 (SARS-CoV-2) on nasopharyngeal RT-PCR swab.

Over the three following days, he had increasing oxygen requirement and was transferred to intensive care unit on the 31st of March 2020 and started on continuous positive airway pressure (CPAP) therapy.

On the 01st of April 2020, he developed dense left sided weakness, paraesthesia and difficulty swallowing which completely resolved after 20 min. A CT acute stroke showed no acute intracranial pathology, but an occluded left vertebral artery. He was diagnosed with transient ischaemic attack and started on dual antiplatelets. He was successfully weaned of CPAP and step down to the ward on the 04th of April 2020.

R. Beyrouti (✉)
Comprehensive Stroke Service, National Hospital for Neurology and Neurosurgery, University College Hospitals NHS Foundation Trust, London, UK
e-mail: Rahma.beyrouti@nhs.net

A. Chandratheva · D. J. Werring
Comprehensive Stroke Service, National Hospital for Neurology and Neurosurgery, University College Hospitals NHS Foundation Trust, London, UK

Stroke Research Centre, UCL Queen Square Institute of Neurology, London, UK
e-mail: arvind.chandratheva@nhs.net; d.werring@ucl.ac.uk

S. K. Gill et al. (eds.), *Stroke Medicine*,
https://doi.org/10.1007/978-3-031-58188-5_22

In the context of persistent oxygen requirement with repeat D-dimer of >80,000 μg/L, a CT pulmonary angiogram was performed on the 05th of April 2020 and demonstrated bilateral pulmonary emboli within the right segmental middle lobe and the left subsegmental lower lobe arteries with no radiographic evidence of right heart strain. It also showed multifocal bilateral subpleural confluent ground-glass changes and consolidation in keeping with classic severe covid-19 infection. A lower limb doppler ultrasound also showed an occlusive deep venous thrombosis in the left posterior tibial vein and the left peroneal vein. He was started on split dose Enoxaparin 60 mg BD and dual antiplatelets were stopped.

He had an MRI head on the 06th of April 2020 (Fig. 22.1) which showed left cerebellar subacute infarct with haemorrhagic transformation and left vertebral artery thrombus with intradural propagation. His neurological examination at the time showed very mild left arm drift and dysmetria. Given the extensive arterial and venous thromboembolic disease, the benefit of continuing low molecular weight heparin (LMWH) outweighed the risk of further cerebellar bleeding. He was then continued on Enoxaparin with close monitoring.

On the 08th of April 2020, 22 days after COVID-19 onset, he developed acute confusion with abbreviated mental test score (AMTS) 5/10 and word finding difficulties. On examination, he was dysphasic, confused with GCS 14/15. He had mild right hemiparesis, bilateral incoordination and right homonymous hemianopia. A CT head showed an acute left posterior cerebral artery (PCA) infarct involving the left lingual gyrus with no evidence of intracerebral haemorrhage. A note was made of well-established left PICA territorial infarct within the posterior fossa. CT angiogram showed an occlusion of the P2 segment of the left PCA with no basilar artery thrombus. MRI head performed 1 day later showed extensive acute left PCA territory infarct involving the thalamus, occipital lobe and posteromedial temporal lobe (Fig. 22.2). Patchy acute infarcts were also shown within the right occipital lobe. Given further multifocal infarcts on full dose anticoagulation, with evidence of a hypercoagulable state, the decision was made to increase Enoxaparin from 60 mg bd to 80 mg bd (2 mg/kg) after discussion with haematology team.

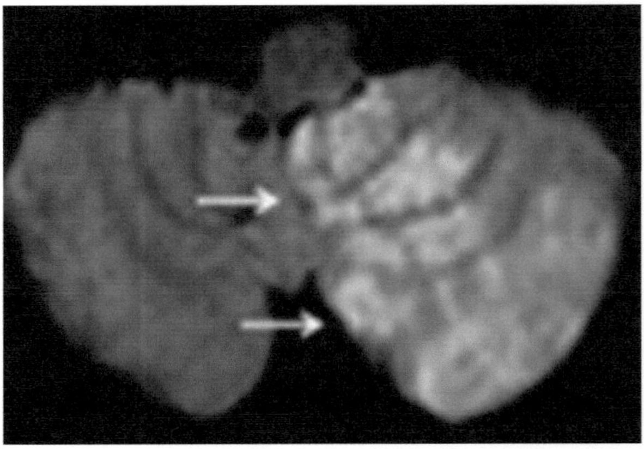

Fig. 22.1 Diffusion-weighted MRI showed acute left posterior-inferior cerebellar artery territory infarction

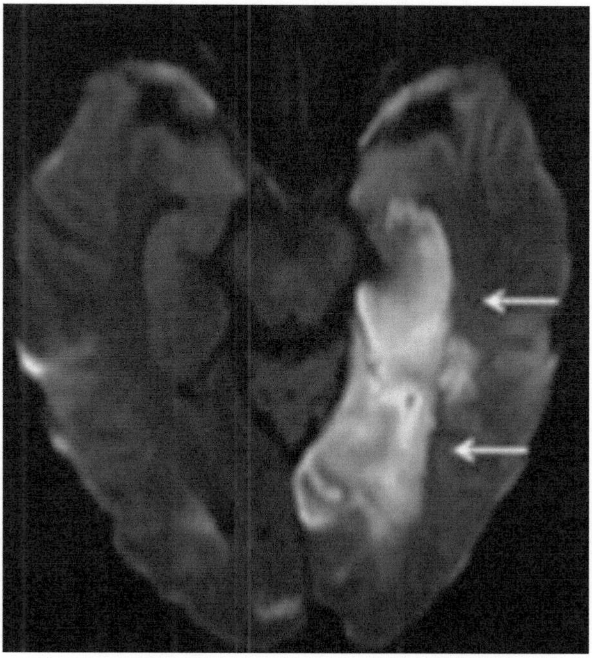

Fig. 22.2 Diffusion-weighted MRI showed bilateral acute posterior cerebral artery territory infarcts despite therapeutic anticoagulation

An MRI dissection protocol showed no evidence of vertebral artery dissection. The echocardiogram was normal with no intracardiac thrombus; a bubble study was negative and cardiac monitoring showed sinus rhythm. Thrombophilia testing showed a positive lupus anticoagulant with medium titre IgM anticardiolipin antibodies, negative IgG anticardiolipin antibodies and low titre IgM and IgG anti-β2-glycoprotein-1 antibodies.

He was previously fit and well with no history of arterial or venous thrombosis. He was a regular scuba diver, swimming outdoors and cycling most days and going to the Gym 3–4 times weekly.

During the course of the following week, he made a good recovery from his COVID-19 pneumonitis and he was discharged to neuro-rehabilitation unit where he made remarkable progress in therapy. Three months after his stoke, his gait and coordination were back to normal. His power was 5/5 throughout. He had residual incomplete right homonymous hemianopia, hemianopic alexia and mildly impaired verbal memory and executive functions. On repeat antiphospholipid test, he had a positive lupus anticoagulant with medium titre IgM anticardiolipin antibodies, negative IgG anticardiolipin antibodies and negative IgM and IgG anti-β2-glycoprotein-1 antibodies. He was switch to Warfarin with an INR target 3–4 under review with Haematology.

Discussion

Coronavirus disease (COVID-19), due to the Acute Respiratory Syndrome Coronavirus 2 (SARS-CoV-2), emerged in late December 2019 and resulted in a rapidly spreading acute respiratory disease epidemic originating in Wuhan, China. On March 11th, 2020, the World Health Organization (WHO) declared COVID-19 a global pandemic due to the constantly increasing number of cases outside China.

Clinical and Radiological Characteristics

As the coronavirus pandemic progressed, it quickly became clear that acute ischaemic stroke (AIS) is the most frequently reported neurological complication of COVID-19. The incidence of AIS among COVID-19 patients varies from 0.9% to 2.7% [1]. Compared with influenza, a known stroke factor, patients with COVID-19 were more likely to have an AIS (odds ratio [OR], 8.1; 95% CI, 2.5–26.6) [2].

AIS associated with COVID-19 appears to have distinct characteristics. A systematic review found that compared to individuals who experienced a stroke without COVID-19, patients with COVID-19 and stroke were younger with a higher frequency of large vessel occlusion [3], while a UK-wide case-control study found that AIS associated with COVID-19 is more often due to large vessel occlusion (LVO) in multiple vascular territories (17.9% vs 8.1%, $p < 0.03$) [4].

Severity and Outcome

The median duration of AIS from onset of COVID-19 symptoms is 6 days (IQR 0 to 14) [4]. However, clinicians should be wary that thrombotic complication such as AIS may be seen in both early and late phases of the infection. AIS has been associated with coronavirus disease severity with a 2.5-fold increased disease severity in patients with COVID-19 [5]. The severity of the infective disease also consistently emerged as an important risk factor for stroke across different studies [6, 7]. In a recent Dutch study, there was a 31% incidence of thrombotic complications in patients with COVID-19 admitted to ICU, mainly consisting of acute pulmonary embolism, deep vein thrombosis and ischemic stroke [8]. In a case-control study from New York, it was observed that patients with concomitant COVID-19 suffered more severe strokes with higher NIHSS score (median NIHSS score 19 vs 8, $p < 0.007$) and higher in-hospital mortality (63.6% vs 9.3%, $p < 0.001$) [9]. In a UK multicentre case-control study, the proportion of ischaemic strokes resulting in death during admission was significantly higher in COVID-19 patients (19.8% vs

6.9%, $p < 0.00003$) with higher median mRS on discharge (4 vs 3, $p < 0.00003$) [4]. In previous systematic reviews, the pooled mortality of COVID-19 patients with AIS varies from 31% to 38% [1, 3].

Pathogenesis

The pathogenesis of cerebrovascular complications in COVID-19 is probably complex. SARS-CoV-2 infection is caused by binding of the viral surface spike protein to the human angiotensin-converting enzyme 2 (ACE2) receptor after activation of the spike protein by transmembrane protease serine 2 [10]. ACE2 is expressed in the lung (principally type II alveolar cells) which appears to be the predominant portal of entry. ACE2 is also highly expressed in myocardium, vascular endothelium, and arterial smooth muscle [11]. Three distinct mechanisms have been proposed to account for the link between Coronavirus infection and acute ischaemic stroke.

Firstly, endothelial damage caused by SARS-CoV-2 binding to the ACE2 receptors largely present in the brain vessels may be responsible of local direct endothelial injury and thrombogenesis [12]. In fact, endothelial cell infection and diffuse endotheliitis have been demonstrated in COVID-19 via histological identification of viral elements within endothelial cells and an accumulation of inflammatory cells and apoptosis [12, 13]. This increases the risk of microthrombosis of small penetrating arteries and large artery occlusion. In addition, disruption of the renin-angiotensin system due to down regulation of endothelial ACE2 receptors and accumulation of angiotensin II promotes oxidative stress and vasoconstriction and aggravates endothelial dysfunction [13, 14].

Secondly, SARS-CoV-2 myocardial invasion via ACE2 receptors is responsible of arrhythmogenic cardiomyopathy and cardiac embolism which may also have a contributory role in COVID-19-related stroke [15]. In an observational study of 138 hospitalized patients with COVID-19, acute cardiac injury was present in 7.2%, and arrhythmia in 16.7% [16]. More recently, another observational study of 191 patients in China showed that 23% were complicated with heart failure and 17% with acute cardiac injury. All of which are factors potentially predisposing patients to AIS [17].

Finally, COVID-19 has been widely associated with coagulopathy with life-threatening thromboembolic events including ischaemic stroke [18]. In fact, SARS-CoV-2 appears to be responsible of a hyperinflammatory state, or cytokine storm associated with the excessive release of pro-inflammatory cytokines, such as TNF-α, IL-1, IL-6, which can cause severe coagulation disorders. Pro-inflammatory cytokines induce endothelial and mononuclear cell activation, promote the release of ultra-long von Willebrand factor (VWF) multimers and the overexpression of tissue factor, and activate the extrinsic coagulation pathway. This leads to increased thrombin generation and hypercoagulable state with increased D-dimers [19]. Additionally, there have been multiple reports of positive antiphospholipid autoantibodies in patients with COVID-19 which may contribute to thrombotic disorders [20, 21]. The real prevalence of these autoantibodies in patients with SARS-CoV-2 remains unclear. The available data seem to indicate that while the percentage of Lupus anticoagulant positivity range is approximately 50–80% of the patients, the positivity for antiphospholipid antibodies is instead significantly lower and higher for anticardiolipin antibodies than anti-β2-glycoprotein-1 antibodies [22].

Treatment

Early prophylactic or therapeutic anticoagulation with LMWH often guided by D-dimer levels could be beneficial to reduce thromboembolism in patients with COVID-19, including those with ischaemic stroke but must be balanced against the risk of haemorrhagic transformation [13]. In a recent randomized controlled trial, an initial strategy of therapeutic-dose anticoagulation with heparin in noncritically ill patients with Covid-19, increased the probability of survival to hospital discharge with reduced use of cardiovascular or respiratory organ support as compared with usual-care thromboprophylaxis. Major bleeding occurred more frequently in the anticoagulation group (1.9% vs. 0.9%) [23]. In contrast to the benefit found in noncritically ill patients, a parallel analysis from the same multiplatform trial showed that empirical therapeutic-dose anticoagulation was not beneficial in critically ill patients (i.e., those receiving ICU-level care at enrollment) [24].

Conclusion

Our case highlights distinct characteristics of ischaemic stroke associated with COVID-19 which occurs in the context of highly prothrombotic state with predominance of large vessel occlusion and multiple vascular territories involvement.

Key Points

- COVID-19 can be associated with a severe coagulopathy which is sometimes associated with life-threatening thromboembolic events including AIS
- The incidence of AIS among COVID-19 patients varies from 0.9% to 2.7%
- AIS associated with COVID-19 is more often due to large vessel occlusion (LVO) affecting multiple vascular territories than non-COVID-19 associated AIS
- The median duration of AIS from onset of COVID-19 symptoms is 6 days (IQR 0 to 14)
- Patients with COVID-19 suffer more severe strokes with higher NIHSS score and higher in-hospital mortality

References

1. Tan YK, Goh C, Leow AST, et al. COVID-19 and ischemic stroke: a systematic review and meta-summary of the literature. J Thromb Thrombolysis. 2020;50(3):587–95. https://doi.org/10.1007/s11239-020-02228-y.
2. Merkler AE, Parikh NS, Mir S, et al. Risk of ischemic stroke in patients with coronavirus disease 2019 (COVID-19) vs patients with influenza. JAMA Neurol. 2020;77(11):1366–72. https://doi.org/10.1001/jamaneurol.2020.2730.
3. Nannoni S, de Groot R, Bell S, Markus HS. Stroke in COVID-19: a systematic review and meta-analysis. Int J Stroke. 2021;16(2):137–49. https://doi.org/10.1177/1747493020972922.
4. Perry RJ, Smith CJ, Roffe C, Simister R, et al. SETICOS collaborators. Characteristics and outcomes of COVID-19 associated stroke: a UK multicentre case-control study. J Neurol Neurosurg Psychiatry. 2021;92(3):242–8. https://doi.org/10.1136/jnnp-2020-324927. Epub 2020 Nov 5
5. Aggarwal G, Lippi G, Michael Henry B. Cerebrovascular disease is associated with an increased disease severity in patients with coronavirus disease 2019 (COVID-19): a pooled analysis of published literature. Int J Stroke. 2020;15:385–9.
6. Lodigiani C, Iapichino G, Carenzo L, Cecconi M, Ferrazzi P, Sebastian T, Kucher N, Studt JD, Clara Sacco C, Alexia B, et al. Humanitas COVID-19 Task Force. Venous and arterial thromboembolic complications in COVID-19 patients admitted to an academic hospital in Milan, Italy. Thromb Res. 2020;191:9–14. https://doi.org/10.1016/j.thromres.2020.04.024.
7. Li Y, Li M, Wang M, et al. Acute cerebrovascular disease following COVID-19: a single center, retrospective, observational study. Stroke Vasc Neurol. 2020;5:279–84.
8. Klok FA, Kruip MJHA, van der Meer NJM, et al. Incidence of thrombotic complications in critically ill ICU patients with COVID-19. Thromb Res. 2020;191:145–7. https://doi.org/10.1016/j.thromres.2020.04.013.
9. Yaghi S, Ishida K, Torres J, Grory BM, Raz E, Humbert K, et al. SARS2-CoV-2 and stroke in a New York healthcare system. Stroke. 2020;51:2002–11. https://doi.org/10.1161/strokeaha.120.030335.
10. Hoffmann M, Kleine-Weber H, Schroeder S, et al. SARS-CoV-2 entry depends on ACE2 and TMPRSS2 and is blocked by a clinically proven protease inhibitor. Cell. 2020;181:271–80.e8.
11. Clerkin KJ, Fried JA, Raikhelkar J, et al. Coronavirus disease 2019 (Covid-19) and cardiovascular disease. Circulation. 2020;141:1648–55.
12. Varga Z, Flammer AJ, Steiger P, Haberecker M, Andermatt R, Zinkernagel AS, et al. Endothelial cell infection and endotheliitis in COVID-19. Lancet Lond Engl. 2020;395(10234):1417–8.
13. Beyrouti R, Best JG, Chandratheva A, Perry RJ, Werring DJ. Characteristics of intracerebral haemorrhage associated with COVID-19: a systematic review and pooled analysis of individual patient and aggregate data. J Neurol. 2021;268:1–11. https://doi.org/10.1007/s00415-021-10425-9. [published online ahead of print, 5 Feb 2021].
14. Bautista-Vargas M, Bonilla-Abadía F, Cañas CA. Potential role for tissue factor in the pathogenesis of hypercoagulability associated with in COVID-19. J Thromb Thrombolysis. 2020;50(3):479–83. https://doi.org/10.1007/s11239-020-02172-x.
15. Guo T, Fan Y, Chen M, Wu X, Zhang L, He T, et al. Cardiovascular implications of fatal outcomes of patients with coronavirus disease 2019 (COVID-19). JAMA Cardiol. 2020;5:811–8. https://doi.org/10.1001/jamacardio.2020.1017.
16. Wang D, et al. Clinical characteristics of 138 hospitalized patients with 2019 novel coronavirus-infected pneumonia in Wuhan, China. JAMA. 2020;323:1061–9.
17. Zhou F, et al. Clinical course and risk factors for mortality of adult inpatients with COVID-19 in Wuhan, China: a retrospective cohort study. Lancet. 2020;395(10229):1054–62.
18. Tang N, Li D, Wang X, Sun Z. Abnormal coagulation parameters are associated with poor prognosis in patients with novel coronavirus pneumonia. J Thromb Haemost. 2020;18(4):844–7.
19. Song Y, Fan H, Tang X, Luo Y, Liu P, Chen Y. The effects of severe acute respiratory syndrome coronavirus 2 (SARS-CoV-2) on ischemic stroke and the possible underlying mechanisms. Int J Neurosci. 2021;133:1–20. https://doi.org/10.1080/00207454.2021.1897588. [published online ahead of print, 26 Mar 2021].

20. Zhang Y, Xiao M, Zhang S, et al. Coagulopathy and antiphospholipid antibodies in patients with Covid-19. N Engl J Med. 2020;382:e38. https://doi.org/10.1056/NEJMc2007575.
21. Beyrouti R, Adams ME, Benjamin L, et al. Characteristics of ischaemic stroke associated with COVID-19. J Neurol Neurosurg Psychiatry. 2020;91:889–91. https://doi.org/10.1136/jnnp-2020-323586.
22. Pineton de Chambrun M, Frere C, Miyara M, Amoura Z, Martin-Toutain I, Mathian A, Hekimian G, Combes A. High frequency of antiphospholipid antibodies in critically-ill COVID-19 patients: a link with hypercoagulability? J Intern Med. 2020; https://doi.org/10.1111/joim.13126. Epub ahead of print.
23. The ATTACC, ACTIV-4a, and REMAP-CAP Investigators. Therapeutic anticoagulation with heparin in noncritically ill patients with Covid-19. N Engl J Med. 2021;385:790–802.
24. The REMAP-CAP, ACTIV-4a, and ATTACC Investigators. Therapeutic anticoagulation with heparin in critically ill patients with Covid-19. N Engl J Med. 2021;385:777–89.

Chapter 23
Lying in Wait—Stroke and a Blistering Rash

Shane Lyons, Aine Merwick, Lucy Blair, Lionel Ginsberg, and Robert Simister

Abbreviations

CSF	Cerebral spinal fluid
CT	Computerised tomography
CTA	Computerised tomography angiography
HZO	Herpes zoster ophthalmicus
MCA	Middle cerebral artery
MRI	Magnetic resonance imaging
VZV	Varicella Zoster Virus

Clinical History

A 31 year old right handed man presents with left hand and left forearm sensory loss and right sided headache.

S. Lyons (✉)
Neurology Department, Tailaghat University Hospital, Dublin, Ireland

A. Merwick
Neurology Department, Cork University Hospital, Cork, Ireland

L. Blair
Hyper Acute Stroke Unit, University College Hospital, London, UK

L. Ginsberg
Department of Neurology, Royal Free Hospital, London, UK

R. Simister
Comprehensive Stroke Service, National Hospital for Neurology and Neurosurgery, UCLH Trust, London, UK

S. K. Gill et al. (eds.), *Stroke Medicine*,
https://doi.org/10.1007/978-3-031-58188-5_23

Over the preceding week he has experienced a flickering 'chequerboard' appearance in both eyes, lasting 1–2 min. The visual disturbance is binocular and is characterised by discrete gaps in his vision. The disturbance is intermittent and on each occasion lasts a number of minutes and then resolves. As it resolves he experiences a headache over the right side of the head. The disturbance occurs 2 or 3 times a day. Around this same time period he also experiences separately an auditory experience in which he hears an echo of his voice that is as real to him as if he had repeated the sentence. This does not occur when others speak to him.

He has a background of herpes zoster ophthalmicus (shingles) in the right trigeminal V1 division, which had been treated with steroids and acyclovir, 7 months previously. The symptoms at the time were characterised as a severe pain around and behind the right eye, with a blistering rash over the right temple. He was treated with aciclovir approximately 2 days after onset of the symptoms. He had some transient visual disturbance at time of the acute infection and subsequently developed a suspected secondary skin infection. As a consequence of this he was referred to see ophthalmology service where he was prescribed a sustained course of topical steroid eye drops and topical antiviral eye drops.

He has no family history of vascular disease and no previous history of thrombotic events, joint problems, smoking, recreational drug use or immunosuppressive illness. He has no history of hypertension, diabetes mellitus or hypercholesterolaemia.

Examination

On examination blood pressure at presentation is 161/100 mmHg, his temperature is 37.4 °C, and heart rate is regular at 97 beats per minute with normal heart sounds, no audible murmur and a regular pulse. There are no skin lesions detected. Fundi are normal and eye movements are full, with no double vision. Visual fields are full to confrontation on bedside testing and the remainder of cranial nerve examination is normal.

Power in the upper and lower limbs is normal: MRC power grade 5/5 throughout. Deep tendon reflexes are symmetrically present. The plantar response is downgoing. There are no sensory deficits. National Institute of Health Stroke Score (NIHSS) is 0 [1].

He scores 28/30 on a Montreal Cognitive Assessment tool cognitive evaluation losing points for delayed recall and attention, as well as having mildly reduced verbal fluency [2].

Investigations

A CT brain is performed, after the left upper limb sensory symptoms have developed and shows an acute/subacute cortical infarct involving the right temporal lobe including the temporal operculum, with further smaller infarcts in the posterior right temporal lobe. CTA shows a high-grade stenosis of the proximal right M1 middle cerebral artery MCA and supraclinoid right internal carotid artery (ICA) stenosis, but with no intracranial occlusion. Aortic arch, subclavian arteries, and vertebral arteries are normal.

MRI shows multiple cortical infarcts within the right MCA territory, involving the temporal lobe, the parieto-occipital junction, and mature cortical damage within the right inferior parietal lobule with some haemosiderin deposition, in keeping with a mature MCA infarct, suggestive of a prior ischaemic event in the same vascular territory (Fig. 23.1).

MRA shows flow attenuation and contrast enhancement in the supraclinoid right internal carotid artery (ICA) extending into proximal right M1 middle cerebral artery (Fig. 23.2).

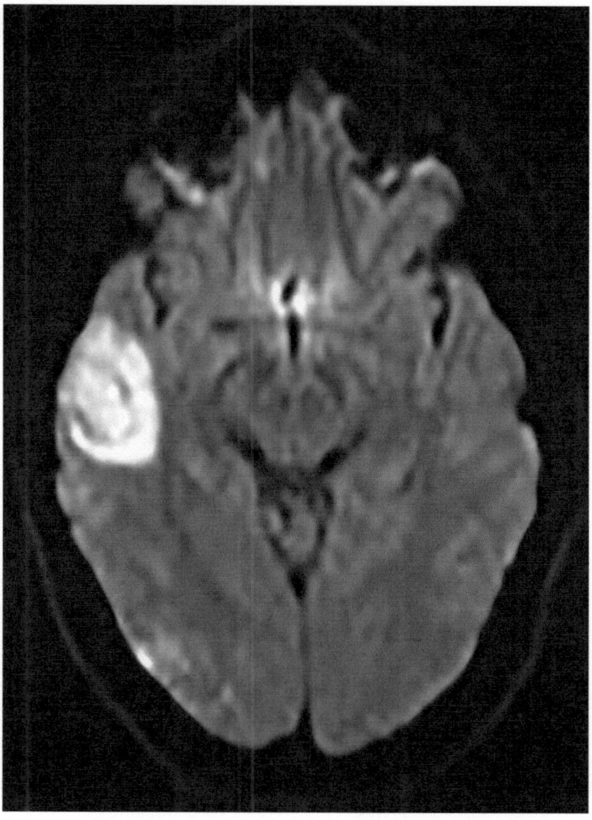

Fig. 23.1 MRI shows multiple cortical infarcts within the right MCA territory, involving the temporal lobe, the parieto-occipital junction

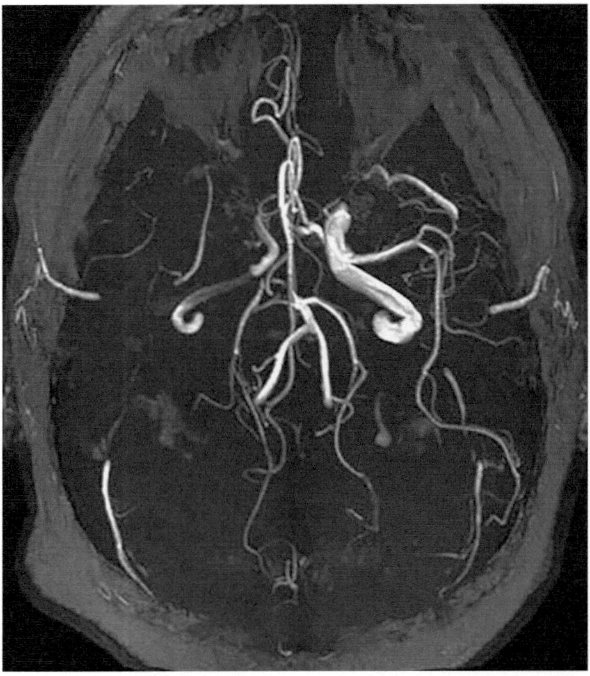

Fig. 23.2 MRA shows flow attenuation in the supraclinoid right internal carotid artery (ICA) extending into proximal right M1 middle cerebral artery

His total cholesterol is 5.8 mmol/litre, HDL1.1 mmol/litre, LDL 4.0 mmol/litre, glucose 5.2 mmol/litre, erythrocyte sedimentation rate (ESR) 8.

Electrocardiograph (ECG) shows sinus rhythm, and cardiac monitoring is also normal. Echocardiography (ECHO) shows normal left ventricular dimensions with good global systolic function and an estimated left ventricular ejection fraction of 69%. No valvular abnormalities, shunt or patent foramen ovale are detected.

Serological tests for thrombophilia, inflammatory markers and autoimmune profiles are negative. HIV, hepatitis B and hepatitis C testing are also negative.

Cerebrospinal fluid (CSF) shows WCC = 0/microliter, protein 0.54 g/L, CSF VZV PCR negative, with a normal opening pressure. CSF VZV IgG is negative. Serum VZV IgG is positive and VZV IgM is negative; suggestive of previous infection.

He is treated acutely with intravenous acyclovir, followed by oral valciclovir, to complete a 21 day course of anti-viral therapy, along with a tapering course of oral steroids starting at 90 mg/kg, reducing by 5 mg. He is also commenced on an antiplatelet agent (clopidogrel 75 mg) and statin (atorvastatin 40 mg).

MRI and MRA 2 months later shows persistent right ICA wall thickening and signal change extending into the right MCA with vessel enhancement and flow attenuation. Positron emission tomography (PET) CT scan performed 3 months after the stroke presentation did not show any enhancement. No stroke recurrence occurs over a period of 18 months follow up and he makes an excellent functional recovery.

Discussion

This case demonstrates some key features of stroke related to VZV vasculopathy. Alternative causes of large vessel vasculopathy including inflammation, connective tissue diseases, other infectious agents, dissection, and premature atherosclerosis were considered. The preceding history of herpes zoster in the ipsilateral trigeminal nerve and carotid artery distribution was considered to be clinically relevant. The presence of infarcts of different ages suggested that there may have been ischaemic events around the time of the initial episode of herpes zoster ophthalmicus with subsequent ischemia prompting hospital attendance.

Primary infection with varicella zoster virus (VZV) results in chickenpox and thereafter the pathogen remains latent in the sensory and autonomic ganglia [3, 4]. Latent infection may reactivate, often decades after the initial infection, particularly if the host is immunocompromised due to medication, disease, or senescence resulting in the blistering dermatomal rash of herpes zoster (HZ). Approximately 50% of people infected with VZV will experience reactivation before 85 years of age [5]. When the trigeminal nucleus is involved a rash of the ipsilateral face is produced giving the classic appearance of herpes zoster ophthalmicus (HZO). VZV is associated with a range of neurological complications including post-herpetic neuralgia, cranial nerve palsies, meningoencephalitis, cerebellitis, myelopathy, multiple ocular disorders, and vasculopathy [6]. Since 1896, when a case of HZO with contralateral hemiplegia was described by Baudouin, VZV has been associated with cerebrovascular disease [7]. The association between stroke and VZV in children is long established. VZV is implicated in 31% of all arterial ischaemic strokes in children and 44% of transient cerebral arteriopathy [8, 9]. The role of VZV in stroke in adults has come to medical attention more recently. Epidemiological studies from Europe, Asia, and the United States have demonstrated an increased risk of stroke and MI in patients with a recent history of HZ, with hazard ratios (HR) between 1.3 and 4.28 [10–12]. The increased risk of stroke is most marked among those less than 40 years of age [12, 13]. A UK clinical practice research database study showed that the stroke risk was increased following HZ compared with baseline unexposed period, then gradually reduced over 6 months: weeks 1–4 (age-adjusted incidence ratios (IR), 1.63; 95% CI, 1.32–2.02), weeks 5–12 (IR, 1.42; 95% CI, 1.21–1.68), and weeks 13–26 (IR, 1.23; 95% CI, 1.07–1.42), with no increase thereafter [14]. HZO in particular is associated with a higher risk of stroke, often ipsilateral to the rash [13, 15].

Several studies have contributed to our understanding of the mechanisms underlying VZV vasculopathy. VZV reactivates in the sensory ganglia and spreads transaxonally to the cerebral arteries where the nerves terminate in the vascular adventitia. In an autopsy series of patients with VZV vasculopathy VZV DNA, VZV antigen, Cowdry A bodies, and herpesvirus particles have been demonstrated within affected arteries [16]. This is followed by transmural spread and subsequent disruption of the vascular anatomy. Histological studies of affected arteries also demonstrate disrupted internal elastic laminae, thickened intima with cells expressing alpha-smooth muscle actin and smooth muscle myosin heavy chain as well as decreased numbers of medical smooth muscle cells [17].

The clinical manifestations of VZV vasculopathy include transient ischaemic attack (TIA), ischaemic stroke, intraparenchymal and subarachnoid haemorrhage, venous sinus thrombosis, aneurysm, spinal cord infarction, and arterial ectasia. Neurological symptoms were preceded by a rash in 63% of cases with a mean time from rash to the development of neurological complications was 4.1 months. 97% of cases demonstrated abnormalities on brain imaging, generally characterised by deep, grey-white matter junction lesions. In half of cases both large and small arteries were involved, while in 37% only small arteries were involved, exclusive large artery involvement was relatively rare at 13% [18]. High resolution MRI has enabled the visualisation of vessel changes. Gadolinium enhancement may be seen in the perforating arteries and stenosis, which may reverse on serial imaging, is demonstrated in affected vessels [19, 20]. Black blood MRI represents an alternative modality to facilitate imaging of vessel wall changed [21].

As we found in our case, CSF pleocytosis is not required to diagnose VZV vasculopathy and only approximately 30% of cases have CSF VZV DNA detected. As we found in our case CSF pleocytosis is not required to diagnose VZV vasculopathy and only approximately 30% of cases have CSF VZV DNA detected. Detection of anti-VZV IgG antibodies in CSF has been reported in up to 93% of patients in one study of adult patients [18]. In paediatric studies up to 100% of children with stroke attributed to primary chicken pox had detectable anti-VZV IgG antibodies in CSF [22].

Peri-infectious and post infectious vasculitis and vasculopathy has been reported in fungal, bacterial and spirochete as well as viral infections (specifically in Lyme disease, tuberculosis, syphilis, and histoplasmosis) [23–26]. An increased peri-infection stroke risk has been described in association with other systemic infections, and infection along with inflammation has been associated with increased atherosclerosis risk [23, 27]. Acute infection (odds ratio 5.1 [3.5–7.3]) has been identified as an independent risk predictors of stroke amongst TIA patients included in the Austrian Stroke registry [29]. A relationship between infection, vasculopathy and stroke in other viral infections e.g. HIV and CMV has also been hypothesised [23, 28, 29] Increased stroke risk in adult and paediatric patients with HIV has been reported, however it may be unclear if HIV directly causes a vasculopathy or if the associated immunosuppression facilitates ongoing infections by organisms known to cause vasculopathy e.g. herpes zoster or syphilis [28, 30–32]. In the setting of suspected VZV vasculopathy, testing for HIV or underlying immunosuppression may be prudent. Differentiating between VZV vasculopathy and co-existent HIV is challenging in practice, although one small case series has suggested deep-seated ischemic infarcts are more frequently seen in VZV vasculopathy than in HIV vasculopathy, amongst patients with HIV [29]. Since the onset of the COVID19 pandemic, an association between SARS2-CoV2 and stroke has been hypothesised [33, 34]. A number of mechanisms have been suggested for the effect of SARS-CoV2 on the vascular endothelium including direct viral infection of endothelial cells via the angiotensin converting enzyme 2 receptor or indirect mechanisms such as cytokine storm. In young people and adolescents a Kawasaki-like disease has been described [35].

The treatment of VZV vasculopathy is challenging as data on optimal treatment is limited. It is suggested that immunocompetent patients are treated with intravenous acyclovir (10–15 mg/kg) three times per day continued for 14 days [35]. Immunocompromised patients or those with recurrent VZV vasculopathy may need a longer course. Given that histologic specimens in VZV vasculopathy demonstrate inflammation within the cerebral arteries some experts suggest a 5 day course of oral prednisolone (1 mg/kg daily) without a taper [35]. However, it has also been hypothesised that steroids may prolong viral infection and there is a lack of robust prospective studies to guide intervention.

The role of VZV in other vascular conditions is debated. An immunohistochemical analysis of temporal artery biopsies in patients with giant cell arteritis (GCA) demonstrated the presence of VZV antigen in 74% of biopsies from patients with GCA compared to 8% of normal biopsies raising the possibility that VZV may play a role in triggering GCA [36]. However, this finding has not been consistently replicated [37].

VZV vasculopathy can present with a wide range of complications including ischaemic stroke, haemorrhage, and venous thrombosis. This potentially treatable vasculopathy requires vigilance as it may occur several months after infection or reactivation. It may also present without in the characteristic rash (zoster sine herpete). Primary infection, and hence the risk of VZV vasculopathy may be prevented through use of the VZV vaccine.

Key Learning Points

- Acute and subacute stroke risk is increased up to five fold following herpes zoster infection.
- CSF features may include pleocytosis, *intrathecally*-produced VZV-*specific IgG*, or abnormal CSF PCR with detection of VZV DNA.
- Treatment with intravenous aciclovir is recommended for 14 days.
- In patients presenting with VZV vasculopathy underlying immunosuppression must be looked for.
- Residual vessel abnormalities may persist or may be first detected months after the acute infection/reactivation.

Key Radiology Learning Points

- VZV vasculopathy manifests as a large artery obliterative vasculopathy that resembles moyamoya syndrome.
- Vessel wall enhancement may be detected.

- Typical angiographic changes include segmental constriction, often with post-stenotic dilatation.
- Deep infarcts are more common than superficial infarction.
- White matter more is commonly affected than grey matter.
- The grey–white matter junctions are commonly affected
- VZV vasculopathy may present also with subarachnoid haemorrhage, cerebral haemorrhage or with carotid dissection.

References

1. Brott T, Adams HP, Olinger CP, Marler JR, Barsan WG, Biller J, Spilker J, Holleran R, Eberle R, Hertzberg V, Rorick M, Moomaw CJ, Walker M. Measurements of acute cerebral infarction: a clinical examination scale. Stroke. 1989;20:864–70.
2. Nasreddine ZS, Phillips NA, Bédirian V, Charbonneau S, Whitehead V, Collin I, Cummings JL, Chertkow H. The Montreal Cognitive Assessment, MoCA: a brief screening tool for mild cognitive impairment. J Am Geriatr Soc. 2005;53(4):695–9.
3. Gilden DH, Vafai A, Shtram Y, Becker Y, Devlin M, Wellish M. Varicella-zoster virus DNA in human sensory ganglia. Nature. 1986;306:478–80.
4. Gilden DH, Gesser R, Smith J, Wellish M, Laguardia JJ, Cohrs RJ, Mahalingam R. Presence of VZV and HSV-1 in human nodose and celica ganglia. Virus Genes. 2001;23:145–7.
5. Hope-Simpson RE. The nature of herpes zoster: a long-term study and a new hypothesis. Proc R Soc Med. 1965;58:9–20.
6. Mueller NH, Gilden DH, Cohrs RJ, Mahalingam R, Nagel MA. Varicella zoster virus infection: clinical features, molecular pathogenesis of disease, and latency. Neurol Clin. 2008;26(3):675-viii.
7. Baudouin E. Les troubles moteurs dans le zona. Grande imprimerie de Troyes; 1920.
8. Askalan R, Laughlin S, Mayank S, Chan A, Mac Gregor D, Andrew M, et al. Chickenpox and stroke in childhood: a study of frequency and causation. Stroke. 2000;32(6):1257–62.
9. Braun KP, Bulder MM, Chabrier S, Kirkham FJ, Uiterwaal CSP, Tardieu M, et al. The course and outcome of unilateral intracranial arteriopathy in 79 children with ischaemic stroke. Brain. 2009;132:544–57.
10. Kang JH, Ho JD, Chen YH, Lin HC. Increased risk of stroke after a herpes zoster attack: a population-based follow-up study. Stroke. 2009;40:3443–8.
11. Patterson BJ, Rausch DA, Irwin DE, Liang M, Yan S, Yawn BP. Analysis of vascular event risk after herpes zoster from 2007 to 2014 US insurance claims data. Mayo Clin Proc. 2019;94(5):763–75.
12. Sreenivasan N, Basit S, Wohlfahrt J, Pasternak B, Munch TN, Nielsen LP, Melbye M. The short- and long-term risk of stroke after herpes zoster—a nationwide population-based cohort study. PLoS One. 2013;8(7):e69156.
13. Breuer J, Pacou M, Gauthier A, Brown MM. Herpes zoster as a risk factor for stroke and TIA. A retrospective cohort study in the UK. Neurology. 2014;82(3):206–12.
14. Langan SM, Minassian C, Smeeth L, Thomas SL. Risk of stroke following herpes zoster: a self-controlled case-series study. Clin Infect Dis. 2014;58(11):1497–503.
15. Lin HC, Chien CW, Ho JD. Herpes zoster ophthalmicus and the risk of stroke: a population-based follow-up study. Neurology. 2010;74:792–7.
16. Gilden DH, Kleinschmidt-DeMasters BK, Wellish M, Hedley-Whyte ET, Rentier B, Mahalingam R. Varicella zoster virus, a cause of waxing and waning vasculitis: the New England Journal of Medicine case 5-1995 revisited. Neurology. 1996;47:1441–6.

17. Nagel MA, Traktinskiy I, Azarkh Y, et al. Varicella zoster virus vasculopathy: analysis of virus-infected arteries. Neurology. 2011;77:364–70.
18. Nagel MA, Cohrs RJ, Mahalingam R, et al. The varicella zoster virus vasculopathies: clinical, CSF, imaging, and virologic features. Neurology. 2008;70(11):853–60.
19. Cheng-Ching E, Jones S, Hui FK, et al. High-resolution MRI vessel wall imaging in varicella zoster virus vasculopathy. J Neurol Sci. 2015;351(1–2):168–73.
20. Yamaguchi Y, Morioka K, Nagasawa H, Wada M. Gadolinium enhancement in perforating arteries in a patient with varicella zoster virus vasculopathy: a case report. J Neurol Sci. 2019 Aug;15(403):122–4.
21. Shah J, Poonawala H, Keay SK, et al. Varicella-zoster virus vasculopathy: a case report demonstrating vasculitis using black-blood MRI. J Neurol Neurophysiol. 2015;6(6):1000342.
22. Miravet E, Danchaivijitr N, Basu H, Saunders DE, Ganesan V. Clinical and radiological features of childhood cerebral infarction following varicella zoster virus infection. Dev Med Child Neurol. 2007;49(6):417–22.
23. Elkind MS. Inflammatory mechanisms of stroke. Stroke. 2010;41(10 Suppl):S3–8.
24. Lebas A, Toulgoat F, Saliou G, Husson B, Tardieu M. Stroke due to Lyme neuroborreliosis: changes in vessel wall contrast enhancement. J Neuroimaging. 2012;22(2):210–2.
25. Chahine LM, Khoriaty RN, Tomford WJ, Hussain MS. The changing face of neurosyphilis. Int J Stroke. 2011;6(2):136–43.
26. Nguyen FN, Kar JK, Zakaria A, Schiess MC. Isolated central nervous system histoplasmosis presenting with ischemic pontine stroke and meningitis in an immune-competent patient. JAMA Neurol. 2013;70(5):638–41.
27. Ferrari J, Knoflach M, Kiechl S, Willeit J, Schnabl S, Seyfang L, et al. Early clinical worsening in patients with TIA or minor stroke: the Austrian Stroke Unit Registry. Neurology. 2010;74:136–41.
28. Nagel MA, Mahalingam R, Cohrs RJ, Gilden D. Virus vasculopathy and stroke: an under-recognized cause and treatment target. Infect Disord Drug Targets. 2010;10(2):105–11.
29. Gutierrez J, Ortiz G. HIV/AIDS patients with HIV vasculopathy and VZV vasculitis: a case series. Clin Neuroradiol. 2011;21(3):145–51.
30. Patsalides AD, Wood LV, Atac GK, Sandifer E, Butman JA, Patronas NJ. Cerebrovascular disease in HIV-infected pediatric patients: neuroimaging findings. Am J Roentgenol. 2002;179(4):999–1003.
31. Schieffelin JS, Williams PL, Djokic D, Anderson JP, Nachman S, Oleske JM. Central nervous system vasculopathy in HIV-infected children enrolled in the Pediatric AIDS Clinical Trials Group 219/219C Study. J Ped Infect Dis. 2013;2(1):50–6.
32. Benjamin LA, Bryer A, Emsley HC, Khoo S, Solomon T, Connor MD. HIV infection and stroke: current perspectives and future directions. Lancet Neurol. 2012;11(10):878–90.
33. Ellul MA, Benjamin L, Singh B, Lant S, Michael BD, Easton A, Kneen R, Defres S, Sejvar J, Solomon T. Neurological associations of COVID-19. Lancet Neurol. 2020;19(9):767–83.
34. Gilden D, Cohrs RJ, Mahalingam R, Nagel MA. Varicella zoster virus vasculopathies: diverse clinical manifestations, laboratory features, pathogenesis, and treatment. Lancet Neurol. 2009;8(8):731–40.
35. Gu SX, Tyagi T, Jain K, et al. Thrombocytopathy and endotheliopathy: crucial contributors to COVID-19 thromboinflammation. Nat Rev Cardiol. 2021;18:194–209.
36. Gilden D, White T, Khmeleva N, Heintzman A, Choe A, Boyer PJ, Grose C, Carpenter JE, Rempel A, Bos N, Kandasamy B, Lear-Kaul K, Holmes DB, Bennett JL, Cohrs RJ, Mahalingam R, Mandava N, Eberhart CG, Bockelman B, Poppiti RJ, Tamhankar MA, Fogt F, Amato M, Wood E, Durairaj V, Rasmussen S, Petursdottir V, Pollak L, Mendlovic S, Chatelain D, Keyvani K, Brueck W, Nagel MA. Prevalence and distribution of VZV in temporal arteries of patients with giant cell arteritis. Neurology. 2015;84(19):1948–55.
37. Verdijk RM, Ouwendijk WJD, Kuijpers RWAM, Verjans GMGM. No evidence of varicella-zoster virus infection in temporal artery biopsies of anterior ischemic optic neuropathy patients with and without Giant cell arteritis. J Infect Dis. 2021;223(1):109–12.

Chapter 24
Stroke in People Living with HIV

Jonathan W. S. Cattrall and Abid Malik

Clinical History

A 58-year-old woman was brought to the Emergency Department having been found on the floor at home. She was last seen well 30 min earlier, but when found had significant left sided weakness and an altered conscious level. During transit, paramedics noted seizure activity characterised by vacant episodes and left sided facial twitching, requiring pharmacological termination. On arrival to the Emergency Department, the patient's conscious level remained low and she required Intensive Therapy Unit (ITU) admission due to airway concerns and a requirement for arterial line monitoring.

Her past medical history included a right cortical ischaemic infarct, well-controlled epilepsy, hypertension, and previous tuberculosis. In addition, she had longstanding Human Immunodeficiency Virus (HIV) infection with poor compliance with antiretroviral medication, and had experienced multiple complications including HIV encephalopathy, cerebral toxoplasmosis, and HIV related end-stage renal failure (ESRF) requiring dialysis.

Empirical treatment with antibiotics and antivirals for a central nervous system infection was initiated, due to seizure activity in the context of uncontrolled HIV.

J. W. S. Cattrall
Department of Brain Sciences, Imperial College London, London, UK

Charing Cross Hospital, Imperial College Healthcare NHS Trust, London, UK
e-mail: j.cattrall@nhs.net

A. Malik (✉)
Charing Cross Hospital, Imperial College Healthcare NHS Trust, London, UK
e-mail: abidmalik@nhs.net

S. K. Gill et al. (eds.), *Stroke Medicine*,
https://doi.org/10.1007/978-3-031-58188-5_24

Examination

On initial review, her GCS was 9 (E4 V2 M3), limiting the examination. The vestibulo-ocular reflex (VOR) was absent, and pupils were 4 mm and unreactive, however corneal reflex was intact. Peripheral tone was normal, and there was flexion to pain with relative bilateral limb weakness in both upper and lower limbs on examination. Flexor plantar responses were present, reflexes in upper limbs were normal, and reflexes in lower limbs were unable to be assessed. Blood pressure on arrival was 220/110 mmHg which was treated with labetalol in 10–20 mg boluses to little effect, therefore a glyceryl trinitrate (GTN) infusion was commenced. During the admission her GCS improved to 14 (E4 V4 M6), however she remained confused and disorientated. On examination later in her inpatient admission, weakness remained in both upper and lower limbs, with more pronounced weakness in her lower limbs bilaterally. It was also noted that the weakness in her right side was more pronounced in comparison to her left, but antigravity power was present in all four limbs. She had no facial weakness as was initially identified and a full range of eye movements.

Investigations

CT head imaging demonstrated bilateral parenchymal haemorrhages located in the right thalamus and left striatocapsular region (Fig. 24.1). There were two additional foci of extra-axial hyperdensity abutting the right cerebellar tentorium. Confluent periventricular white matter signal abnormalities were identified, in addition to volume loss and multiple mature infarcts (Fig. 24.1). CT angiogram showed calcification of the left horizontal MCA with a focal distal narrowing, in addition to irregularity of the distal right MCA. There was also narrowing of the P1 segment of the left posterior cerebral artery. No aneurysmal abnormalities were noted. A later MRI scan of the brain with contrast identified the previously noted bleeds. In addition, diffuse white matter T2/Flair hyperintensity was demonstrated throughout both hemispheres, in addition to numerous background mature infarcts within the deep grey structures and brainstem. There was also extensive background microhaemorrhages predominantly with a central distribution. The findings were consistent with longstanding HIV infection and poorly controlled hypertension (Fig. 24.2).

Blood test results on admission showed a normal full blood count, with no initial rise in inflammatory markers, and a renal profile which was indicative of ESRF. A raised cholesterol was also identified (total cholesterol 7.8 mmol/L, LDL 4.42 mmol/L, HDL 2.6 mmol/L, triglycerides 1.72 mmol/L). Initial blood gases showed a mixed respiratory and metabolic acidosis which rapidly improved. The patient had a low CD4 T-cell count of 21 cells/mm^3, and had an HIV viral load of 51 copies/ml. The most recent CD4 count before this was 6 years prior and was 249 cells/mm^3. Further infection related investigations, the results of which were obtained over a number of days during the admission, gradually provided additional

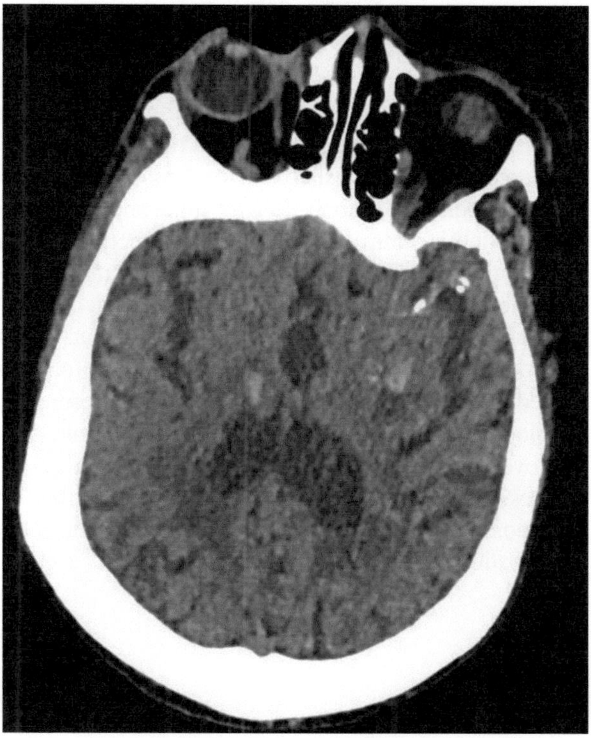

Fig. 24.1 CT head without contrast demonstrated an acute right thalamic haemorrhage and acute left striatocapsular haemorrhage

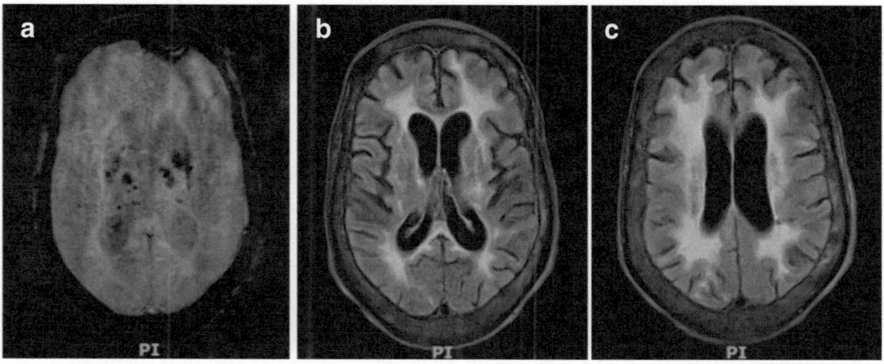

Fig. 24.2 (**a**) Susceptibility-weighted imaging (SWI) shows high burden of microhaemorrhages centrally, consistent with hypertensive disease and HIV vasculopathy. (**b**, **c**) T2-weighted MRI (BLADE, dark fluid) imaging shows white matter abnormalities in both hemispheres, in addition to brain atrophy, both associated with a positive HIV status

evidence against an opportunistic infection as the cause of the presentation. Blood culture results were negative for bacterial growth, in addition to negative syphilis blood serology. A lumbar puncture (LP) produced clear and colourless cerebrospinal fluid (CSF) with a normal glucose (3.7 mmol/L) and protein (0.45 g/L) level, and no pleocytosis (<1 white cell per mm^3, 5 red cells per mm^3). A full CSF viral screen, including an additional screen for JC virus, was negative, as were CSF tests for fungal antigens. The CSF HIV viral load was 42 copies/mL indicating no viral escape. Bacterial cultures of CSF showed no early growth at 5 days, and none at 6 weeks for acid-fast bacilli. Two electroencephalograms were conducted during admission, both showing continuous diffuse slow activity and lateralised periodic discharges (LPDs) with sharp wave morphology over the right temporal and parietal regions, frequently associated with spike and polyspike activity.

Although a central nervous system infection was initially suspected due to the presentation of seizure activity in the context of marked immunosuppression and HIV, there was no convincing evidence of concomitant infection or HIV escape on imaging or CSF investigations. The parenchymal haemorrhages were thought to be due to a combination of hypertensive disease on a background of chronic HIV related vasculopathy. Antimicrobials were therefore stopped and treatment focused on blood pressure control and continued monitoring. The patient subsequently improved and was discharged from ITU after 9 days of admission. Despite making progress on the ward with no further seizures, after 5 days the patient developed a pneumonia and rapidly deteriorated. This hospital acquired infection ultimately led to the patient's death.

Discussion

This case is an example of a haemorrhagic stroke on a background of previous ischaemic infarcts, attributed largely to longstanding poorly controlled HIV and hypertensive disease. There is now strong evidence of the association between HIV infection and the increased risk of both ischaemic and haemorrhagic stroke [1–3]. Multiple mechanisms by which HIV infection can directly or indirectly increase the risk of cerebrovascular disease have been described, the majority of which can be categorised into secondary infective causes, HIV vasculopathy, cardioembolic causes and coagulopathies [2]. The phenomena of immune reconstitution inflammatory syndrome (IRIS) when starting or restarting anti-retroviral therapy (ART) has also been established as a likely mechanism for ischaemic stroke [4].

In the acute phase, people living with HIV (PLWH) that present with a stroke, in particular those with low CD4 counts and those presenting with seizures, should be thoroughly investigated for concomitant infections, as numerous opportunistic infections commonly associated with untreated HIV can lead to both ischaemic and haemorrhagic stroke. For example, tuberculous meningitis may cause vasculitis and in addition can lead to stenosis or degradation of the vessels via proliferative or necrotising processes respectively, both with the potential to cause a stroke [5].

In the presented case, HIV vasculopathy and uncontrolled hypertension were thought to be the aetiological drivers of the bilateral haemorrhages, which is supported by the imaging findings presented in Fig. 24.2. HIV vasculopathy encompasses atherosclerotic disease, non-atherosclerotic vessel disease, vasculitis and small vessel disease [6]—chronic vasculopathic changes, in this case affecting the small vessels bilaterally, has resulted in the rupture of weakened vessel walls, likely occurring following a hypertensive episode. Intracranial imaging such as MRI can be valuable in diagnosing HIV vasculopathy by highlighting the white matter abnormalities or microhaemorrhages typical of the disease, [7] as can neurovascular imaging, which may highlight vasculitic changes pointing to an inflammatory cause, or vascular abnormalities in the form of fusiform aneurysms [8].

In addition to the direct effects of the HIV virus, PLWH frequently also have additional vascular risk factors, such as higher rates of hypertension in those receiving ART [9] and higher rates of smoking which contribute to the overall risk of stroke [6, 10, 11].

The clinical presentation of stroke in PLWH is generally the same to that of HIV negative individuals [3]. Likewise, treatment of ischaemic or haemorrhagic stroke in patients with HIV will in most part be similar to that of the HIV negative population, with consideration of the important nuances in aetiology that may need appropriate management. Clinicians should ensure colleagues with expertise in treating PLWH are involved early in the clinical course, especially with regards to starting or restarting ART therapy and treating infective HIV complications leading to stroke. Evidence for thrombolysis in patients with HIV is not available from trials, however retrospective studies indicated a similar risk of death in PLWH as in HIV negative patients [12, 13]. Evidence for or against endovascular therapy in PLWH remains limited [6].

The case demonstrates the multifaceted link between HIV and cerebrovascular disease, both directly, through the HIV infection, here causing an HIV vasculopathy, and indirectly, through the impact on other cardiovascular risk factors such as hypertension in those receiving ART. Key clinical and radiological considerations are summarised below.

Key Clinical Learning Points

- Acute central nervous system infection is a key differential in patients with HIV presenting with alterations in conscious level and seizure activity, warranting full investigation, however HIV is also known to increase risk of ischaemic and haemorrhagic stroke.
- Patients living with HIV are vulnerable to multiple causes of cerebrovascular disease including opportunistic infections, HIV vasculopathies, cardioembolic events, coagulopathies and IRIS, in addition to an increased risk of traditional risk factors for stroke.
- Effective management of HIV with anti-retroviral therapy is essential to reduce the risk of neurological sequalae of the disease including stroke, though this is a complex interaction as ART itself may be implicated in the pathophysiology of stroke.
- Management of traditional risk factors for stroke may require increased attention and alternative strategies in patients with HIV.
- Early input from HIV specialists should be considered both during the acute presentation of stroke and at outpatient follow-up.

Key Radiological Learning Points

- Early plain CT head should not be delayed in patients with HIV presenting with clinical features of stroke, regardless of suspicion of infective aetiology.
- Intracranial imaging provides valuable evidence to support HIV vasculopathy including: MRI with or without contrast, to assess microhaemorrhage burden and white matter abnormalities; CT angiography, valuable in identifying fusiform aneurysms; and advanced imaging techniques such as black-blood MRI, which better characterise vasculitic disease.

References

1. Benjamin LA, Bryer A, Emsley HC, Khoo S, Solomon T, Connor MD. HIV infection and stroke: current perspectives and future directions. Lancet Neurol. 2012;11(10):878–90.
2. Benjamin L, Khoo S. Chapter 15—HIV infection and stroke. In: Brew BJ, editor. Handbook of clinical neurology [Internet]. Elsevier; 2018. p. 187–200. (The Neurology of HIV Infection; vol. 152). Available from: https://www.sciencedirect.com/science/article/pii/B9780444638496000153. Cited 23 Nov 2022.
3. Corbett C, Brey N, Pitcher RD, O'Hagan S, Esterhuizen TM, Chow FC, et al. Prevalence and characteristics of HIV-associated stroke in a tertiary hospital setting in South Africa. Neurology. 2022;99(9):e904–15.
4. Benjamin LA, Allain TJ, Mzinganjira H, Connor MD, Smith C, Lucas S, et al. The role of human immunodeficiency virus–associated vasculopathy in the etiology of stroke. J Infect Dis. 2017;216(5):545–53.
5. Lammie GA, Hewlett RH, Schoeman JF, Donald PR. Tuberculous cerebrovascular disease: a review. J Infect. 2009;59(3):156–66.
6. Feinstein MJ, Hsue PY, Benjamin LA, Bloomfield GS, Currier JS, Freiberg MS, et al. Characteristics, prevention, and management of cardiovascular disease in people living with HIV: a scientific statement from the American Heart Association. Circulation. 2019;140(2):e98–124.
7. Su T, Wit FWNM, Caan MWA, Schouten J, Prins M, Geurtsen GJ, et al. White matter hyperintensities in relation to cognition in HIV-infected men with sustained suppressed viral load on combination antiretroviral therapy. AIDS. 2016;30(15):2329–39.
8. Thawani JP, Nayak NR, Pisapia JM, Petrov D, Pukenas BA, Hurst RW, et al. Aneurysmal vasculopathy in human-acquired immunodeficiency virus-infected adults: imaging case series and review of the literature. Interv Neuroradiol. 2015;21(4):441–50.
9. Masenga SK, Hamooya BM, Nzala S, Kwenda G, Heimburger DC, Mutale W, et al. Patho-immune mechanisms of hypertension in HIV: a systematic and thematic review. Curr Hypertens Rep. 2019;21(7):56.
10. Estrada V, Bernardino JI, Masiá M, Iribarren JA, Ortega A, Lozano F, et al. Cardiovascular risk factors and lifetime risk estimation in HIV-infected patients under antiretroviral treatment in Spain. HIV Clin Trials. 2015;16(2):57–65.
11. Tron L, Lert F, Spire B, Dray-Spira R, Group the AV study. Tobacco smoking in HIV-infected versus general population in France: heterogeneity across the various groups of people living with HIV. PLoS One. 2014;9(9):e107451.

12. Sweeney EM, Thakur KT, Lyons JL, Smith BR, Willey JZ, Cervantes-Arslanian AM, et al. Outcomes of intravenous tissue plasminogen activator for acute ischaemic stroke in HIV-infected adults. Eur J Neurol. 2014;21(11):1394–9.
13. Abdel Razek MA, Gutierrez J, Mampre D, Cervantes-Arslanian A, Ormseth C, Haussen D, et al. Intravenous thrombolysis for stroke and presumed stroke in HIV-infected adults: a retrospective, multicenter U.S. study. Stroke. 2018;49(1):228–31.

Chapter 25
Posterior Circulation Transient Ischaemic Attack

Zhengyue Grace Yang and Arvind Chandratheva

Clinical History

A 70-year-old man attended the emergency department. He had dizziness which he described as a sense of the room moving every time he turned. The onset was acute whilst sitting eating breakfast. He had vomited twice. There was no deafness, tinnitus, headache or speech disturbance. He denied previous episodes of dizziness on getting up or turning in bed. He had a preceding episode of transient diplopia lasting 10 min the day before. He has a background of hypertension, diabetes and hypothyroidism for which he was on treatment. He denied any recent medication changes and there was no history of falls or head injury.

Examination

On arrival he was alert, BP 170/99, noted to have mild dysarthria, able to walk independently but unsteady tandem gait. He had horizontal nystagmus bilaterally but head impulse tested negative. There was no skew deviation and hearing was normal. Remainder of examination was normal. His examination improved over 1 h in the emergency department.

Z. G. Yang
UCL Medical School, London, UK
e-mail: grace.yang.19@ucl.ac.uk

A. Chandratheva (✉)
UCLH, London, UK
e-mail: arvind.chandratheva@nhs.net

S. K. Gill et al. (eds.), *Stroke Medicine*,
https://doi.org/10.1007/978-3-031-58188-5_25

Investigations

A CT head scan was normal and CT angiogram revealed left vertebral atherosclerosis with >50% stenosis. MRI head revealed a DWI positive hyperintensity with restriction on ADC consistent with acute ischaemia in the left cerebellum. 12 lead ECG showed normal sinus rhythm. He was diagnosed with a recurrent posterior circulation TIA and commenced on Aspirin and Clopidogrel 75 mg with 300 mg loading dose, Atorvastatin 80 mg and antihypertensives increased.

Discussion

Approximately 20% of all strokes are preceded by transient ischaemic attacks (TIA) [1, 2]. 20% of all TIAs occur in the posterior circulation [3]. Diagnosis of TIA is based on symptoms obtained from history, risk factors, and corresponding brain scans. Posterior circulation TIA can be difficult to diagnose as isolated brainstem transient neurological attacks (TNAs) such as vertigo, diplopia, isolated dysarthria for which patients may not seek medical attention are more common in posterior circulation TIA [4]. Additionally, these symptoms can be the consequence of other diseases such as migraine, epilepsy and vestibular disorder [5]. About half of patients assessed for suspected TIA will have another diagnosis [1], highest among patients presenting without motor and speech symptoms, or with isolated atypical transient symptoms (TS) such as unusual cortical visual deficit, dysarthria, diplopia, vertigo/unsteadiness and partial sensory deficit [2]. But TIA should still be considered as 16% of posterior circulation stroke were preceded by TIA of which 92% were transient isolated brainstem symptoms (non-consensus TIA) [6, 7]. Moreover there was no significant difference in 1-year risk of stroke between isolated atypical TS, isolated typical TS and non-isolated TS patients [6]; overall TIA diagnosis will increase by about 50% with the designation of non-consensus TIAs as cerebrovascular events [7].

Of those with atypical TS, positive DWI lesion MRI was highest in those with dysarthria and partial sensory deficit, however, in general, posterior circulation stroke are less likely to present with DWI positive MRI [1, 4]. This may be due to lower DWI sensitivity in the brainstem and cerebellum [6].

Positive DWI lesions are associated with an increased 7-day and 3-month risk of stroke [8]. Other factors include TIA duration and atrial fibrillation. DWI positive TIA is present in approximately 40–50% of TIAs and is dependent on timing of imaging and location [4, 8]. Absence of a lesion on DWI does not rule out ischemia. Appropriate history of a sudden onset focal neurological event in the context of relevant clinical risk factors and identifying a causative underlying aetiology are key.

High risk of recurrence following TIA can be associated with certain clinical characteristics e.g. $ABCD^2 > 4$, imaging findings e.g. acute cerebral ischaemia on imaging, and identification of high risk underlying aetiology e.g. cardiac embolism, small vessel disease and ≥50% symptomatic atherosclerotic stenosis [6, 9].

However, $ABCD^2$, which generates a recurrent stroke risk score using clinical features such as age, hypertension, weakness and speech disturbance, duration of symptoms, diabetes mellitus, (additional dual-TIA category for $ABCD^3$), are not recommended to be used in isolation for triaging TIA patients, as 20% with a score below 4 required emergency treatment consideration (≥50% symptomatic intracranial stenosis, cardiac embolism) [10] and 22% of recurrent strokes occurred in patients with $ABCD^2$ score below 4 [11]. Adding brain imaging (ABCD2-I and ABCD3-I) modestly improves discrimination yet brain imaging is not available in general practice or for paramedics, situations when these risk scores could be used [8].

Stroke specialist assessment should be on the same day as presentation, and treatment started immediately [1]. The EXPRESS study showed that early initiation of treatments after TIA (dual antiplatelet agents, statins, blood pressure lowering drugs and endarterectomy as required) was associated with 80% relative risk reduction of early recurrent stroke without increase in intracerebral haemorrhage [12].

Of all strokes that occurred within 30 days after a TIA, 42% were in the first 24 hours, emphasising the importance of emergency assessment and treatment. Hyperacute risk of stroke, at 6-, 12-, and 24-h after first TIA are 1.2%, 2.1% and 5.1% respectively [13]. Meta-analysis of acute risk of stroke showed stroke risk of 3.1% and 5.2% at 2- and 7-days respectively, and this figure was lower in patients seen in specialist stroke services treated on an emergency basis [2, 9].

The 90 day risk is up to 3 times higher in patients with symptomatic vertebrobasilar (VB) stenosis [9, 14], with doubled risk for intracranial than extracranial stenosis [14] ≥50% arterial VB stenosis is found more commonly in patients with non-consensus TIA symptoms than classic TIA symptoms [7]. Unlike anterior circulation TIA where carotid revascularisation is effective for those with ≥50% symptomatic carotid artery stenosis [1], current standard care for symptomatic VB large artery stenosis is medical therapy [9, 15]. Further work is required to determine whether stenting may have a role.

Maximal medical treatment includes dual antiplatelet treatment with aspirin and clopidogrel. The CHANCE trial compared aspirin and clopidogrel dual-therapy to aspirin monotherapy initiated within 24 h for 21 days in patients with high-risk TIA or minor stroke showed greater efficacy of dual antiplatelet therapy. A reduction of subsequent stroke risk by 32%, with no difference in bleeding or haemorrhagic stroke rates [16]. However, patients in the study were highly selected and the epidemiology of stroke in this trial's population (Chinese) is different to Western European populations; the proportion of patients on antihypertensives, statins and diabetes treatments are lower [16], and polymorphisms associated with incomplete metabolism of clopidogrel is common in Asian populations [17]. The POINT trial, compared clopidogrel and aspirin dual antiplatelet therapy versus aspirin initiated within 12 h for 90 days. There was a 25% relative risk reduction of stroke but a 13% relative risk increase of major haemorrhage compared to aspirin monotherapy, which may be due to the longer duration dual antiplatelet therapy and larger loading dose compared to CHANCE [17]. There is also the suggestion that DAPT could reduce stroke-related disability [18]. Both trials excluded patients with cardioembolic TIA. These trials show that clopidogrel and aspirin dual therapy may be beneficial for patients who are at high risk for recurrent ischemia, with a NNT of 40 for recurrent stroke [19]. However, caution in duration longer than 21 days as highlighted in POINT and MATCH due to increase in risk of haemorrhage [20, 21].

In antiplatelet therapy, aspirin and dipyridamole dual-therapy is more beneficial than aspirin alone [12], however the ESPRIT study suggest that it has a small absolute benefit cost-effectiveness [22]. In the PRoFESS study, this dual-therapy had poorer tolerance and non-significant increase in intracranial haemorrhage compared to clopidogrel [20]. Clopidogrel was superior to aspirin when reducing stroke, MI and vascular death risk, shown in the CAPRIE trial [20].

In addition to antihypertensives targeting blood pressure <130/80 and diabetic control, patients should be started on a statin; SPARCL randomised control trial showed that for recent TIA patients without known coronary heart disease, 80 mg of atorvastatin per day reduce the 5 years risk of strokes by 16% compared to placebo, with a NNT of 45 [23].

Atrial fibrillation is the commonest cardiac arrhythmia increasing risk of ischemic stroke [24] hence 12-lead ECG must be performed. In AF patients, thrombus is more fibrin-rich than platelet-rich, so anticoagulation therapy with warfarin, or direct oral anticoagulants which avoid warfarin associated drug–diet interactions, do not require anticoagulation monitoring and have 50% relative risk reduction of intracerebral haemorrhage, should be started [24, 25].

Key Clinical Learning Points

- 20% of strokes are preceded by TIA and those presenting in the posterior circulation are often atypical transient neurological symptoms e.g. isolated dysarthria, vertigo or diplopia
- Posterior circulation TIA with MRI DWI positive are associated with high risk of recurrence but MRI is less sensitive in the posterior circulation
- Predictors of recurrent stroke include certain clinical characteristics e.g. ABCD2 > 4, imaging findings e.g. DWI positive and identification of certain underlying aetiology e.g. AF and symptomatic vertebrobasilar >50%
- Short term dual antiplatelet treatment with Aspirin and Clopidogrel after loading dose can reduce risk of recurrent stroke
- Treatment strategy should include antihypertensives targeting <130/80 (unless otherwise contraindicated) and high intensity statin therapy particularly important for those with large artery atherosclerosis

Key Radiological Learning Points

- Although lower in sensitivity for posterior circulation TIA, DWI positive lesion is present in 40–50% of TIAs
- Look for vertebrobasilar stenosis >50% using CT angiography

References

1. Coutts SB. Diagnosis and management of transient ischemic attack. Continuum. 2017;23(1, Cerebrovascular Disease):82–92. https://doi.org/10.1212/CON.0000000000000424.
2. Giles MF, Rothwell PM. Risk of stroke early after transient ischaemic attack: a systematic review and meta-analysis. Lancet Neurol. 2007;6(12):1063–72. https://doi.org/10.1016/S1474-4422(07)70274-0.
3. Markus HS, van der Worp HB, Rothwell PM. Posterior circulation ischaemic stroke and transient ischaemic attack: diagnosis, investigation, and secondary prevention. Lancet Neurol. 2013;12(10):989–98. https://doi.org/10.1016/S1474-4422(13)70211-4.
4. Paul NLM, Simoni M, Rothwell PM. Transient isolated brainstem symptoms preceding posterior circulation stroke: a population-based study. Lancet Neurol. 2013;12:65–71. https://doi.org/10.1016/S1474-4422(12)70299-5.
5. Chandratheva A, Werring D, Kaski D. Vertebrobasilar insufficiency: an insufficient term that should be retired. Pract Neurol. 2021;21:2–3. [Available from: https://pn.bmj.com/content/practneurol/21/1/2.full.pdf?casa_token=A9p3QVb-gY8AAAAA:J7XErDVOU1tMkr7FhgdtRYl31UZNI5TW-k3zdjuKr_IZ5QUfLUZATpgs-K_C-eW2t8IpmT0sJKI].
6. Lavallée PC, Sissani L, Labreuche J. Clinical significance of isolated atypical transient symptoms in a cohort with transient ischemic attack. Stroke. 2017;48(6):1495–500. https://doi.org/10.1161/nriSTROKEAHA.117.016743.
7. Tuna MA, Rothwell PM. Diagnosis of non-consensus transient ischaemic attacks with focal, negative, and non-progressive symptoms: population-based validation by investigation and prognosis. Lancet. 2021;397:902–12. https://doi.org/10.1016/S0140-6736(20)31961-9.
8. Bhatt A, Jani V. The ABCD and ABCD2 scores and the risk of stroke following a TIA: a narrative review. ISRN Neurol. 2011;2011:518621. https://doi.org/10.5402/2011/518621.
9. Gulli G, Marquardt L, Rothwell PM, et al. Stroke risk after posterior circulation stroke/transient ischemic attack and its relationship to site of vertebrobasilar stenosis. pooled data analysis from prospective studies. Stroke. 2013;44:598–604. https://doi.org/10.1161/STROKEAHA.112.669929.
10. Amarenco P, Labreuche J, Lavallée PC. Does ABCD2 score below 4 allow more time to evaluate patients with a transient ischemic attack? Stroke. 2009;40:3091–5. https://doi.org/10.1161/STROKEAHA.109.552042.
11. Amarenco P, Lavallée PC, Labreuche J. One-year risk of stroke after transient ischemic attack or minor stroke. N Engl J Med. 2016;374:1533–42. https://doi.org/10.1056/NEJMoa1412981.
12. Rothwell PM, Giles MF, Chandratheva A. Effect of urgent treatment of transient ischaemic attack and minor stroke on early recurrent stroke (EXPRESS study): a prospective population-based sequential comparison. Lancet. 2007;370:1432–42. https://doi.org/10.1016/S0140-6736(07)61448-2.
13. Rothwell PM, Warlow CP. Timing of TIAs preceding stroke. Time window for prevention is very short. Neurology. 2005;64(5):817–20. https://doi.org/10.1212/01.WNL.0000152985.32732.EE.
14. Gulli G, Khan S, Markus HS. Vertebrobasilar stenosis predicts high early recurrent stroke risk in posterior circulation stroke and TIA. Stroke. 2009;40:2732–7. https://doi.org/10.1161/STROKEAHA.109.553859.
15. Compter A, van der Worp HB, Schonewille WJ. Stenting versus medical treatment in patients with symptomatic vertebral artery stenosis: a randomised open-label phase 2 trial. Lancet Neurol. 2015;14(6):606–14. https://doi.org/10.1016/S1474-4422(15)00017-4.
16. Wang Y, Wang Y, Zhao X, et al. Clopidogrel with aspirin in acute minor stroke or transient ischemic attack. N Engl J Med. 2013;369:11–9. https://doi.org/10.1056/NEJMoa1215340.
17. Johnston S, Easton J, Farrant M, et al. Clopidogrel and aspirin in acute ischemic stroke and high-risk TIA. N Engl J Med. 2018;379:215–25. https://doi.org/10.1056/NEJMoa1800410.
18. Cucchiara B, Elm JJ, Easton D, et al. Disability after minor stroke and transient ischemic attack in the POINT trial. Stroke. 2020;51:792–9. https://doi.org/10.1161/STROKEAHA.119.027465.

19. Long B, Gottlieb M, Zehtabchi S. Antiplatelet agents for preventing early recurrence of ischemic stroke or transient ischemic attack. The NNT [Internet]. The NNT Group. 2021; Available from: https://www.thennt.com/nnt/antiplatelet-agents-preventing-early-recurrence-ischemic-stroke-transient-ischemic-attack/. Updated 2021; cited 21 May 2021.
20. Gouya G, Arrich J, Wolzt M. Antiplatelet treatment for prevention of cerebrovascular events in patients with vascular diseases. a systematic review and meta-analysis. Stroke. 2014;45(2):492–503. https://doi.org/10.1161/STROKEAHA.113.002590.
21. Diener HC, Bogousslavsky J, Brass LM. Aspirin and clopidogrel compared with clopidogrel alone after recent ischaemic stroke or transient ischaemic attack in high-risk patients (MATCH): randomised, double-blind, placebo-controlled trial. Lancet. 2004;364:331–7. https://doi.org/10.1016/S0140-6736(04)16721-4.
22. Halkes PH, van Gijn J, Kappelle LJ, et al. Aspirin plus dipyridamole versus aspirin alone after cerebral ischaemia of arterial origin (ESPRIT): randomised controlled trial. Lancet. 2006;367:1665–73. Available from: https://www.acpjournals.org/doi/pdf/10.7326/ACPJC-2006-145-3-057.
23. The Stroke Prevention by Aggressive Reduction in Cholesterol Levels (SPARCL) Investigators. High-dose atorvastatin after stroke or transient ischemic attack. N Engl J Med. 2006;355:549–59. https://doi.org/10.1056/NEJMoa061894.
24. Lip G. The role of aspirin for stroke prevention in atrial fibrillation. Nat Rev Cardiol. 2011;8:602–6. https://doi.org/10.1038/nrcardio.2011.112.
25. Steiner T, Weitz JI, Veltkamp R. Anticoagulant-associated intracranial hemorrhage in the era of reversal agents. Stroke. 2017;48:1432–7. https://doi.org/10.1161/STROKEAHA.116.013343.

Chapter 26
Stroke Mimicking Peripheral Neuropathy or Myelopathy: Bilateral Medial Medullary Infarct

Aytakin Khalil and Paul Bentley

Clinical History

A 53 year old man presented with weakness and numbness in all four limbs that developed over 12 h. He initially felt shoulder "heaviness" at 2 AM before falling asleep. He then awoke at 7.30 AM, with tingling and numbness between the left knee and foot, as well as mild weakness in the left leg. After 2 h he developed left upper limb numbness, which gradually spread from shoulder to hand. Over the following hour, he developed right lower limb numbness, followed by right arm numbness, which is when he presented to hospital (11 AM). Weakness and numbness intensified in all limbs progressively during the course of the day until 7 PM when symptoms plateaued. He later also reported back pain, difficulty passing urine, and extreme fatigue since the previous day. He had a symptomatic COVID19 infection 3 weeks earlier, and ongoing fatigue. He was a smoker, but had no other past medical history, and was not taking medications.

A. Khalil
Imperial College London NHS Healthcare Trust, London, UK
e-mail: aytakin.khalil@nhs.net

P. Bentley (✉)
Imperial College London NHS Healthcare Trust, London, UK

Department of Brain Sciences, Imperial College London, London, UK
e-mail: p.bentley@imperial.ac.uk

S. K. Gill et al. (eds.), *Stroke Medicine*,
https://doi.org/10.1007/978-3-031-58188-5_26

Examination

He was alert and orientated. There was flaccid pyramidal-pattern weakness in all four limbs, slightly worse on the left side, which progressed over 5 h (initial Medical Research Council power grading: 2–4/5; later: 0–1/5). Deep tendon reflexes were brisk throughout, and plantar reflexes were extensor bilaterally. Light touch sensation was reduced to elbows, in upper limbs bilaterally; to knee in the left leg, and from foot to T10 level on the right. Pain and joint position sensations were intact, but vibration sensation was absent below the anterior iliac spine on the left. Neck flexion was slightly weak. Five hours after clinical presentation, (10 h from symptom onset), upbeat nystagmus and slightly dysphonic speech were noted on repeat examination. Vital signs were normal and he was apyrexial.

Investigations

Unenhanced computerized tomography of the head was normal. Computed tomography angiogram of intracranial and carotid arteries did not show stenosis or occlusion. Arterial blood gas at 8 PM showed PO2 7.7 kPa (normal 10–13 kPa) and PaCO2 6.2 (normal 4.7–6.0 kPa). Magnetic resonance imaging (MRI) of the brain and whole spine with post-contrast sequences was arranged. MRI brain diffusion-weighted sequence showed a wedge-shaped area of restricted diffusion involving the ventral medulla on either side of midline (Fig. 26.1). There was no pathological contrast enhancement. Contrast-enhanced MRI whole spine was normal. COVID-19 PCR test was positive on admission. D-dimer level on Day 4 was 11,028 ng/mL Lupus antibody was negative. CT pulmonary angiogram on Day 4, requested due to new hypoxia, showed extensive bilateral pulmonary emboli.

Diagnosis of ischemic stroke was confirmed on MRI brain, roughly 10 h from onset. Presentation to hospital was in any case beyond 4.5 h from onset, and so intravenous thrombolysis would have been inappropriate even if diagnosis had been made earlier. Treatment was initially Aspirin 300 mg, that was switched to treatment-dose low molecular weight heparin on Day 4 when pulmonary embolism was diagnosed.

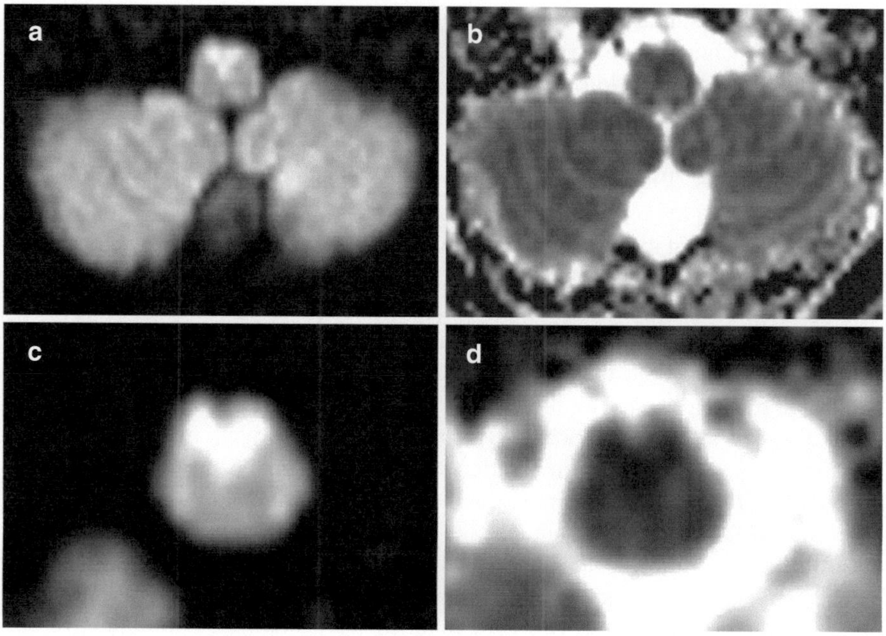

Fig. 26.1 Axial diffusion weighted image (**a**, **c**) and apparent diffusion coefficient (ADC) map (**b**, **d**) show "Y" or "heart" shape restricted diffusion in medial medullary region

Discussion

Medial medullary infarction is rare, accounting for one-quarter of medullary infarctions; which themselves account for only 7% of brainstem ischaemic strokes; while brainstem ischaemic strokes as a whole account for 10% of all ischaemic strokes [1–3]. The case we present is even more unusual in showing *bilateral* medial medullary infarction, which occurs in ~15% of medial medullary infarctions [4]. However, the importance of this condition lies in the fact that its clinical presentation is atypical for stroke, and so easily mistaken for alternative neurological diagnoses, leading to incorrect or delayed treatments. In our case, presentation was initially mild, then progressive over the course of a half-day, before resulting in severe quadriparesis. Presentation by the patient, and clinical diagnosis, were both delayed beyond the recommended time for thrombolysis administration—that is more often seen in posterior, than anterior, circulation strokes, because clinical features of the former are more ambiguous [5, 6]. Yet, disability and mortality caused by brainstem ischaemic strokes, especially when bilateral [7, 8], is significantly higher than other ischaemic strokes, making it all the more imperative that revascularisation treatments are initiated early. Clinicians need to be cautious though about over-reliance on MRI in the acute situation to confirm a diagnosis of stroke, since this may be falsely negative, especially for small brainstem lesions [9].

The medial medullary syndrome was first described by Dejerine as a triad of: (1) contralateral hemiparesis sparing the face; (2) contralateral loss of deep (joint position and vibration) sensation; and (3) ipsilateral hypoglossal paralysis. This follows from the neuroanatomy of the medial medulla, which contains the following structures, from ventral to dorsal, corresponding to the above three signs: (1) corticospinal tract pyramids; (2) medial lemniscus tract (continuation of the spinal cord dorsal columns); and (3) hypoglossal nucleus and nerve.

One of the largest case series of medial medullary infarctions (n = 86) found that the classical Dejerine Triad of signs is not typical [5]. While hemiparesis, and hemisensory disturbance do occur in the majority of cases; ipsilateral tongue weakness is rare. Instead, tongue movements are more often clumsy, or show deviation in a contralesional direction, due to involvement of more rostral, corticobulbar fibres within the pyramids, prior to, or at the level of decussation. Furthermore, although deep sensation was the commonest type of sensory impairment, many patients also show impaired pinprick and temperature sensation that can be attributed to involvement of the spinoreticulothalamic system, that is located medially to the spinothalamic tracts. Other common clinical features of medial medullary infarction are dysarthria and vertigo—both found in the majority; as well as ataxia, ipsilesional nystagmus (and/or internuclear ophthalmoplegia or skew deviation), and dysphagia in 25%. Ataxia and vertigo can be explained by lesioning of midline-crossing "climbing fibres" between inferior olives and inferior cerebellar peduncles; and given strong inputs from vestibular nuclei into inferior olives.

Additional distinguishing clinical patterns of medial medullary infarction, that set it relatively apart from more typical stroke syndromes are:

1. Gradual onset. In medial medullary ischaemic strokes causing severe weakness, progression over several days occurred in two-thirds [5]. This may be explained by the commonest pathology of medial medullary infarction being atherosclerotic occlusion of perforators; or small-vessel disease, as opposed to thromboembolism [5].
2. Upbeat nystagmus is commoner than with strokes in other locations [10, 11], due to involvement of the nucleus intercalatus of Staderini, that is adjacent to the hypoglossal nucleus in the dorsal medial medulla [12], Vertical nystagmus results from dysfunction of the superior vestibular nucleus—ventral tegmental tract (VTT) pathway and/or medial longitudinal fasciculus (MLF) [12]; most commonly due to strokes in the caudal medulla; and less commonly by lesions affecting the ventral pons or the midbrain interstitial nucleus of Cajal [10, 11].
3. Ipsilesional hemiparesis can occur because of caudal lesions, affecting corticospinal pathways *below* the pyramidal decussation [13];
4. Central post-stroke pain is commoner than with other stroke locations [5].

The arterial blood supply to the medial medulla is provided by perforating branches of the anterior spinal artery (Fig. 26.2). These branches of the anterior spinal artery penetrate into medial portions of the medulla alternating to the right and left. Bilateral lesions arise either because of occlusion of the anterior spinal artery, or because some penetrating arteries occasionally bifurcate into right and left branches

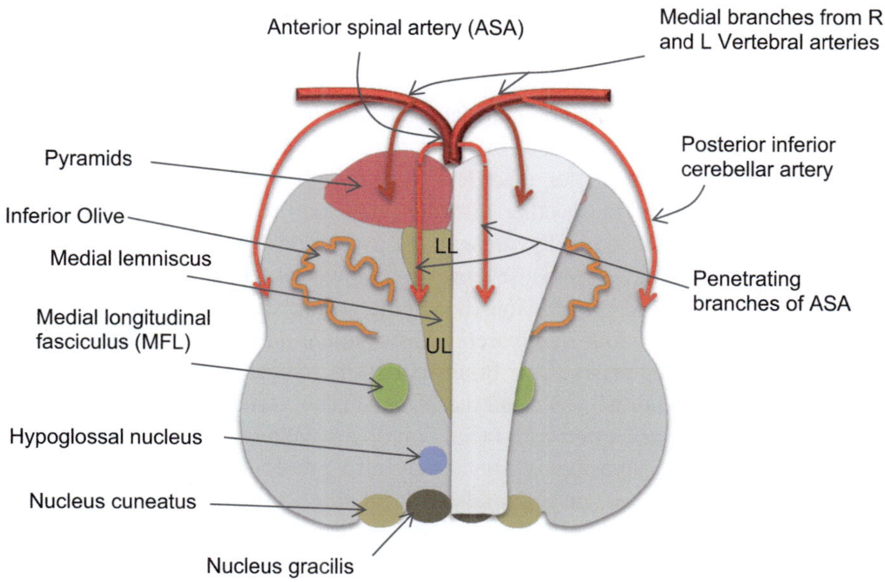

Fig. 26.2 Schematic illustration of medulla structures (on the left), blood supply and medial medulla infarct territory (on the right). Structure involved in the current case are pyramids, medial lemniscus, and likely MLF, nuclei cuneatus and gracilis (dorsal tracts). Sensory dermatomal representation of lower and upper limbs (LL, UL) within medial lemniscus indicated

[5]. Importantly, a vertebral artery occlusion is unlikely to result in medial medullary infarction because of dual blood supply. By contrast, vertebral artery occlusions are likely to cause lateral medullary infarction, because the lateral medulla is supplied via only a single artery: namely, posterior inferior cerebellar artery.

A particularly challenging aspect of the described case was that medial medullary infarction occurred bilaterally, resulting in progressive quadriparesis, thus mimicking either cervical myelopathy or a neuromuscular disorder such as Guillain Barre syndrome or myasthenia gravis. In a systematic review of 37 cases of bilateral medial medullary infarction [7], quadriparesis occurred in 65%, while tongue weakness, that is uncommon in unilateral medial medullary infarction, occurred in 40%. Respiratory failure occurred in 25%; while long-term outcomes were dependency in two-thirds; and death in a quarter. In the current case, quadriparesis (with sensory involvement), occurred progressively in a “N-pattern” rising from leg to arm on one side, then the other. This resembles a pattern described in 20% of bilateral medial medullary infarcts [7], where weakness progressed from hemiparesis to quadriparesis within 72 h. The observation that numbness of legs occurred before arm numbness, implies, based on somatotopic brainstem maps (Fig. 26.2), that ischaemia affected progressively, ventral, before dorsal, medial lemniscus. Since ventral areas are closest to the source of the arterial supply this indicates that more distal areas may be relatively protected by collaterals, and affected only with prolonged ischaemia. This interpretation is supported by noting that the anatomical extent of medial medullary infarcts consists in >95% of cases of either small ventral lesions, or full-thickness ventral and dorsal lesions (i.e. dorsal-only lesions are very rare) [5, 14, 15]. Moreover, medial medullary infarcts have caused paraparesis, but never isolated bi-brachial or isolated bulbar/facial sensorimotor impairment [7].

Having pointed out features of bilateral medial medullary stroke that overlap with peripheral neuromuscular disorders, it is worth highlighting the opposite conundrum: features of these other disorders that may resemble stroke. Guillain Barre syndrome (GBS) typically presents as ascending symmetric, lower-motor neuron pattern of weakness over several days or weeks. However, GBS variants include those with rapid progression (becoming severe within <24 h) [16]; those with asymmetric (including hemiparetic) distributions [17]; upper motor neuron pattern of deep-tendon reflexes, or brainstem signs indicative of GBS-associated "Bickerstaff's encephalitis" [18]; and the Miller-Fisher variant, which entails ophthalmoplegia, and ataxia, often with facial or bulbar weakness that may be mistaken for brainstem stroke. Myasthenia gravis may also present acutely, fluctuate, and show asymmetric features, or signs falsely localising to the posterior circulation, e.g. ataxia due to proximal leg weakness, or pseudo-internuclear ophthalmoplegia; while earlier transient episodes may resemble TIAs [19]. Other disorders to consider with acute brainstem signs are Wernicke's encephalopathy (that is common, and should be treated if there is a history of alcohol excess) and botulism (that is rare; but should be thought of if autonomic dysfunction occurs e.g. hypersalivation, diarrhoea, pupillary paralysis). Finally, high cervical cord lesions must be considered in cases of rapid-onset quadriparesis. However, the classical progression of weakness with foramen magnum lesions is in a "round the clock" pattern (e.g. leg-arm-arm-leg); while high cord lesions typically start either as a hemicord or central cord syndromes (causing respectively, dissociated sensory loss; or bibrachial weakness or cape-like sensory impairment). These differ from the "N-pattern" of sensorimotor progression described in the current case, and sequential hemiparesis described in other medial medullary infarct cases [7, 8]. Sensory examination with a cord lesion usually identifies a truncal sensory level; whereas brainstem sensory impairment, is generally confined to the extremities (especially distally), reflecting the higher sensitivity and larger cortical representation of these body parts [20].

A final observation from our case is that COVID-19 infection related coagulopathy was likely a contributing factor of both ischemic stroke and pulmonary artery embolism [21].

Key Clinical Learning Points

- Bilateral medial medullary infarction is rare, and presents atypically for stroke, but is potentially treatable if diagnosed sufficiently early.
- Bilateral brainstem strokes can present subacutely, and progress over hours or days, mimicking common peripheral neuromuscular emergencies such as Guillain Barre syndrome and myasthenia gravis, or high cervical cord lesions.

- Vertical nystagmus and tongue weakness should be looked for, since they are relatively specific signs of medial medullary stroke.
- Central neurological signs may accompany peripheral neuromuscular emergencies, falsely indicating stroke.

Key Radiological Learning Points

- MRI may be normal in early brainstem infarction and should not be relied upon to exclude stroke.
- A classical radiological feature of bilateral medial medullary infarct is a "Y" or "heart" shape diffusion restriction in the medial medullary region.
- Vertebral arteries often appear normal in medial medullary infarction since the commonest responsible lesions are atheromatous occlusion of perforating branches, distal to the anterior spinal artery; or small vessel disease. By contrast, lateral medullary infarcts are more often due to vertebral artery disease or embolism.

References

1. Ortiz de Mendivil A, Alcalá-Galiano A, Ochoa M, Salvador E, Millán JM. Brainstem stroke: anatomy, clinical and radiological findings. Semin Ultrasound CT MR. 2013;34(2):131–41. https://doi.org/10.1053/j.sult.2013.01.004. PMID: 23522778
2. Tao LS, Lin JJ, Zou M, Chen SF, Weng YY, Chen KY, Hu BL. A comparative analysis of 375 patients with lateral and medial medullary infarction. Brain Behav. 2021;11(8):e2224. https://doi.org/10.1002/brb3.2224. Epub 14 Jun 2021. PMID: 34124854; PMCID: PMC8413826.
3. Kameda W, Kawanami T, Kurita K, Daimon M, Kayama T, Hosoya T, Kato T, Study Group of the Association of Cerebrovascular Disease in Tohoku. Lateral and medial medullary infarction: a comparative analysis of 214 patients. Stroke. 2004;35(3):694–9. https://doi.org/10.1161/01.STR.0000117570.41153.35. Epub 12 Feb 2004. PMID: 14963274.
4. Kuruvilla A, Bhattacharya P, Rajamani K, Chaturvedi S. Factors associated with misdiagnosis of acute stroke in young adults. J Stroke Cerebrovasc Dis. 2011;20(6):523–7. https://doi.org/10.1016/j.jstrokecerebrovasdis.2010.03.005. Epub 17 Aug 2010. PMID: 20719534.
5. Kim JS, Han YS. Medial medullary infarction: clinical, imaging, and outcome study in 86 consecutive patients. Stroke. 2009;40(10):3221–5. https://doi.org/10.1161/STROKEAHA.109.559864. Epub 23 Jul 2009. PMID: 19628797.
6. Sommer P, Seyfang L, Posekany A, Ferrari J, Lang W, Fertl E, Serles W, Töll T, Kiechl S, Greisenegger S. Prehospital and intra-hospital time delays in posterior circulation stroke: results from the Austrian Stroke Unit Registry. J Neurol. 2017;264(1):131–8.
7. Hu F, Nie H, Bai Y, Liang X, Li L, Shen Y. The stroke mechanism, clinical presentation, and radiological feature of bilateral medial medullary infarction. Neurol Sci. 2022;43(12):6881–8. https://doi.org/10.1007/s10072-022-06382-4. Epub 9 Sep 2022. PMID: 36083535.
8. Pongmoragot J, Parthasarathy S, Selchen D, Saposnik G. Bilateral medial medullary infarction: a systematic review. J Stroke Cerebrovasc Dis. 2013;22(6):775–80. https://doi.org/10.1016/j.jstrokecerebrovasdis.2012.03.010. Epub 26 Apr 2012. PMID: 22541608.

9. Bentley P. Magnetic resonance imaging for acute minor neurological symptoms: good for ruling stroke in, not out. JAMA Neurol. 2020;77(6):775–6. https://doi.org/10.1001/jamaneurol.2020.0661. PMID: 32310256.
10. Kim JS, Yoon B, Choi KD, Oh SY, Park SH, Kim BK. Upbeat nystagmus: clinicoanatomical correlations in 15 patients. J Clin Neurol. 2006;2(1):58–65. https://doi.org/10.3988/jcn.2006.2.1.58. Epub 20 Mar 2006. PMID: 20396486; PMCID: PMC2854944.
11. Kakar P, Kamdar A, Prabhudev H, Buddha S, Kaski D, Bentley P. Diagnostic confusion resolved by being upbeat. JRSM Cardiovasc Dis. 2012;1(2):1–6.
12. Pierrot-Deseilligny C, Milea D. Vertical nystagmus: clinical facts and hypotheses. Brain. 2005;128(6):1237–46.
13. Bassetti C, Bogousslavsky J, Mattle H, Bernasconi A. Medial medullary stroke: report of seven patients and review of the literature. Neurology. 1997;48(4):882–90. https://doi.org/10.1212/wnl.48.4.882. PMID: 9109872.
14. Kim JS, Kim HG, Chung CS. Medial medullary syndrome. Report of 18 new patients and a review of the literature. Stroke. 1995;26(9):1548–52. https://doi.org/10.1161/01.str.26.9.1548. PMID: 7660396.
15. Hong YH, Zhou LX, Yao M, Zhu YC, Cui LY, Ni J, Peng B. Lesion topography and its correlation with etiology in medullary infarction: analysis from a multi-center stroke study in China. Front Neurol. 2018;9:813. https://doi.org/10.3389/fneur.2018.00813. PMID: 30319537; PMCID: PMC6170644.
16. Steiner I, Wirguin I, Blumen SC, Dano M, Raphaeli G, Schwartz I, et al. "Hyperacute" Guillain-Barré Syndrome. Eur Neurol. 2008;59(1–2):88–90.
17. Hu M, Li X, Wong HY, Feng XG, Wang YZ, Zhang GR. Asymmetric limb weakness in Guillain-Barré syndrome: three case reports. World J Clin Cases. 2022;10(6):1896–902. https://doi.org/10.12998/wjcc.v10.i6.1896. PMID: 35317159; PMCID: PMC8891786.
18. Odaka M, Yuki N, Yamada M, Koga M, Takemi T, Hirata K, Kuwabara S. Bickerstaff's brainstem encephalitis: clinical features of 62 cases and a subgroup associated with Guillain-Barré syndrome. Brain. 2003;126(Pt 10):2279–90. https://doi.org/10.1093/brain/awg233. Epub 7 Jul 2003. PMID: 12847079.
19. Libman R, Benson R, Einberg K. Myasthenia mimicking vertebrobasilar stroke. J Neurol. 2002;249(11):1512–4. https://doi.org/10.1007/s00415-002-0858-2. PMID: 12420089.
20. Lee SH, Kim DE, Song EC, Roh JK. Sensory dermatomal representation in the medial lemniscus. Arch Neurol. 2001;58(4):649–51. https://doi.org/10.1001/archneur.58.4.649. PMID: 11295997.
21. AlSheef M, Zaidi ARZ, Abonab M, Obaid M, Bawazir K, Zaidi SZA, Kullab GJ, Alawfi S, Enani M. Dual catastrophe of COVID-19: massive pulmonary embolism and stroke in a previously healthy young patient: a case report. J Infect Public Health. 2021;14(5):647–50. https://doi.org/10.1016/j.jiph.2021.01.009. Epub 30 Jan 2021. PMID: 33857723; PMCID: PMC7847184.

Chapter 27
Acute Vestibular Syndrome Following Anterior Inferior Cerebellar Artery (AICA) Occlusion

Eduardo San Pedro Murillo, Nehzat Koohi, and Diego Kaski

Case Report

Clinical History

A 69-year-old man presented with sudden collapse caused by multiple simultaneous infarcts in the posterior circulation territory. Investigations revealed paroxysmal atrial fibrillation and ischemic cardiopathy, without significant stenosis at the supra-aortic vessels. Therefore, the stroke was presumably of cardioembolic origin, and the patient was thus anticoagulated with rivaroxaban. He recovered partially, his clinical sequelae mainly being a complex ophthalmoplegia, an ill-defined gait impairment and pseudobulbar syndrome. One year after the event, a brain MRI scan demonstrated chronic ischemic lesions affecting the entire left cerebellar hemisphere, right rostral midbrain and caudal pons, and more modest injury at the right cerebellar hemisphere and occipital lobe.

Aged 73 he then presented with an abrupt-onset, 2-week history of left-sided hearing loss. When specifically questioned, he also acknowledged coinciding deterioration of his gait impairment with tendency to fall toward to the left side to which he had not given much importance because of being already impeded in this respect.

E. S. P. Murillo
Department of Neurology, University Hospital "12 de Octubre", Madrid, Spain

N. Koohi · D. Kaski (✉)
Centre for Vestibular and Behavioural Neuroscience, Department of Clinical and Movement Neurosciences, Institute of Neurology, University College London, London, UK

The Ear Institute, University College London, London, UK

Neuro-otology Department, University College London Hospitals, London, UK
e-mail: n.koohi@ucl.ac.uk; d.kaski@ucl.ac.uk

S. K. Gill et al. (eds.), *Stroke Medicine*,
https://doi.org/10.1007/978-3-031-58188-5_27

On further questioning, there were no precipitating factors and no other neurological complaints.

Examination

The bedside neuro-otological examination revealed left sided hearing loss and signs of left vestibular hypofunction. The former included: abnormal head-impulse test to the left. The nystagmus, although difficult to fully characterise given the existing complex ophthalmoplegia, appeared to be essentially a right-beating most marked on right gaze, following Alexander's law, and attenuated with fixation. Otherwise, the neurological exam was at patient's baseline.

Investigations

Audio-Vestibular Testing

To assess peripheral and central auditory function, pure-tone audiometry (PTA), tympanometry, acoustic reflex thresholds (ART), transient-evoked otoacoustic emissions (TEOAEs), and auditory brainstem responses (ABR) were performed. PTA revealed age-related mild high-frequency sensorineural hearing loss in the right ear and mild to moderate high-frequency sensorineural hearing loss in the left ear (Fig. 27.1). Tympanometry measures were within normal limits bilaterally

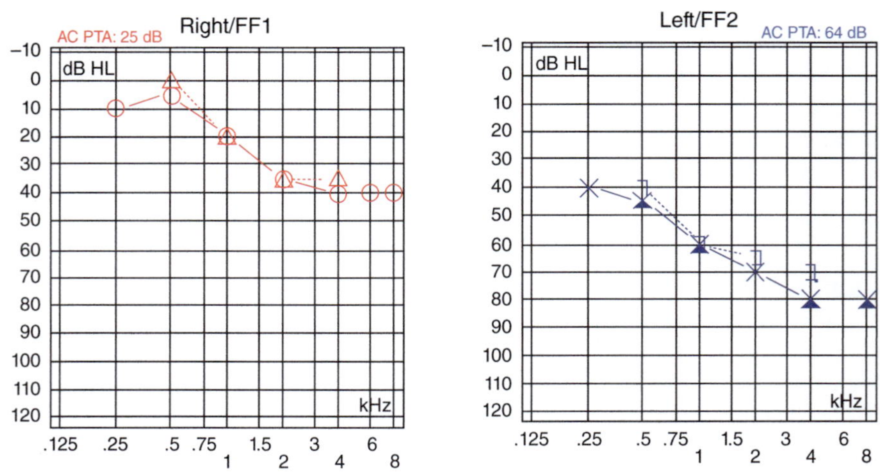

Fig. 27.1 Pure tone audiometry (PTA) of the right (red) and left (blue) ears. Red and blue lines represent the less intense tone perceived by the patient for each frequency. Both air (blue X and red O) and bone (red Δ and blue]) conductions are equally involved, sensorineural pattern. High-frequencies are bilaterally affected, suggesting an age-related process. However, left ear is clearly more impaired

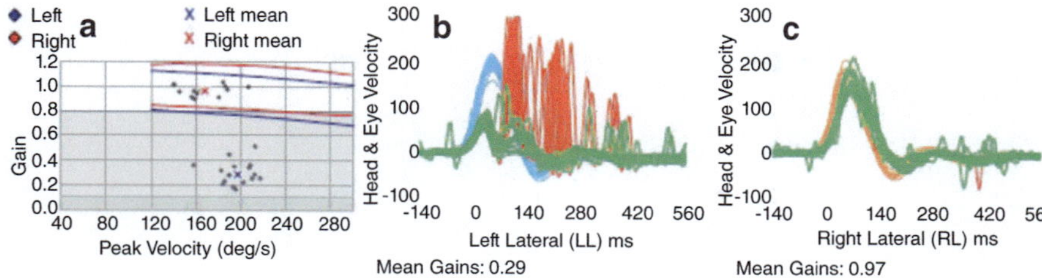

Fig. 27.2 Video head impulse test (vHIT) A. the mean gain of the left vestibulo-ocular reflex (VOR) in the left side (blue X) is clearly below de normal interval (blue lines) while the mean gain of the right VOR is within the normal limits. B. In the left side, the VOR (green line) is defective, its curve lacking the normal morphology (present on the right side C). It is compensated with corrective saccades (red line B)

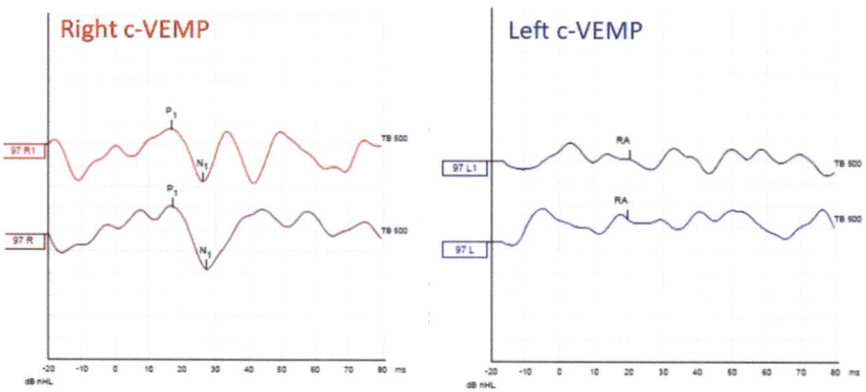

Fig. 27.3 Cervical vestibular evoked myogenic potentials (c-VEMPS). The c-VEMP was clearly present on the right (red) (note the clear P1 and N1 deflections). However, the c-VEMP was impossible to obtain consistently on the left (no P1 or N1 discernible from background)

confirming no middle ear involvement. ART revealed brainstem pattern of hearing impairment. TEOAEs were reduced in the right ear and absent in the left, consistent with PTA findings. Ipsi lateral ABR demonstrated absent responses with poor morphology in the left ear, and present responses but delayed interpeak latencies consistent with damage at the pons. Vestibular tests included video head impulse test (vHIT) and cervical vestibular evoked myogenic potentials (c-VEMP). vHIT identified reduced mean vestibulo-ocular reflex gains for the left horizontal canal (Fig. 27.2) and cVEMP showed present responses on the right and absent responses on the left (Fig. 27.3).

Neuroimaging

A new MRI did not demonstrate any new ischemic lesions (Fig. 27.4).

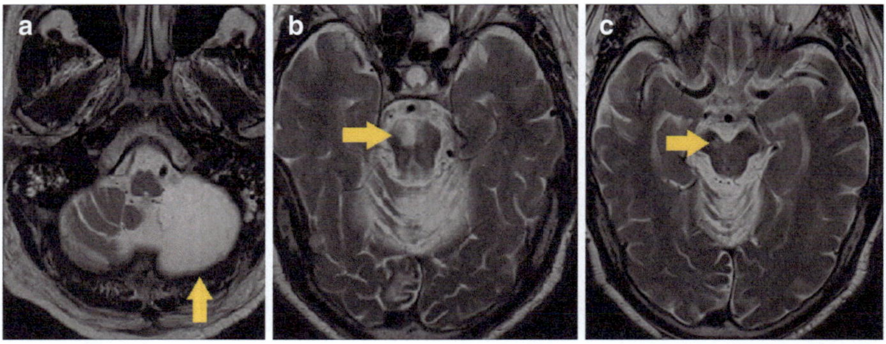

Fig. 27.4 A new brain MRI did not demonstrate any new ischemic lesions. Three axial T2 slices are displayed, demonstrating chronic ischemic changes in concordance with the past known ischemic events in A. left cerebellar hemisphere. B. right caudal pons. C. right rostral midbrain.

Discussion

Acute audio-vestibular symptoms are most commonly associated with a benign peripheral (inner ear) pathology [1–4]. Thus, in the absence of additional neurological symptoms or signs suggesting central nervous system (CNS) involvement, a stroke might not be considered as a possible explanation [3, 4]. Ischemic posterior circulation stroke in the territory of the anterior inferior cerebellar artery (AICA) is the leading cause of acute audiovestibular loss. Approximately 10% of ischaemic strokes in the territory of AICA show audio-vestibular symptoms in isolation and patients may have normal brain MRIs on initial presentation. Up to 30% of these might be a prodromal event in the previous 10 days [1, 2]. This possibility is commonly overlooked, delaying correct management which could prevent further ischemic events [3, 4], as was the case with our patient. To make a correct diagnosis, the clinical picture is as important as imaging [5, 6]. The different manifestations of the ischaemic stroke in the AICA territory with respect to more benign peripheral (inner ear) pathology are based on facts of vascular anatomy, which are subsequently discussed.

Blood Supply of the Audio-Vestibular System

Vascular ischemic lesions in the territory of the AICA account for the great majority of strokes that develop audio-vestibular symptoms exclusively or in combination [1, 2]. This is because the vestibulo-cochlear labyrinth vascular supply is dependent on the internal auditory artery (IAA), which is in approximately a 90% of cases a terminal branch of the AICA, being in the remaining 10% a branch of the posterior inferior cerebellar artery [7–9]. The IAA (Fig. 27.5) gives two main divisions, the common cochlear and anterior vestibular arteries (CCA and AVA) [7, 9]. The CCA

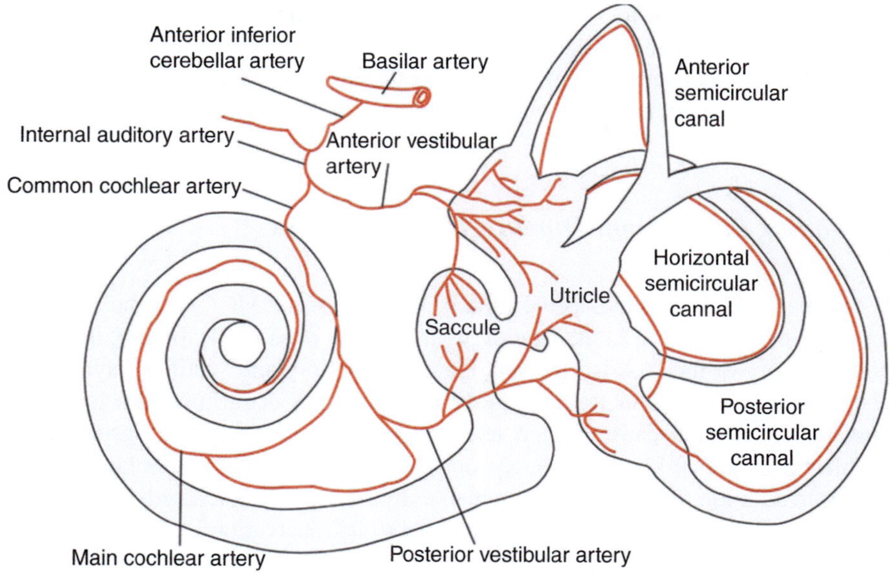

Fig. 27.5 Vascular anatomy of the internal auditory artery (IAA), a branch of the anterior inferior cerebellar artery (AICA), and its branches. These supply the inner ear labyrinth, vestibule and cochlea, structures responsible for movement and auditory perception respectively

then branches in the main cochlear and vestibulocochlear arteries (MCA and VCA), the latter further subdividing in the cochlear ramus (CR) and the posterior vestibular artery (PVA) [7, 9]. Subsequently, the relevance of this anatomical facts with regard to the possible manifestations of ischaemic strokes in the AICA territory are discussed.

Hearing Impairment Due to AICA Infarction

The first thing to do when localizing the lesion responsible for the hearing impairment is to determine whether the hearing loss is unilateral or bilateral. Afferent fibres, after relying in the cochlear nucleus in the inferolateral pons, project to more proximal structures of the auditory pathway in a bilateral way and in equal amount [10]. Therefore, unilateral hearing impairment must have its origin in the cochlear nucleus or more peripheral to it. All these structures are almost always irrigated by the AICA [7–10]. In our case, the patient complaints of unilateral left hearing loss pointed towards a peripheral origin. The pure-tone audiometry, otoacoustic emissions and auditory brainstem-evoked responses supported this hypothesis demonstrating an asymmetrical hearing impairment confirming an involvement of the left ear auditory function [5]. The cochlea has a tonotopic organization, with higher-frequency tones detected at the base and lower-frequency tones toward the apex. The MCA supplies the apical three fourths of the cochlea, causing predominantly low-frequency hearing loss. The remaining basal cochlea is irrigated by the CR, hence producing the inverse pattern in pure-tone audiometry, with relative preservations of lower-frequency tones [7, 9, 10] In our patient, the hearing loss across all frequencies in the left ear suggested the occlusion of at least both CR and MCA.

Vestibular Impairment Due to AICA Infarction

When the MCA is affected, as the PVA is a branch of the MCA, vestibular symptoms are to be expected in association with auditory ones [7, 9]. In fact, the complete territory of the IAA is involved, therefore auditory and vestibular symptoms coexist [2, 7, 9]. This fact allows to differentiate IAA occlusion from inner ear dysfunction of viral cause, which tends to present as an isolated vestibular or cochlear impairment [2]. Accordingly, our patient showed clear vestibular manifestations in addition to auditory ones, which are subsequently discussed.

The vestibule vascular irrigation is parallel to its innervation [7, 9]. The AVA is homologous to the superior division of the vestibular nerve, both supplying the utricle, superior part of the saccule, and the ampulae of the superior and horizontal semicircular canals [7, 9]. The PVA is homologous to the inferior division of the vestibular nerve, both supplying the inferior part of the saccule and the ampulae of the inferior semicircular canals [7, 9] . Both the PVA and AVA are usually simultaneously affected causing a sudden loss of function in the whole vestibule [6, 7, 9]. As a result, two main consequences arise. First, vestibular hyporreflexia, evident as a corrective saccade in the head-impulse test toward the side of the lesion. Second, an asymmetry in the vestibular afferent tone which arises from both abnormal afferent semicircular canal and otolith signals, and is responsible for vertigo [6, 7, 9]. For unclear reasons, the component attributed to the otolith organs is usually subtle, consisting solely of a deviation of the subjective vertical visual without skew deviation [6, 7, 9]. We were unable to demonstrate any of them in our patient. More pronounced, as was the case with our patient is the component causing vertigo derived from the hypofunction of all semicircular canals in combination, which accounts for veering toward the affected side and a horizontal-rotatory jerk nystagmus beating towards the affected ear in the plane of perceived movement [6, 7, 9].

Central Nervous System Involvement Due to AICA Infarction

When the ischaemic stroke in the AICA territory is fully stablished, signs of involvement at other levels of the CNS are found [1]. This is because before ending in the IAA, the AICA also gives branches that supply the inferolateral portion of the pons and anteroinferior cerebellum including the flocculus and dentate nucleus [11, 12]. However, during the hyperacute phase, this involvement may be subtle, being easily overlooked if not specifically searched for [11, 12]. Thus, in addition to audio-vestibular symptoms, one should explore the presence of cerebellar signs including ipsilateral limb dysmetria, and features of pontine involvement, such as Horner's syndrome, ipsilateral facial hypoesthesia, and contralateral thermoalgic hypoesthesia, but with involvement of the VII instead of lower cranial nerves [11, 12]. Less common findings are ipsilateral gaze palsy, dysphagia and contralateral hemiparesis [11, 12]. In our patient, there was no evidence, neither clinical nor radiological, of involvement of the CNS apart from his long-standing sequela due to the earlier stroke some years before.

Differential Diagnosis and Role of Imaging

As previously stated, 10% of the ischaemic strokes in the territory of AICA show audio-vestibular symptoms in isolation, and up to a third of these cases display prodromal episodes consisting of isolated audio-vestibular symptoms, preceding the ischemic event in up to 10 days [1, 2]. This is attributed to a higher vulnerability of the labyrinth with respect to the remaining structures supplied by the AICA, due to its high-energy requirements, and the fact that the IAA is a terminal branch with scarce collaterals [6–9, 13–15]. Both the TIA-like prodromal episodes and the stablished IAA stroke can mimic benign peripheral (inner ear) vestibular disorders such as Ménière's disease and acute vestibular neuritis [3, 4]. It is of utmost importance to distinguish between a benign cause from a sinister episode preceding a stroke [3, 4]. With this respect, the presence of vascular risk factors is an important diagnostic clue. These account for the a priori probability of suffering a vascular event, and when being present, should raise our index of suspicion of an AICA stroke accounting for acute audio-vestibular symptoms despite occurring in isolation [3, 4]. This was the case in our patient, whose past medical history indicated a very high probability of suffering a new ischemic event, warranting the need to consider stroke as a likely explanation for his hearing impairment.

When the pons or cerebellum are affected, radiological confirmation of AICA infarct is often possible. However, MRI in the hyperacute phase (<24 h) might be inconclusive, as with the other posterior fossa ischemic lesions, which are normal in up to 20% of instances [15]. These can be overcome by repeated imaging, as our case exemplifies, when only the IAA is affected, the MRI is not capable of demonstrating ischemia of this structure [3, 4].

In summary, the diagnosis of ischaemic stroke in the territory of AICA must rely on clinical grounds. It is based on the presence of compatible neurological findings (i.e. audio-vestibular symptoms in up to a third of cases without involvement of the CNS) with a course typical of stroke (abrupt-onset) in a patient with vascular risk factors. It must be differentiated from other peripheral causes. Taking all these things into consideration when facing a patient who presents with audio-vestibular symptoms is essential to minimize the risk of missing an ischaemic stroke in the territory of AICA [1–4].

Key Clinical Learning Points

- Up to one third of AICA strokes present with prodromal episodes consisting of isolated audio-vestibular symptoms, easily mistaken with more being peripheral (inner ear) pathol ogy.
- These symptoms are due to IAA involvement (most vulnerable to ischemia), which supplies the labyrinth (inner ear). Thus, audio-vestibular investigations may show a peripheral origin.
- Stroke imaging is also often unhelpful to make the differential diagnosis, which has to be therefore clinical. The following characteristics should make us suspect an AICA infarction:
- According to vascular anatomy, either part of the labyrinth can be selectively involved. However, vestibulo-cochlear involvement is the rule, in contrast with viral neuritis.
- Signs of involvement of the CNS (ipsilateral: limb dysmetria, Horner's, facial hypoesthesia or palsy; and contralateral: body thermoalgic hypoesthesia). These might be absent.
- A course typical of stroke (abrupt-onset), in a patient with high a priori vascular risk.

Key Radiological Learning Points

- When involving the CNS, AICA strokes may display ischemia on MRI in the inferolateral pons and anteroinferior cerebellum including the flocculus and dentate nucleus.
- Diffusion-weighted MRI of hyper-acute (<24 h) ischemic lesions of the posterior fossa, including AICA strokes, are often unrevealing. In this case, repeated imaging is advised.
- AICA strokes limited to the territory of the IAA (the most vulnerable to ischemia), cannot be demonstrated either by MRI or other imaging technique. In this cases, diagnosis is clinical.

References

1. Kim HA, Lee H. Recent advances in understanding audiovestibular loss of a vascular cause. J Stroke. 2017;19(1):61–6. https://doi.org/10.5853/jos.2016.00857.
2. Lee H, Kim JS, Chung EJ, Yi HA, Chung IS, Lee SR, Shin JY. Infarction in the territory of anterior inferior cerebellar artery: spectrum of audiovestibular loss. Stroke. 2009;40(12):3745–51. https://doi.org/10.1161/STROKEAHA.109.564682. Epub 24 Sep 2009. PMID: 19797177.
3. Lee H. Audiovestibular loss in anterior inferior cerebellar artery territory infarction: a window to early detection? J Neurol Sci. 2012;313(1–2):153–9. https://doi.org/10.1016/j.jns.2011.08.039. Epub 13 Oct 2011. PMID: 21996273.
4. Kim JS, Cho KH, Lee H. Isolated labyrinthine infarction as a harbinger of anterior inferior cerebellar artery territory infarction with normal diffusion-weighted brain MRI. J Neurol Sci. 2009;278(1–2):82–4. https://doi.org/10.1016/j.jns.2008.12.002. Epub 9 Jan 2009. PMID: 19135217.

5. Lee H, Sohn SI, Jung DK, Cho YW, Lim JG, Yi SD, Lee SR, Sohn CH, Baloh RW. Sudden deafness and anterior inferior cerebellar artery infarction. Stroke. 2002;33(12):2807–12. https://doi.org/10.1161/01.str.0000038692.17290.24. PMID: 12468774.
6. Grad A, Baloh RW. Vertigo of vascular origin. Clinical and electronystagmographic features in 84 cases. Arch Neurol. 1989;46(3):281–4. https://doi.org/10.1001/archneur.1989.00520390047014. PMID: 2919982.
7. Mazzoni A. Internal auditory canal arterial relations at the porus acusticus. Ann Otol Rhinol Laryngol. 1969;78(4):797–814. https://doi.org/10.1177/000348946907800413. PMID: 5799404.
8. Mazzoni A. Internal auditory artery supply to the petrous bone. Ann Otol Rhinol Laryngol. 1972;81(1):13–21. https://doi.org/10.1177/000348947208100103. PMID: 5009813.
9. Mazzoni A. The vascular anatomy of the vestibular labyrinth in man. Acta Otolaryngol Suppl. 1990;472:1–83. https://doi.org/10.3109/00016489009121137. PMID: 2239254.
10. Häusler R, Levine RA. Auditory dysfunction in stroke. Acta Otolaryngol. 2000;120(6):689–703. https://doi.org/10.1080/000164800750000207. PMID: 11099144.
11. Amarenco P, Roullet E, Hommel M, Chaine P, Marteau R. Infarction in the territory of the medial branch of the posterior inferior cerebellar artery. J Neurol Neurosurg Psychiatry. 1990;53(9):731–5. https://doi.org/10.1136/jnnp.53.9.731. PMID: 2246654; PMCID: PMC1014248.
12. Amarenco P, Hauw JJ. Cerebellar infarction in the territory of the anterior and inferior cerebellar artery. A clinicopathological study of 20 cases. Brain. 1990;113(Pt 1):139–55. https://doi.org/10.1093/brain/113.1.139. PMID: 2302529.
13. Lee H, Cho YW. Auditory disturbance as a prodrome of anterior inferior cerebellar artery infarction. J Neurol Neurosurg Psychiatry. 2003;74:1644–8.
14. Perlman HB, Kimura RS, Fernandez C. Experiments on temporal obstruction of the internal auditory artery. Laryngoscope. 1959;69(6):591–613. https://doi.org/10.1288/00005537-195906000-00001. PMID: 13673604.
15. Sparaco M, Ciolli L, Zini A. Posterior circulation ischemic stroke-a review part II: imaging and acute treatment. Neurol Sci. 2019;40(10):2007–15. https://doi.org/10.1007/s10072-019-03936-x. Epub 24 May 2019. PMID: 31127426.

Chapter 28
The Difference Between Looking and Seeing at 2 am

Murva Asad, Aneliya Takova, and Richard Perry

Clinical History

A 59-year-old right-handed man had recent diagnoses of cardiomyopathy, valvular disease, and atrial fibrillation treated with rivaroxaban. He went to bed as normal at 10.30 pm. When he got up at midnight to go to the bathroom, he immediately fell to the floor. His family noted that he was then unable to speak or move his left side.

Examination

On arrival in hospital at 2.03 am he had very severe neglect of his left side, with forced gaze deviation to the right, and he also appeared to have a left-sided visual field defect. He had no movement against gravity with his left arm or leg, and left hemisensory loss. When he tried to speak, he made incomprehensible sounds, even when speaking in his native language of Albanian. With an interpreter he could follow basic one-step commands. He appeared to be confused and agitated. His National Institutes of Health Stroke Scale score was 20 [1].

M. Asad (✉) · R. Perry
Department of Neurology, National Hospital for Neurology and Neurosurgery, London, UK
e-mail: murva.asad@nhs.net; richard.perry2@nhs.net

A. Takova
National Hospital for Neurology and Neurosurgery, London, UK
e-mail: aneliya.takova@nhs.net

S. K. Gill et al. (eds.), *Stroke Medicine*,
https://doi.org/10.1007/978-3-031-58188-5_28

Investigations and Clinical Progress

His blood glucose was normal (5.8 mmol/L), and ECG confirmed atrial fibrillation. His initial CT head did not show any evidence of acute ischaemia or haemorrhage, although the right terminal carotid appeared hyperdense, consistent with acute thrombosis (Fig. 28.1a). The clinical diagnosis was stroke, but thrombolysis was contraindicated because he had taken a dose of rivaroxaban at 6pm the previous evening and his anti-Xa level was 337 ng/mL.

A CT angiogram was performed, with a strong suspicion that this would show a right middle cerebral artery occlusion. The images showed occlusion of the whole right internal carotid artery (ICA) from just above its origin, but there was excellent filling of the right middle cerebral artery (MCA) and anterior cerebral artery (ACA), due to collateral supply via a substantial anterior communicating artery (ACom), so initially there did not seem to be a potential target for mechanical thrombectomy (Fig. 28.1b).

The anterior third of the right posterior communicating artery (PCom) did not fill with contrast (Fig. 28.1b) but the significance of this observation was not immediately apparent, in a patient with an occluded right ICA and what appeared clinically to be an anterior circulation syndrome (severe left-sided weakness, neglect and a language disturbance).

After discussion with an interventional neuroradiologist, he was sent back to the Neuroradiology Department for a CT perfusion scan. The images demonstrated normal perfusion of the right anterior circulation, but a large perfusion deficit in the right posterior cerebral artery (PCA) territory (Fig. 28.2). On further

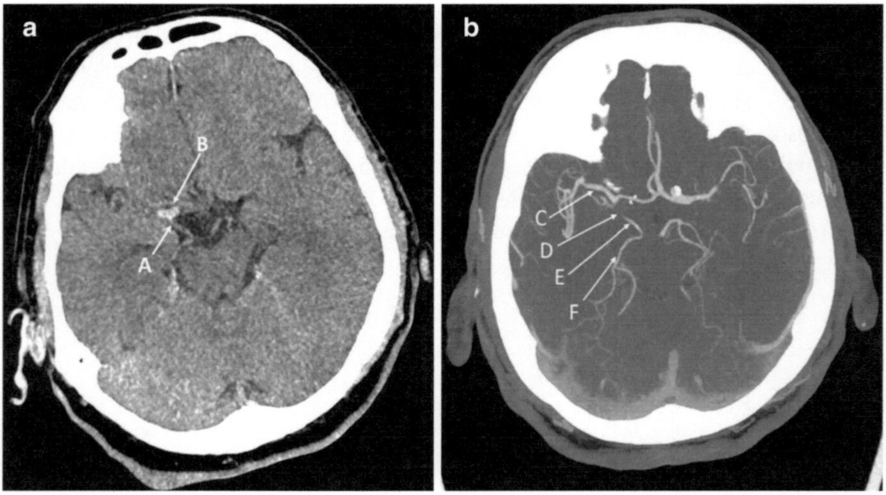

Fig. 28.1 (**a**) Non-contrast CT head showing hyperdense thrombus in the right ICA (B) occluding the origin of the right PCom (A). (**b**) CT angiogram of the intracranial vessels showing a patent right MCA (C) and a filling defect (D) in the anterior third of a large calibre PCom (E) which is primarily supplying the PCA (F) i.e. foetal PCA

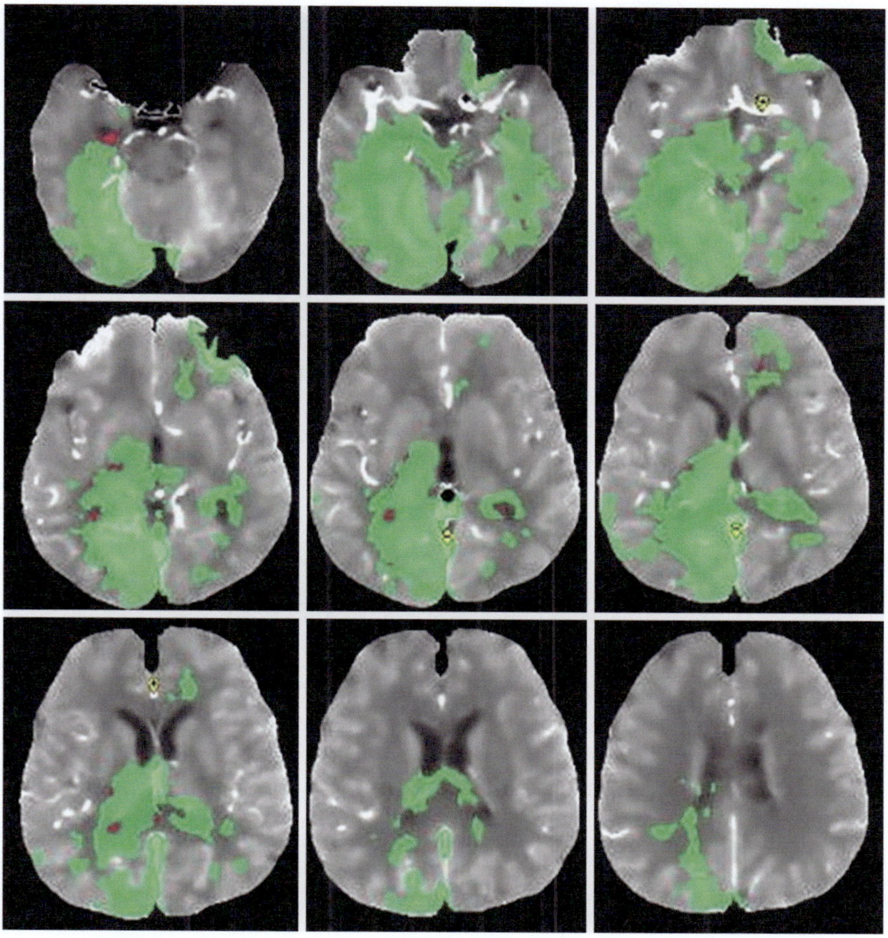

Fig. 28.2 CT perfusion scan demonstrating a relative cerebral blood flow (rCBF) <30% (i.e., core) volume of 2 ml in red and a time to peak of the residual function (T_{max}) >6 s (i.e., penumbra) volume of 181 ml in green the right PCA territory. The defects on the contralateral side were felt to be related to collateral flow and the ICA terminus occlusion altering haemodynamics

review of the CT angiogram, it was apparent that the P1 segment of the right PCA was very slender, indicating the presence of a partial foetal origin to the right PCA, i.e., the dominant supply to this vessel was from the anterior circulation via the PCom.

We concluded that thrombus from the occluded right ICA had propagated into the PCom, and the occlusion of this vessel was the cause of his stroke. The patient proceeded to mechanical thrombectomy, and a large thrombus was removed from the terminal portion of the right ICA and from the right PCom, using a combination of aspiration and deployment of a stent retriever. On waking-up from the procedure, the patient was able to move his left side.

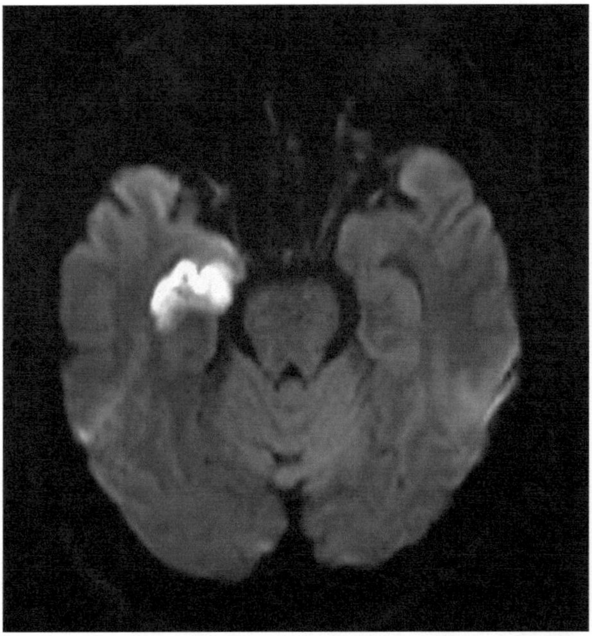

Fig. 28.3 Magnetic resonance diffusion-weighted imaging showing an area of restriction in the right medial temporal lobe representing the final volume of infarct after endovascular thrombectomy

The patient made a good recovery (Fig. 28.3). By the time of discharge 6 days later from the Hyperacute Stroke Unit to the local Acute Stroke Unit, there was no evidence of neglect and he had regained full power and normal visual fields. Neuropsychological assessment demonstrated deficits in visual recognition memory and sustained attention, for which cognitive rehabilitation was recommended.

Discussion

The term "foetal" PCA usually refers to both partial foetal PCA (where a hypoplastic P1 segment connects the PCA to the basilar artery) or complete foetal PCA (where a P1 segment is not visible). In both cases, the PCA is supplied primarily by the PCom derived from the internal carotid artery. It is estimated that around 30% of people have unilateral foetal PCA configuration and up to 9% have a bilateral configuration [2]. Early in embryonic development the ICAs initially supply the PCAs before the vertebrobasilar system develops and the "adult" (most common) configuration is formed; the "foetal" PCA is a persistence of that earlier configuration [3].

This case demonstrates an important implication of this common variant: occlusion or significant stenosis of the ipsilateral ICA can cause PCA territory infarction which is otherwise usually a result of vertebrobasilar disease. Our patient presented with what was initially thought to be a middle cerebral artery syndrome including severe left-sided neglect with gaze deviation to the right, left hemiparesis and hemisensory loss and a speech disturbance which appeared to be dysphasia. However, the CT angiogram revealed an occluded right ICA but excellent filling of the right MCA via the anterior communicating artery, prompting us to reevaluate. CT perfusion scan of the brain subsequently drew attention to the right PCA territory, and the significance of our patient's foetal PCA anatomy became apparent, allowing us to proceed to timely mechanical thrombectomy. Although the left homonymous hemianopia was a clinical clue to the true location of the infarct, this sign is difficult to interpret in the context of severe neglect, which can mimic a hemianopia.

Following multiple studies published in 2015 [4–8], mechanical thrombectomy of anterior circulation large vessel occlusion is now well recognised to improve functional outcomes in stroke and has become standard of care. Fewer data are available on mechanical thrombectomy in foetal PCA or PCom occlusions. One multicentre retrospective review of 25 cases of foetal PCA or PCom occlusions found thrombectomy to be safe and feasible [9].

The DEFUSE-III and DAWN trials have previously demonstrated the influence of CT perfusion on identifying the penumbra in acute stroke and selecting thrombectomy candidates in extended windows, but CT perfusion may also be useful in localisation and diagnosis, as in this challenging case where PCA territory ischaemia mimicked that of the MCA [10, 11]. One study has suggested that 17.8% of PCA strokes may clinically mimic MCA stroke to varying degrees when severe motor deficit, visuospatial neglect, and aphasia (due to thalamic involvement) are present [12]. In the hyperacute setting, the non-contrast CT brain may be normal or subtle early ischaemic changes in the posterior circulation may be missed if the clinician is focused on the anterior circulation. The CT perfusion can be a useful tool in guiding the clinician to the relevant vessel occlusion.

Identifying this variant neurovascular anatomy is also important in patients with PCA territory infarction in the context of foetal PCA and ipsilateral ICA stenosis, as they may benefit from carotid endarterectomy to reduce future stroke risk [13]. ICA stenosis in the presence of foetal PCA anatomy may also be considered a cause of unilateral "multi-territory" infarcts involving both the ipsilateral MCA and PCA territories [14].

This case underscores the clinical significance of foetal posterior cerebral artery anatomy in the context of acute stroke, highlighting the importance of recognising and addressing this common variant for accurate diagnosis and timely intervention.

Key Clinical Learning Points

- Variant vascular anatomy is important to be aware of and, in the case of persistent foetal PCA, is common.
- Occlusion of the internal carotid artery can cause a posterior cerebral artery territory stroke if there is foetal anatomy of the PCA.
- Posterior cerebral artery infarction may mimic middle cerebral artery infarction with hemiparesis, neglect, and language disturbances.

Key Radiological Learning Points

- Can guide mechanical thrombectomy by highlighting the potentially viable tissue.
- CT perfusion can also be helpful in diagnosis and localisation of acute stroke.
- Mechanical thrombectomy of the foetal PCA is potentially feasible and safe and can be associated with improved functional outcomes.

References

1. Lyden PD, Lu M, Levine SR, Brott TG, Broderick J. A modified National Institutes of Health Stroke Scale for use in stroke clinical trials: preliminary reliability and validity. Stroke. 2001;32(6):1310–7.
2. van Raamt AF, Mali WPTM, van Laar PJ, van der Graaf Y. The foetal variant of the circle of Willis and its influence on the cerebral collateral circulation. Cerebrovasc Dis. 2006;22(4):217–24.
3. Padget DH. The development of the cranial arteries in the human embryo. Contributions to embryology. Carnegie Inst. 1948;32:205–61.
4. Campbell BCV, Mitchell PJ, Kleinig TJ, Dewey HM, Churilov L, Yassi N, et al. Endovascular therapy for ischemic stroke with perfusion-imaging selection. N Engl J Med. 2015;372(11):1009–18. https://doi.org/10.1056/nejmoa1414792.
5. Berkhemer OA, Fransen PSS, Beumer D, van den Berg LA, Lingsma HF, Yoo AJ, et al. A randomized trial of intraarterial treatment for acute ischemic stroke. N Engl J Med. 2015;372(1):11–20. https://doi.org/10.1056/nejmoa1411587.
6. Goyal M, Demchuk AM, Menon BK, Eesa M, Rempel JL, Thornton J, et al. Randomized assessment of rapid endovascular treatment of ischemic stroke. N Engl J Med. 2015;372(11):1019–30. https://doi.org/10.1056/nejmoa1414905.
7. Saver JL, Goyal M, Bonafe A, Diener H-C, Levy EI, Pereira VM, et al. Stent-retriever thrombectomy after intravenous T-pa vs. T-pa alone in stroke. N Engl J Med. 2015;372(24):2285–95. https://doi.org/10.1056/nejmoa1415061.
8. Jovin TG, Chamorro A, Cobo E, de Miquel MA, Molina CA, Rovira A, et al. Thrombectomy within 8 hours after symptom onset in ischemic stroke. N Engl J Med. 2015;372(24):2296–306. https://doi.org/10.1056/nejmoa1503780.
9. Abdalkader M, Sahoo A, Dmytriw AA, Brinjikji W, Dabus G, Raz E, et al. Mechanical thrombectomy of the foetal posterior cerebral artery. Stroke. 2021;1(1):115. https://doi.org/10.1161/svin.121.000115.

10. Albers GW, Marks MP, Kemp S, Christensen S, Tsai JP, Ortega-Gutierrez S, et al. Thrombectomy for stroke at 6 to 16 hours with selection by perfusion imaging. N Engl J Med. 2018;378(8):708–18. https://doi.org/10.1056/nejmoa1713973.
11. Nogueira RG, Jadhav AP, Haussen DC, Bonafe A, Budzik RF, Bhuva P, et al. Thrombectomy 6 to 24 hours after stroke with a mismatch between deficit and infarct. N Engl J Med. 2018;378(1):11–21. https://doi.org/10.1056/nejmoa1706442.
12. Maulaz AB, Bezerra DC, Bogousslavsky J. Posterior cerebral artery infarction from middle cerebral artery infarction. Arch Neurol. 2005;62(6):938. https://doi.org/10.1001/archneur.62.6.938.
13. Mann L, Preece R, Haslam L, Paravastu SCV, Bulbulia RA, Kulkarni SR. Posterior cerebral circulation stroke secondary to foetal origin of posterior communicating artery: an indication for carotid endarterectomy. EJVES Vasc Forum. 2020;50:7–11. https://doi.org/10.1016/j.ejvsvf.2020.12.022.
14. Yang JH, Choi H-Y, Nam HS, Kim SH, Han SW, Heo JH. Mechanism of infarction involving ipsilateral carotid and posterior cerebral artery territories. Cerebrovasc Dis. 2007;24(5):445–51. https://doi.org/10.1159/000108435.

Chapter 29
Thalamic Infarct and Beyond

Talal Al-Mayhani

A 57-year-old right-handed woman, with background of migraine, hypertension and hypercholesterolemia, was brought to the Emergency Stroke Unit (ESU) after her family found her confused on waking up in the morning. For 2 days prior to this presentation, she had had headache that was similar to her usual migraine, but was associated with non-specific numbness in the left hand.

Examination and Localization

The patient was brought to the ESU by ambulance and walked in without need for assistance. She was awake, and following commands, oriented to place, but not to time or person. She had word finding difficulty, was perseverating and struggled to recall the details of the history, with notable frustration.

There were athetotic movements and on and off dystonic posturing in the fingers of the outstretched left hand, along with left hemibody hypoaesthesia affecting the face, arm and leg. Right upper quadrantanopia was also detected. The vital signs were within normal range.

The examination findings raised the possibility of multifocal lesions: the left hemibody sensory loss localizes to the right thalamus and, less commonly, right parietal lobe (cortical sensory loss). The right upper quadrantanopia localizes to the optic radiation in the left temporal lobe, and the association with the encephalopathic picture of memory deficit further supports such localization.

T. Al-Mayhani (✉)
National Hospital for Neurology and Neurosurgery, London, UK
e-mail: talal.al-mayhani@nhs.net

S. K. Gill et al. (eds.), *Stroke Medicine*,
https://doi.org/10.1007/978-3-031-58188-5_29

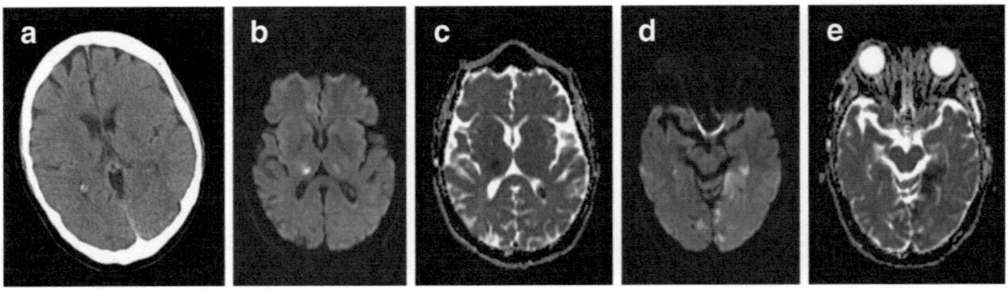

Fig. 29.1 (**a**) Axial CT head with no contrast showing small area of hypodensity in the right thalamus. An equivocal hypodensity can also be appreciated in the left occipital lobe. (**b**, **c**) Axial MRI head DWI and ADC sequences showing area of restricted diffusion in the right thalamus, indicating acute ischaemic lesion. (**d**, **e**) Axial MRI head DWI and ADC sequences showing multifocal areas of restricted diffusion in the left medial temporal lobe, and bilateral occipital lobes

Investigations and Management

The routine blood tests were unremarkable. The ECG showed a new and persistent atrial fibrillation. The plain CT head revealed an equivocal hypodensity in the right thalamus (Fig. 29.1a), and CT angiogram excluded large vessel occlusion. MRI head showed multifocal areas of restricted diffusion in the right thalamus (Fig. 29.1b, c) left medial temporal and bilateral occipital lobes (Fig. 29.1d, e). The patient was commenced initially on dual anti-platelets while she was an inpatient and then was discharged on apixaban.

Discussion

Historically, the thalamus was considered the seat of senses, while the striatum was the seat of motor function. Since Deuchene electrical experiments on the cerebral cortex, cortico-centrism has dominated the neuroscience [1]. Nowadays there is movement away from the thalamus as a "sensory station" to more central and active role in modulating and integrating the motor, sensory and cognitive functions.

Part of the diencephalon, the thalamic complex, in neuroanatomical terms, consists of a number of interlinked structures including the epithalamus, dorsal thalamus, metathalamus, ventral thalamus (including subthalamus) and hypothalamus [1]. It is important to note that the clinical "thalamus" that the clinicians usually refer to is in fact the neuroanatomical "dorsal thalamus", usually combined with the metathalamus (i.e. medial and lateral geniculate bodies). For simplicity and for the sake of this discussion, the term "thalamus" will be used in its common and clinical sense, rather than its neuroanatomical sense (i.e. dorsal thalamus). Although the details of the micro-neuroanatomical nomenclature can be different between different authorities, it is generally accepted that the thalamus is formed of complex of more than 35 nuclei, classified into 8 main groups (anterior, medial, lateral, etc.), the details of which are beyond the scope of this chapter. The interested reader, however, may consult the elegant description provided elsewhere [1, 2].

Clinically, the thalamus can be damaged by various pathologies (neoplastic, infective, etc.), including vascular ones: ischaemic stroke forming up to 4% of total cases cerebral ischaemic events, haemorrhagic stroke forming up to 3% of total cases of intracerebral bleeding, and rarely by cerebral deep venous thrombosis [3].

Briefly, there are 4 main thalamic vascular territories supplied by different arteries as follows [3, 4]:

- Polar artery (AKA. premammillary artery of Foix and Hillemand, tuberthalamic of Bogousslawsky): a branch of the posterior communicating artery. It can be absent in up to 40% of individuals. Stroke due to lesion in this artery results in anterior thalamic syndrome characterized by language and memory disturbance, abulia and apathy.
- Paramedian arteries (AKA. perforating, thalamo-subthalamic): a branch of the posterior cerebral artery (usually P1), it may co-supply the rostral midbrain and cerebellar peduncles. It may also have a unilateral stem in third of cases (artery of Percheron). Stroke due to lesion in paramedian arteries results in medial thalamic syndrome characterized by clouded consciousness (even coma), memory disturbance, abulia, apathy and vertical gaze palsy [4].
- Thalamogeniculate artery: a branch of the posterior cerebral artery (usually P2). Stroke due to lesion in this artery results in lateral thalamic syndrome characterized by sensory and motor dysfunction.
- Posterior choroidal artery: a branch of the posterior cerebral artery (usually P2). Stroke due to lesion in this artery results in posterior thalamic syndrome characterized by attention, visual and ocular motor dysfunction, speech disturbance, dystonia and amnesia.

The artery of Percheron, an anatomical variant, deserves a special discussion; as compromise of the blood supply through this artery can account for 4–18% of thalamic infarcts, and 0.1–2% of ischemic stroke [5]. The artery of Percheron ischaemic stroke affects usually the bilateral medial thalamic territories, with the classical triad of vertical gaze palsy (65% of patients), memory impairment (58% of patients) and fluctuating coma (42% of patients) [4].

The clinical presentation of thalamic stroke can be protean, and although it is plausible to talk about 4 broad syndromes that correspond to the vascular territories described above, the symptoms and signs do overlap and do vary. For instance, in the hyperacute stage, secondary vasogenic oedema may result in local dysfunction beyond the affected thalamic territory, and beyond the thalamus itself, leading to complex combination of clinical features.

Although classical features can raise suspicion of thalamic stroke such as hemihypesthaesia, involuntary movements (la main thalamique), thalamic astasia, anaesthaesia dolorosa and/or ophthalmoplegia (sunset sign in upgaze palsy), the clinical features may not follow the typical classical textbook description of stroke, meaning that many cases can easily be missed or misdiagnosed.

Due to the shared blood supply, the association of thalamic stroke with extra-thalamic infarcts within the posterior circulation territories is not uncommon.

The thalamus is closely interconnected with the limbic system via the mamillo-thalamic tract, and the anterior thalamus forms part of the historical circuit of Papez, along with well-established neural circuits connecting the thalami and the medial temporal lobes, with major involvement in memory [6]. The vascular supply of the medial temporal lobe derives from the posterior cerebral artery, with variable collaterals from the anterior circulation. In particular, the hippocampus formation is supplied by the anterior and posterior hippocampal arteries [7].

The prognosis of thalamic stroke is considered generally favourable, and many patients that present with disordered consciousness show reasonable recover. Some patients with thalamic stroke, however, may be left with element of memory dysfunction or ophthalmoplegia. Another notable complication is the development of central pain (Dejerine-Roussy syndrome) that can affect 7–25% of patients with ischaemic or haemorrhagic thalamic stroke, especially when the lateral territory supplied by the thalamogeniculate artery is occluded [1].

Clinical Key Learning Points

- The presentations of thalamic stroke can be subtle or difficult to recognize
- Thalamic infarcts can present with decreased level of arousal—especially when bilateral
- Post stroke pain can be persistent and difficult to manage

Radiology Key Learning Points

- Diffusion weighted MRI imaging with confirm ischaemic stroke when carried out in the 14 days post stroke onset
- There may be areas of ischaemia also seen in other areas of the posterior circulation e.g. occipital lobe

References

1. Jones EG. The thalamus. 2nd ed. Cambridge: Cambridge University Press; 2007.
2. Nieuwenhuys J, Voogd J, Huijzen C. The human central nervous system. 4th ed. New York: Springer; 2008.
3. Schmahmann JD. Vascular syndromes of the thalamus. Stroke. 2003;34(9):2264–78.
4. Reilly M, et al. Bilateral paramedian thalamic infarction: a distinct but poorly recognized stroke syndrome. QJM. 1992;82(1):63–70.
5. Lazarro N, et al. Artery of percheron infarction: imaging patterns and clinical spectrum. AJNR Am J Neuroradiol. 2010;31(7):1283–9.
6. Kafkas A, et al. Thalamic-medial temporal lobe connectivity underpins familiarity memory. Cereb Cortex. 2020;30(6):3827–37.
7. Powell R, Hughes T. A chamber of secrets. Pract Neurol. 2014;14(6):440–5.

Chapter 30
Beware the Basilar: A Case of Stuttering Stroke Symptoms and an Unusual Aftermath

Howell T. Jones and Fiona Humphries

Clinical History

A 60-year-old right-handed male retired computer programmer developed sudden onset dysarthria and left sided face, arm and leg weakness at home after a 2 days history of feeling less steady while walking and was brought by ambulance to the Emergency Stroke Unit at the National Hospital for Neurology and Neurosurgery. He had a past medical history of hypertension, hypercholesterolemia and type two diabetes mellitus and was previously independent and had normal mobility.

Examination

On initial assessment he was alert and orientated. His temperature was 37.0 °C, blood pressure 180/107 mmHg and his pulse was regular at 80 beats/min. His pupils were equal and reactive, eye movements were normal and visual fields full to confrontation. There was a left upper motor neurone seventh cranial nerve palsy and and he was dysarthric but not aphasic. There was mild weakness the left arm and leg with (MRC score 4) in a pyramidal distribution and both of these limbs were also ataxic. Deep tendon reflexes were present with reinforcement in all four limbs with an extensor plantar response on the left. Sensation was normal as was the remainder of the physical examination.

H. T. Jones · F. Humphries (✉)
Department of Stroke Medicine, The National Hospital for Neurology and Neurosurgery, London, UK
e-mail: howell.jones@nhs.net; fhumphries@nhs.net

S. K. Gill et al. (eds.), *Stroke Medicine*,
https://doi.org/10.1007/978-3-031-58188-5_30

Initial Investigations

Blood samples sent on arrival showed a microcytic anaemia with normal renal and liver profiles. Serum glucose was 30 mmol/L and subsequent HbA1c 134 mmol/mol. Electrocardiography illustrated normal sinus rhythm with left axis deviation and met the criteria for left ventricular hypertrophy. A plain CT brain demonstrated no evidence of acute infarction or haemorrhage. CT angiography showed non-significant stenosis of the carotids and a basilar artery that was small in calibre and difficult to visualise; this was thought to be constitutional due to bilateral foetal origin of the posterior cerebral arteries. His BP then rose to 230/120 mmHg and intravenous labetolol was given with the aim of administering tPA, however BP control was not achieved within the 4.5 h thrombolysis window. A dose of aspirin 300 mg was administered rectally and he was commenced on a variable rate insulin infusion.

Progression of the Case

One hour after initial assessment his symptoms progressed and he became anarthric with a dense left hemiparesis (MRC grade 1) and new weakness in the right leg (MRC grade 3). A repeat CT brain was undertaken which showed an ill-defined hypodensity within the brainstem in the region of the right pons. Eight hours later there was a further deterioration with dense bilateral facial weakness, anarthria and airway compromise with worsened bilateral lower limb weakness (now MRC grade 0 on the left and MRC grade 2 on the right) and plantar response was now extensor bilaterally.

Urgent MRI brain and MR angiogram of the intracranial and extracranial vessels demonstrated areas of restricted diffusion bilaterally in the pons in keeping with acute infarction (Fig. 30.1). The angiography demonstrated reduced signal at the transition of the V3/V4 segments of the left vertebral artery (Fig. 30.2) and the basilar artery demonstrated either reduced or absent flow. The newly diagnosed basilar thrombus was discussed with interventional neuroradiology colleagues and the decision was made not to proceed with mechanical thrombectomy. Anticoagulation with a treatment dose of low molecular weight heparin (Enoxaparin) based on weight was commenced and aspirin was stopped. The low molecular weight heparin was split into twice daily dosing to reduce risk of bleeding.

During the proceeding 12 h the patient demonstrated markedly worsening bulbar weakness signs of aspiration pneumonia. He became hypoxic and was commenced on high-flow nasal cannula (HFNC) oxygen and antibiotic therapy. The following day he required admission to the intensive care unit (ICU) and was intubated. It was felt that his profound bilateral bulbar weakness would prevent successful extubation so a percutaneous tracheostomy was inserted on the second day of admission without complication and he was stepped down to the stroke ward four days later.

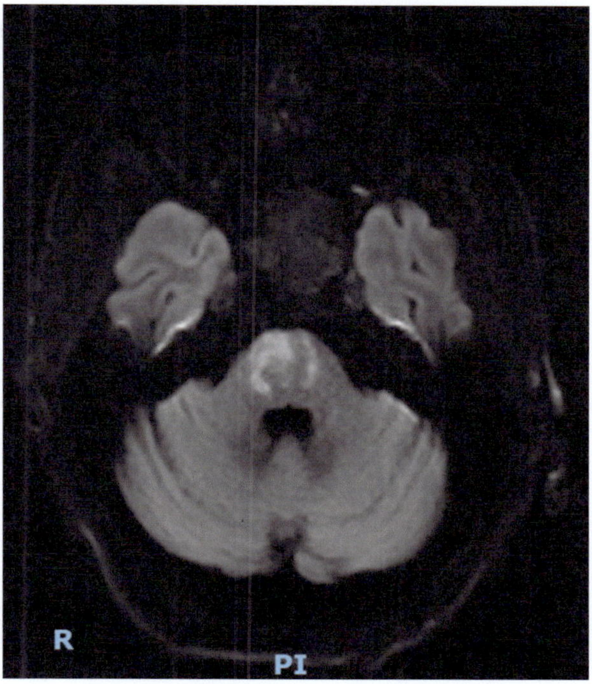

Fig. 30.1 DWI axial image showing bilateral acute pontine infarcts

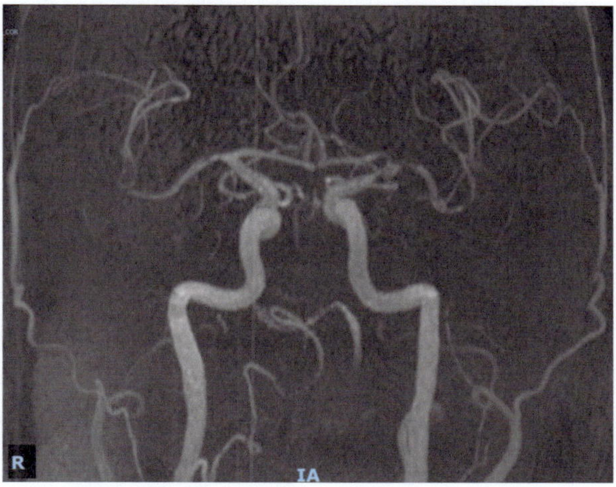

Fig. 30.2 MRA TOF image illustrating reduced signal at left V3/V4 consistent with acute thrombus

He underwent repeat CT angiography which showed the ongoing presence of clot in the basilar artery so anticoagulation was continued for a total of three weeks until serial CT angiography demonstrated recanalization of the vessel. Following this he was managed with three weeks of dual antiplatelet therapy with aspirin and clopidogrel followed by long term clopidogrel monotherapy.

An Unexpected Complication

Soon after stepdown to the stroke ward he began to report abdominal discomfort and rectal pain and defaecation and passing flatus. The rectum was empty on digital examination and bowel movements were small and infrequent despite a combination of stimulant and osmotic laxatives. A catheter had been placed in the bladder on admission and was then removed but that patient went into acute urinary retention so a catheter was reinserted. Following this procedure the patient reported worsening rectal pain and was treated empirically with antibiotics for a urinary tract infection. When symptoms did not improve an ultrasound of the abdomen was undertaken which showed no evidence of abscess formation or obstruction of the kidneys, ureters or bladder but did show an enlarged prostate (35 cc) and after discussion with the urology team a decision was made to commence antibiotics for prostatitis. Despite antimicrobials the patient required increasing doses of opioid analgesia to manage the pain and underwent MRI which excluded a prostatic abscess but demonstrated a dilated rectum of a maximum 8 cm in the anteroposterior plane compatible with neurogenic megarectum.

He was initiated on a neurogenic bowel management regimen involving oral laxatives and rectal suppositions but he developed bilious vomiting. An abdominal X-ray (Fig. 30.3) and subsequent CT scan of the abdomen showed marked faecal loading in the large bowel and distension of the entire small bowel and a diagnosis of acute colonic pseudo-obstruction was made. Advice was sought from the general surgeons and he was managed with a total dose of 2 mg neostigmine with good effect.

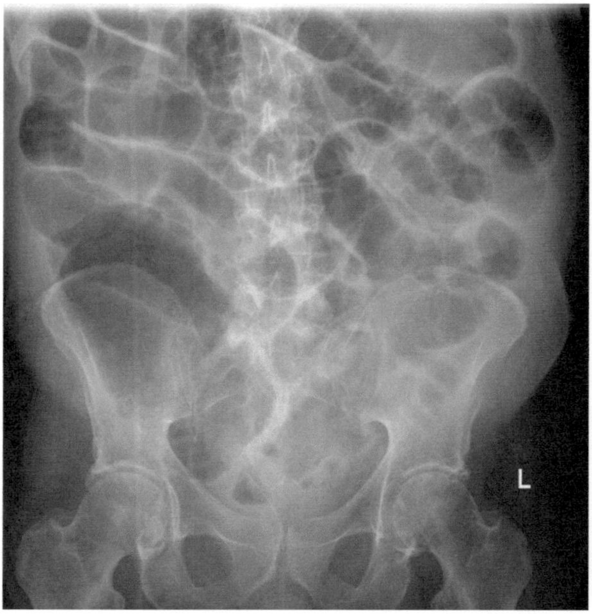

Fig. 30.3 Abdominal X-ray demonstrating signs of acute colonic pseudo-obstruction with dilated bowel loops

Discussion

Basilar Artery Occlusion Syndrome

Strokes affecting the posterior circulation account for 20% of ischaemic strokes and basilar artery occlusion (BAO) make up only 1–4% of ischaemic stroke cases [1].

Clinical Presentation

While ischaemic strokes affecting the anterior circulation typically present with an acute onset of focal symptoms patients with BAO can present in an acute and subacute fashion and may have a prolonged prodromal phase.

Acute BAO symptoms tend to present as a combination of focal motor weakness such as hemiparesis or quadriparesis with altered consciousness [2]. Around half of patients have brainstem signs such as truncal or appendicular ataxia, pupillary abnormalities, nystagmus, extraocular movement abnormalities, hearing loss or pseudobulbar manifestations such as facial palsy, dysphonia, dysarthria, and dysphagia [2]. One of the most feared consequences of BAO is that of 'locked-in syndrome' where bilateral pontine infarction results in a paralysed patient with only limited vertical eye movement and a mortality rate of 75% [3].

In contrast to anterior circulation stroke syndromes BAO can present with symptoms that evolve over hours to days and can be described as insidious or stuttering in nature. Patients with BAO may initially present with an isolated hemiplegia prior to developing brainstem signs or a decreased level of consciousness in a syndrome that this has been dubbed 'herald hemiparesis' [4].

Another important feature of BAO is that many patients report recurrent prodromal symptoms in the days to weeks before their stroke with shortening periods of latency as the stroke looms [5, 6]. The most commonly reported prodromal symptoms are vertigo and nausea followed by headache and neck pain [7, 8]. Other symptoms may include visual loss or diplopia, dysarthria, ataxia, transient limb weakness or numbness or even unilateral or bilateral jerking or posturing episodes that may be mislabelled as epileptiform in nature [7–9].

Aetiology

The aetiology of BAO can be atherosclerosis, thromboembolism or vascular dissection. Atherosclerosis and embolic disease both can affect the vertebrobasilar junction, the mid portion of the basilar is most commonly affected by atherosclerosis, whilst emboli tend to lodge in the distal third particularly at the top of the basilar artery [1]. Dissection tends to occur in the extracranial vertebral arteries and rarely affects the intracranial vessels [1]. Rarer causes of BAO may include vasculitides such as Behçet's, infections such as neurospyhillis, and damage to vessels due to cervical spine or basal skull fracture or cervical instability [10–13], and a proportion of cases remain cryptogenic [1].

Imaging

Rapid access to neuroimaging is essential in cases of suspected BAO to establish the location of the vascular occlusion and to determine whether suitability for hyperacute treatments such as tPA and mechanical thrombectomy.

The gold standard imaging to confirm BAO is cerebral catheter angiography but is now rarely used as a diagnostic technique due to its invasive nature and improved access to non-invasive angiography [1]. CT head (CTH) is the first imaging modality of choice and its primary purpose in BAO cases is to exclude haemorrhage as its sensitivity for detecting ischemia in the posterior fossa is low. In 50–70% of BAO cases CTH will demonstrate a hyperdense basilar artery, though the sensitivity and specificity of this sign are low [14–16] and if BAO is suspected CT angiography of the intracranial and extracranial neck vessels is recommended [17]. Current recommendations state that CT angiography should not be delayed to await renal function in patients with no history of renal dysfunction as to not delay potential hyperacute treatments [17].

MRI is the best imaging modality for confirming an acute stroke in the posterior fossa with diffusion-weighted imaging (DWI) sequencing often demonstrating acute ischaemia within seconds of arterial occlusion [18–20]. Nevertheless, it is important to note that DWI negative strokes are twice as likely in the posterior circulation compared to the anterior circulation and clinical reasoning should take precedence in such cases [20]. MR angiography can illustrate the site of vascular occlusion non-invasively [18] and cerebral microbleeds seen on gradient recalled echo (GRE-T2*) or susceptibility weighted imaging (SWI) MRI sequences may point towards an underlying aetiology that affects the small and large vessels concurrently such as hypertension [18, 19].

Doppler ultrasound of the vertebral arteries can only comment on the presence and direction of blood flow and is less sensitive than both CT or MR angiography with limted use in BAO [18, 19, 21, 22].

In summary, prompt CT and CT angiography of the head and neck vessels should be undertaken in patients with suspected BAO. If inconclusive and the clinical suspicion remains high acute MRI and MR angiography should be considered.

Management

BAO is a potentially life threatening condition and patients should be managed in a dedicated stroke centre that includes interventional neuroradiology, neurosurgery and neurointensive care. Successful management of BAO requires a multidisciplinary approach with medical, nursing, physiotherapy, occupational therapy, speech and language therapy, dietetics and neuropsychology input from the start of the patient stroke journey.

Hyperacute treatments include intravenous thrombolysis (IVT), intra-arterial thrombolysis (IAT) and mechanical thrombectomy (MT). IVT is recommended in BAO within 4.5 h of symptoms and meet the required inclusion/exclusion criteria as it increases recanalization rates and reduce morbidity and mortality [17, 23]. IAT also improves recanalization and reduces morbidity and mortality although is much less commonly administered [17, 24]. MT is recommended for patients with large vessel occlusion who present up to 6 h after the onset of symptoms and who meet other relevant criteria, but in in BAO MT may be offered up to 24 h after the onset of symptoms, although the evidence for MT in BAO is less prominent than in anterior circulation stroke [17, 25, 26]. In patients who do not meet criteria for IVT or MT then treatment with high dose antiplatelet therapy such as aspirin or clopidogrel should be commenced [17].

The presence of a free floating thrombus (FFT) on CT or MR angiography in the context of BAO presents a management challenge. There have been no randomised controlled trials comparing standard antiplatelet therapy with anticoagulation, but data demonstrate that the latter is often used in both carotid and posterior circulation FFT despite the lack of evidence to support this management strategy [17, 27].

Patients with BAO are particularly sensitive to fluctuations in blood pressure and generally blood pressure should only be controlled if there is a strong indication such as post tPA management, and intravenous fluids or even vasopressors may be required should neurological symptoms be blood pressure dependant [1]. After the hyperacute phase blood pressure should be optimised slowly over weeks rather than days as secondary prevention [17].

Patients with BAO are at risk of airway compromise due to reduced consciousness level or diaphragmatic involvement and may require intubation or tracheostomy insertion to allow for mechanical ventilation [28]. They should also be monitored for signs of raised intracranial pressure due to cerebellar or brainstem oedema causing compression of the fourth ventricle, which typically peaks at day three to five after infarction and may require neurosurgical intervention in selected cases [1].

The acute phase of management of BAO mirrors that of other stroke syndromes with investigations to determine the aetiology such as bloodwork including full blood count, coagulation screen, fasting lipids and glycated haemoglobin A1c [17]. Patients should also undergo cardiac investigations such as an electrocardiogram to evaluate for atrial fibrillation and if normal to consider either continuous cardiac monitoring as well an echocardiogram (+/-bubble study) to assess for cardiac causes of emboli such as patent foramen ovalve, intraventricular thrombi or masses or valvular vegetations [17]. Anticoagulation should be considered at an appropriate time should a relevant indication such as atrial fibrillation be identified [17]. Other investigations for rarer causes should be tailored on a case by case basis. The remainder of focus following BAO is as with any stroke on rehabilitation and patient goal setting with an aim or regaining function and managing disability.

Prognosis

BAO has a high morbidity and mortality rate with a mortality rate of up to 80% if left untreated and 40% even if recanalization is achieved [23, 29]. For those patients who survive around two thirds will have persistent severe deficits with only 30% of patients who receive hyperacute IVT or IAT regaining a good level of function [23, 29].

Complications such as infections particularly aspiration pneumonia, thrombo-embolic disease, contractures, pressure ulcers, bladder or bowel dysfunction and depression are common [30]. The risk of recurrent stroke is between 10% and 15% [31].

A Brief Overview of Neurogenic Bowel

Neurogenic bowel refers to loss of the normal sensory and/or motor function of the bowel due to either a central or peripheral neurological cause resulting in colonic dysfunction [32]. Three forms are recognised depending on the location of the neural pathway disruption; reflex neurogenic bowel from an upper motor neuron type lesion; areflexic or flaccid from a lower motor neuron type lesion; or mixed [32, 33].

Pontine infarcts can disrupt the sympathetic and parasympathetic pathways responsible for defaecation causing the reflex or upper motor neuron form of neurogenic bowel resulting in impairment of both the co-ordination of peristaltic waves and the relaxation of the external sphincter and pelvic floor muscles [33–36].

Neurogenic bowel primarily causes constipation, ranging from simple constipation to more serious manifestations such as faecal impaction, acute colonic pseudo-obstruction or the chronic complication of megacolon/megarectum. Constipation can in turn lead to haemorrhoids, anal fissures and tears, rectal prolapse, faecal incontinence and [37].

Acute colonic pseudo-obstruction (ACPO) is also known as by its eponymous name Ogilvie syndrome after British surgeon William Heneage Ogilvie was first described in 1948 [38]. ACPO is a condition where gross dilatation of the colon is present in the absence of mechanical obstruction and is typically seen in older people following surgery or those with underling neurological, infectious or inflammatory conditions, though its pathophysiology is still unclear [39]. The diagnosis can prove difficult and is often based upon clinical and radiological evidence, with early recognition required to avoid serious complications such as colonic ischemia or perforation [40].

The management for ACPO is broad and ranges from gastric and rectal decompression, intravenous hydration and electrolyte correction and treating any underlying condition, through to medical, endoscopic and surgical interventions [39, 40]. One medical therapy is the drug neostigmine.

Neostigmine and Its Role in the Management of Acute Colonic Pseudo-Obstruction

Neostigmine is a reversible acetylcholinesterase inhibitor that inhibits the hydrolysis of acetylcholine whilst also stimulating nicotinic and muscarinic receptors to produce contraction in the colonic smooth muscle and increased peristalsis and is administered in intravenous form [41]. A recent meta-analysis of four studies (127 patients) showed that neostigmine was effective in resolving ACPO with only one dose in 89.2% of cases compared to 14.65% of controls ($P < 0.001$, NNT = 1 [95% CI 1–2]) [42].

Side effects of neostigmine include bronchospasm, bradycardia and hypotension and cardiac monitoring is recommended. It should only be administered where immediate medical support is available and note should be taken that atropine can be administered if significant bradycardia occurs [39]. Patients who are potentially at higher risk of side effects are those with a history of bronchospasm, ischemic heart disease, chronic kidney disease or who are on beta blocker therapy [43]. Risks can be reduced by opting for an infusion of neostigmine as opposed to an intravenous bolus and using lower starting doses in those with the aforementioned risk factors [43].

In summary neostigmine is an approved treatment in patients with ACPO and the benefit from one or two doses often outweighs the potential risks and it should be considered for patients who develop ACPO following pontine stroke [39].

Key Clinical Learning Points

- Whilst some patients with BAO may present with acute motor and bulbar dysfunction patients may present with stuttering symptoms over hours to days.
- Patients with BAO may first present with unilateral weakness and then progress to include brainstem signs or reduced consciousness. This is known as a herald hemiparesis.
- Other prodromal symptoms include neck pain, headache, dizziness, diplopia, dysarthria or ataxia.
- The aetiology of BAO can be atherosclerosis, thromboembolism or vascular dissection, and the location of the BAO can be helpful in determining the most likely mechanism of occlusion
- IVT and IAT have been shown to reduce morbidity and mortality in patients with BAO. The evidence for MT in BAO is less strong than for anterior circulation large vessel occlusion but it can be considered up to 12–24 h after the onset of symptoms due to the significant mortality associated with BAO.
- BAO can result in the development of neurogenic bowel due damage to the pontine defaecation centre
- For patients who develop acute colonic pseudo-obstruction as a result of neurogenic bowel a neostigmine infusion is typically a safe and effective treatment.

Key Radiological Learning Points

- CT remains the first line investigation for patients presenting with symptoms of BAO in order to exclude haemorrhage or other pathology. However, it is vital to remember that CT imaging is less sensitive in detecting early ischemia in the posterior fossa.
- Early use of CT angiography is recommended to detect a filling defect within the basilar artery for patients presenting with symptoms of BAO as the presence of a hyperdense basilar artery on plain CT has poor sensitivity and specificity.
- MRI remains the best modality for assessing ischaemia in the posterior fossa as diffusion-weighted imaging (DWI) can detect acute brainstem or cerebellar infarction within seconds of arterial occlusion. Therefore rapid access to MR imaging in cases of suspected BAO is paramount if CT imaging is non diagnostic.
- Constipation is common following a stroke, and patients with pontine strokes are at risk of neurogenic bowel. For those with significant pain or symptoms of intestinal obstruction there should be a low threshold for abdominal imaging to exclude acute colonic pseudo-obstruction.

References

1. Demel SL, Broderick JP. Basilar occlusion syndromes: an update. Neurohospitalist. 2015;5(3):142–50.
2. Ausman JI, Liebeskind DS, Gonzalez N, Saver J, Martin N, Villablanca JP, et al. A review of the diagnosis and management of vertebral basilar (posterior) circulation disease. Surg Neurol Int. 2018;9:106.
3. Nikić PM, Jovanović D, Paspalj D, Georgievski-Brkić B, Savić M. Clinical characteristics and outcome in the acute phase of ischemic locked-in syndrome: case series of twenty patients with ischemic LIS. Eur Neurol. 2013;69(4):207–12.
4. Fisher CM. The 'herald hemiparesis' of basilar artery occlusion. Arch Neurol. 1988;45(12):1301–3.
5. Voetsch B, DeWitt LD, Pessin MS, Caplan LR. Basilar artery occlusive disease in the New England Medical Center Posterior Circulation Registry. Arch Neurol. 2004;61(4):496–504.
6. Ferbert A, Brückmann H, Drummen R. Clinical features of proven basilar artery occlusion. Stroke. 1990;21(8):1135–42.
7. Grad A, Baloh RW. Vertigo of vascular origin. Clinical and electronystagmographic features in 84 cases. Arch Neurol. 1989;46(3):281–4.
8. Savitz SI, Caplan LR. Vertebrobasilar disease. N Engl J Med. 2005;352(25):2618–26.
9. Ropper AH. 'Convulsions' in basilar artery occlusion. Neurology. 1988;38(9):1500–1.
10. Akman-Demir G, Serdaroglu P, Tasçi B. Clinical patterns of neurological involvement in Behçet's disease: evaluation of 200 patients. The Neuro-Behçet Study Group. Brain. 1999;122(11):2171–82.
11. Oshima K, Sakaura H, Iwasaki M, Nakura A, Fujii R, Yoshikawa H. Repeated vertebrobasilar thromboembolism in a patient with severe upper cervical instability because of rheumatoid arthritis. Spine J. 2011;11(2):1–5.

12. Sugrue PA, Hage ZA, Surdell DL, Foroohar M, Liu J, Bendok BR. Basilar artery occlusion following C1 lateral mass fracture managed by mechanical and pharmacological thrombolysis. Neurocrit Care. 2009;11(2):255–60.
13. Bäuerle J, Zitzmann A, Egger K, Meckel S, Weiller C, Harloff A. The great imitator–still today! A case of meningovascular syphilis affecting the posterior circulation. J Stroke Cerebrovasc Dis. 2015;24(1):1–3.
14. Connell L, Koerte IK, Laubender RP, Morhard D, Linn J, Becker HC, et al. Hyperdense basilar artery sign-a reliable sign of basilar artery occlusion. Neuroradiology. 2012;54(4):321–7.
15. Goldmakher GV, Camargo EC, Furie KL, Singhal AB, Roccatagliata L, Halpern EF, et al. Hyperdense basilar artery sign on unenhanced CT predicts thrombus and outcome in acute posterior circulation stroke. Stroke. 2009;40(1):134–9.
16. Mortimer AM, Saunders T, Cook JL. Cross-sectional imaging for diagnosis and clinical outcome prediction of acute basilar artery thrombosis. Clin Radiol. 2011;66(6):551–8.
17. Powers WJ, Rabinstein AA, Ackerson T, Adeoye OM, Bambakidis NC, Becker K, et al. Guidelines for the early management of patients with acute ischemic stroke: 2019 update to the 2018 guidelines for the early management of acute ischemic stroke: a guideline for healthcare professionals from the American Heart Association/American Stroke Association. Stroke. 2019;50(12):e344–418.
18. Campbell BC, Parsons MW. Imaging selection for acute stroke intervention. Int J Stroke. 2018;13(6):554–67.
19. Safdarian M, Rohani M. Basilar artery thrombosis on brain MRI. Neurohospitalist. 2018;8(3):3.
20. Simonsen CZ, Madsen MH, Schmitz ML, Mikkelsen IK, Fisher M, Andersen G. Sensitivity of diffusion- and perfusion-weighted imaging for diagnosing acute ischemic stroke is 97.5%. Stroke. 2015;46(1):98–101.
21. Biedert S, Winter R, Staudacher T, Betz H, Reuther R. Doppler sonography in basilar artery occlusion. Neuroradiology. 1985;27(5):430–3.
22. Sugrue G, O'Reilly MK, Byrne D, Crockett MT, Murphy S, Kavanagh EC. CT cervicocerebral angiography in acute stroke. Can we justify aortic arch imaging? Ir J Med Sci. 2019;188(2):661–6.
23. Schonewille WJ, Wijman CA, Michel P, Rueckert CM, Weimar C, Mattle HP, et al. Treatment and outcomes of acute basilar artery occlusion in the Basilar Artery International Cooperation Study (BASICS): a prospective registry study. Lancet Neurol. 2009;8(8):724–30.
24. Smith WS. Intra-arterial thrombolytic therapy for acute basilar occlusion: pro. Stroke. 2007;38(2):701–3.
25. Singer OC, Berkefeld J, Nolte CH, Bohner G, Haring HP, Trenkler J, et al. Mechanical recanalization in basilar artery occlusion: the ENDOSTROKE study. Ann Neurol. 2015;77(3):415–24.
26. Kwak HS, Park JS. Mechanical thrombectomy in basilar artery occlusion: clinical outcomes related to posterior circulation collateral score. Stroke. 2020;51(7):2045–50.
27. Bhatti AF, Leon LR Jr, Labropoulos N, Rubinas TL, Rodriguez H, Kalman PG, et al. Free-floating thrombus of the carotid artery: literature review and case reports. J Vasc Surg. 2007;45(1):199–205.
28. Bösel J. Use and timing of tracheostomy after severe stroke. Stroke. 2017;48(9):2638–43.
29. Schonewille WJ, Algra A, Serena J, Molina CA, Kappelle LJ. Outcome in patients with basilar artery occlusion treated conventionally. J Neurol Neurosurg Psychiatry. 2005;76(9):1238–41.
30. Langhorne P, Stott DJ, Robertson L, MacDonald J, Jones L, McAlpine C, et al. Medical complications after stroke: a multicenter study. Stroke. 2000;31(6):1223–9.
31. Chen CJ, Chuang TY, Hansen L, Dutta S, Ding D, Buell TJ, et al. Predictors of 30-day mortality after endovascular mechanical thrombectomy for acute ischemic stroke. J Clin Neurosci. 2018;57:38–42.
32. Chung EA, Emmanuel AV. Gastrointestinal symptoms related to autonomic dysfunction following spinal cord injury. Prog Brain Res. 2006;152:317–33.
33. Emmanuel A. Neurogenic bowel dysfunction. F1000Res. 2019;8:800.

34. Camilleri M, Bharucha AE. Gastrointestinal dysfunction in neurologic disease. Semin Neurol. 1996;16(3):203–16.
35. Krogh K, Mosdal C, Laurberg S. Gastrointestinal and segmental colonic transit times in patients with acute and chronic spinal cord lesions. Spinal Cord. 2000;38(10):615–21.
36. Nino-Murcia M, Stone JM, Chang PJ, Perkash I. Colonic transit in spinal cord-injured patients. Investig Radiol. 1990;25(2):109–12.
37. Musco S, Bazzocchi G, Martellucci J, Amato MP, Manassero A, Putignano D, et al. Treatments in neurogenic bowel dysfunctions: evidence reviews and clinical recommendations in adults. Eur J Phys Rehabil Med. 2020;56(6):741–55.
38. Ogilvie H. Large-intestine colic due to sympathetic deprivation; a new clinical syndrome. Br Med J. 1948;2(4579):671–3.
39. De Giorgio R, Knowles CH. Acute colonic pseudo-obstruction. Br J Surg. 2009;96(3):229–39.
40. Saunders MD. Acute colonic pseudo-obstruction. Best Pract Res Clin Gastroenterol. 2007;21(4):671–87.
41. De Giorgio R, Barbara G, Stanghellini V, Tonini M, Vasina V, Cola B, et al. Review article: The pharmacological treatment of acute colonic pseudo-obstruction. Aliment Pharmacol Ther. 2001;15(11):1717–27.
42. Valle RGL, Godoy FL. Neostigmine for acute colonic pseudo-obstruction: a meta-analysis. Ann Med Surg. 2014;3(3):60–4.
43. Delgado-Aros S, Camilleri M. Pseudo-obstruction in the critically ill. Best Pract Res Clin Gastroenterol. 2003;17(3):427–44.

Chapter 31
An Unusual PRESentation of Stroke

Kerala L. Adams-Carr, Jon Kennedy, and Robert F. Miller

History

A 55-year-old woman with a background of essential tremor and HIV, on antiretroviral therapy, was admitted from clinic with progressive visual disturbance that had started the evening before. She described that she was able to detect someone's presence in front of her but was unable to see them. She could use her phone but took some time to identify the correct numbers when dialling. Her partner reported that she had been bumping into objects on her left-hand side.

The day prior to her presentation she had been discharged from her local hospital where she had been an inpatient for 5 days. She had been admitted with abdominal pain and had a generalised tonic-clonic seizure later that day. She had investigations including a CT head, lumbar puncture, and an MRI brain, and was treated with levetiracetam. During this period she reported a mild occipital headache, and supine blood pressure at times was noted to rise to over 200/100. She was started on amlodipine. Her blood pressure readings stabilised and she was discharged home.

Her HIV diagnosis had been made 18 months prior, at which time she had a viral load of 167,000 with a CD4 count of 5. She commenced antiretroviral therapy (Descovy and dolutegravir, later Truvada and dolutegravir). Abdominal imaging detected multifocal retroperitoneal and mesenteric lymphadenopathy. Multidrug resistant *Mycobacterium kansasii* was cultured from her sputum, and *Mycobacterium avium* complex (MAC) from a lymph node biopsy. She was treated for these non-tuberculous mycobacterial (NTM) infections with 18 months of antimicrobials. Treatment was complicated by recurrent paradoxical reactions (immune

K. L. Adams-Carr (✉) · J. Kennedy · R. F. Miller
Royal Free Hospital, Royal Free London NHS Foundation Trust, University College London, London, UK
e-mail: kerala.adams-carr1@nhs.net; jonathan.kennedy@nhs.net; robert.miller@ucl.ac.uk

S. K. Gill et al. (eds.), *Stroke Medicine*,
https://doi.org/10.1007/978-3-031-58188-5_31

reconstitution inflammatory syndrome: IRIS) with fever, abdominal pain, and lymph node enlargement. These were managed with tapering courses of prednisolone. She stopped steroids 5 weeks prior to admission, and completed NTM treatment 2 weeks prior. She was taking co-trimoxazole prophylaxis.

Examination

On examination fundoscopy was normal and pupils were equal and reactive to light. Visual acuity was reduced to 6/24 on the right and 6/48 on the left. She had a left homonymous hemianopia. She also had evidence of oculomotor apraxia, using a head thrust to generate horizontal saccades; and optic ataxia, greater on the left than the right. On further cognitive testing she was found to have intact object and face recognition but neglected objects on the left side. She had difficulty recognising the beach scene but was able to describe it in parts, suggestive of simultanagnosia. She was unable to do simple subtractions and exhibited left-right disorientation and finger agnosia. She had dressing apraxia and ideomotor apraxia, worse on the left than right. She was able to read single words but not sentences. Upper and lower limb examination revealed a bilateral upper limb postural and action tremor and a no-no head tremor, in keeping with her longstanding history of essential tremor. Gait was unsteady and she struggled to tandem walk. The remainder of her neurological examination was normal, with symmetrically present reflexes and downgoing plantars.

In summary, she exhibited features of Balint and Gerstmann syndromes, a left homonymous hemianopia, left sided neglect, and an ataxic gait.

Investigations

Blood tests were within normal ranges except for a longstanding lymphopenia and mildly deranged liver function. Electrolytes including calcium and magnesium were normal. HIV viral load remained undetectable and CD4 count was 58.

CT head (Fig. 31.1) on admission showed bilateral white matter hypoattenuation within the parietal and occipital lobes. There was involvement of the cortex in the right parietal lobe and both occipital lobes. CT venogram showed no evidence of venous sinus thrombosis, and intracranial CT angiogram showed incidental aplasia of the right anterior cerebral artery, but no evidence of dissection, thrombus, or focal vessel narrowing.

An MRI head (Fig. 31.2) demonstrated high T2 signal in the white matter of the parieto-occipital lobes bilaterally with cortical involvement in the right parietal and occipital lobes. There was high signal on diffusion weighted imaging (DWI) (Fig. 31.3) and corresponding low apparent diffusion coefficient (ADC) values within the right superior frontal lobe, the right occipital lobe, and the right cerebellar hemisphere suggestive of acute ischaemic infarcts.

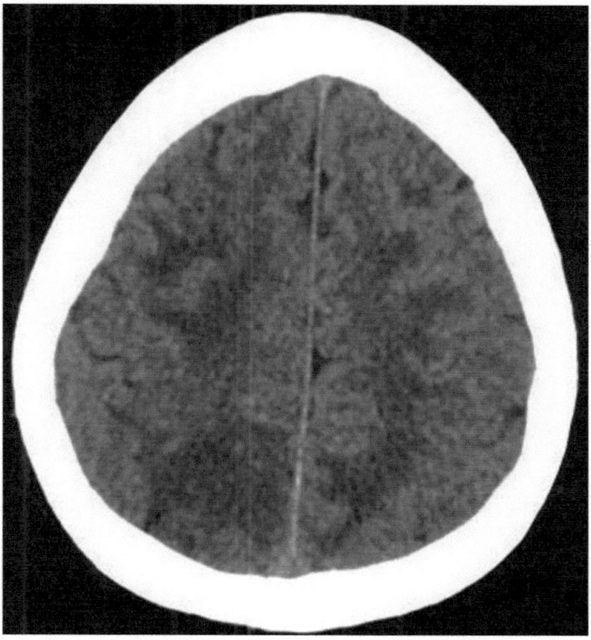

Fig. 31.1 CT head on admission demonstrating hypoattenuation within predominantly white matter, but with cortical involvement in the right occipital region

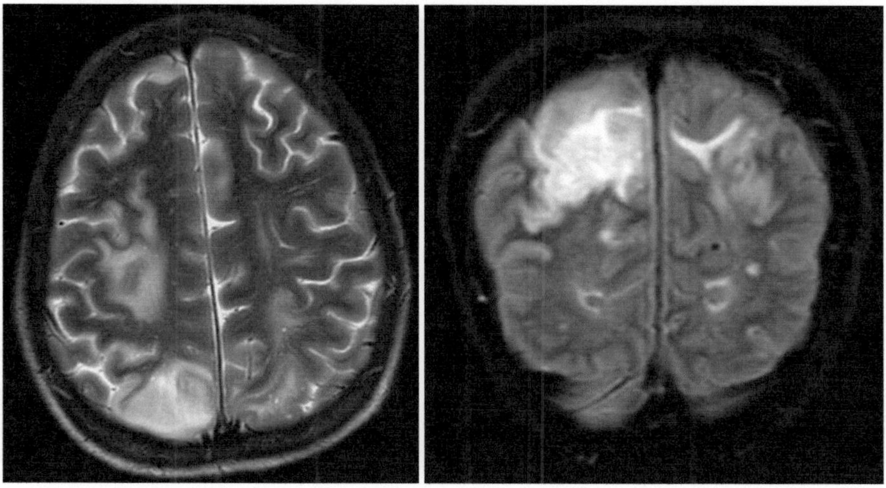

Fig. 31.2 T2 axial images showing hyperintensity within the white matter of the parietal and occipital regions, greater on the right than left. Additional cortical involvement seen in the right occipital lobe. Coronal section

A lumbar puncture showed a normal opening pressure of 7, and was acellular (wcc < 1) with a normal CSF/serum glucose ratio (3.1/5.3) and protein of 0.46. Acid-fast bacilli were not seen. John Cunningham (JC) virus, VZV, HSV-1 and 2, CMV, EBV, parechovirus and enterovirus were not detected with PCR testing.

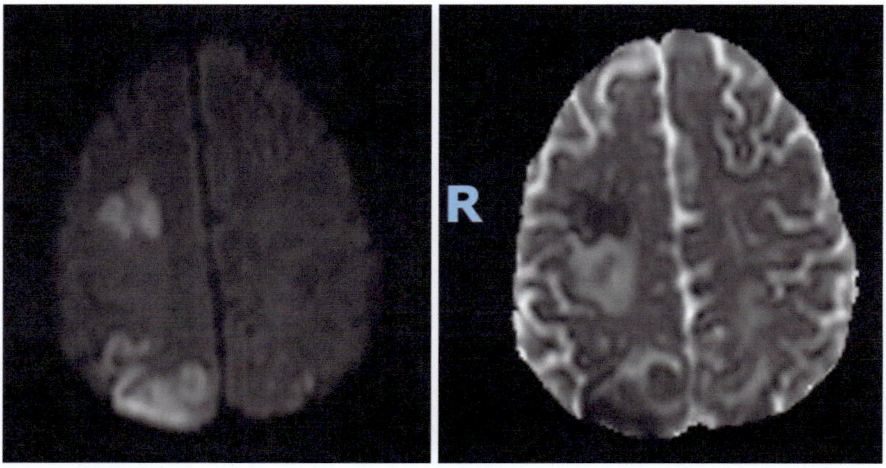

Fig. 31.3 DWI axial section on the left, and ADC on the right. Acute infarction demonstrated within the right frontal and occipital lobes

Oligoclonal bands were positive in the CSF and negative in the serum. CSF cytology was normal.

CT abdomen and pelvis with contrast demonstrated a peripherally enhancing collection in the left psoas muscle and low attenuation retroperitoneal lymph nodes. These were biopsied under CT guidance and histology demonstrated a reactive histiocyte-rich inflammatory process with no Acid-fast bacilli seen and no microorganisms grown on culture. Bacterial 16s and fungal 18s ribosomal RNA PCR were negative.

Investigations for secondary hypertension took place including renal Doppler and MR angiogram of the renal arteries, which excluded renal artery stenosis. A 9am cortisol was normal (355), as were thyroid function tests and plasma catecholamines. Urinary catecholamines showed an isolated abnormality of a mildly raised normetadrenaline level (3.52 micromol/24 h), which was thought not to be significant but will be repeated. A transthoracic echocardiogram was normal.

Clinical Course

A follow up MRI brain scan with contrast 2 weeks later showed improving T2 signal changes with resolution of DWI restriction. There was gyriform enhancement within the right frontal and occipital lobes and bilateral parietal lobes (Fig. 31.4).

Blood pressure stabilised with amlodipine and this was then weaned as propranolol was introduced, given it had previously proven an effective treatment for her essential tremor.

Clinically she improved during her admission and was discharged after 2 weeks. On follow up 1 month later she felt almost back to baseline but was aware of some

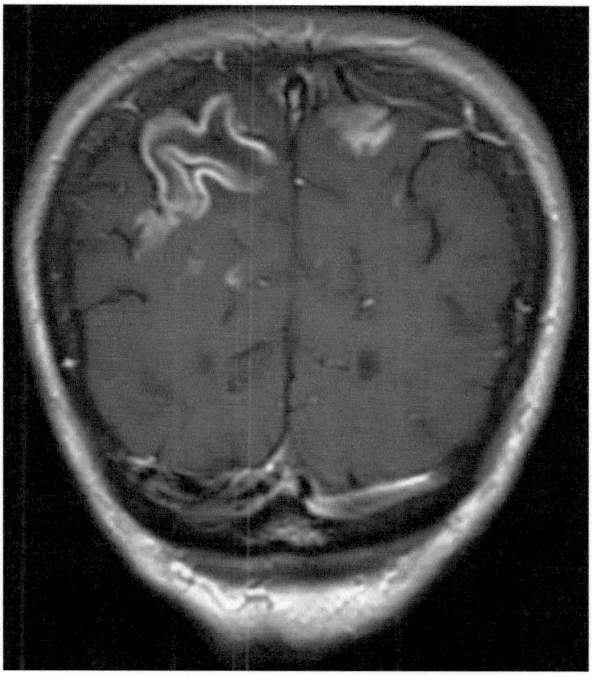

Fig. 31.4 MRI brain, T1 post gadolinium contrast, coronal view. Gyriform enhancement seen within the right parietal lobe

difficulties with vision on the left. She had a persistent left homonymous hemianopia on examination.

Discussion

Posterior reversible encephalopathy syndrome (PRES), or reversible posterior leukoencephalopathy syndrome (RPLS), was first comprehensively described in a 1996 case series [1]. It constitutes a clinical and radiological syndrome of subacute onset, most commonly precipitated by hypertension or cytotoxic medications. It typically presents with headache, visual changes, altered consciousness and seizures, with MRI features of vasogenic oedema affecting predominantly the white matter of the posterior parietal and occipital lobes. Changes can also occur within the frontal and temporal lobes, basal ganglia, cerebellum, and brainstem. The original case series described a fully reversible syndrome without cerebral infarction. However, although rare, it is now understood that PRES can progress to ischaemic infarction, as in this case, or haemorrhage. These complications account for much of the morbidity associated with the condition.

Hypertension is the most common precipitant of PRES, present in around 80% of cases [1, 2]. When blood pressure is acutely raised beyond the limits of cerebral autoregulation, it is proposed that hyperperfusion occurs with increased capillary hydrostatic pressure leading to extravasation of fluid and vasogenic oedema [3]. In cases such as this, where hypertension appears to follow the onset of symptoms, it may occur as a secondary consequence of end organ hypoperfusion in a Cushing-like response to increase perfusion pressure [4].

There have been multiple case reports of PRES in patients with HIV, often in the presence of other possible precipitants such as raised blood pressure, sepsis or renal dysfunction. However, HIV infection may play an independent role in the pathogenesis of PRES, a theory supported by two case reports in which HIV was the only identified risk factor [5, 6]. It is proposed that altered immune system function in HIV may contribute to endothelial dysfunction through activated T cells and cytokine release. Although antiretroviral therapy suppresses viral load and improves endothelial dysfunction, abnormal levels of cerebrovascular reactivity and systemic inflammation are thought to persist [7]. Interestingly there have been at least three other cases reported of patients with HIV and MAC infection, with or without accompanying IRIS, developing PRES [7–9]. It may be that atypical mycobacterial infection and IRIS contribute to the development of endothelial dysfunction and PRES through systemic inflammation and cytokine release.

Infarction, though rare, can occur, particularly affecting watershed areas [10] and causing predominantly visual and perceptual deficits. MR imaging may show hyperintense lesions on DWI due to T2 shine through, but corresponding low ADC values indicate true infarction [11, 12].

There are two main hypotheses behind the ischaemia seen in PRES. One is the 'neuropeptide theory' which suggests that the release of inflammatory cytokines such as TNF alpha and IL-1 upregulates endothelin-1 and other potent vasoconstrictors leading to vasospasm and subsequent ischaemia [3]. This theory is supported by studies conducting catheter and MR angiography and MR perfusion imaging which show widespread or focal vasoconstriction (similar to that seen in reversible cerebral vasoconstriction syndrome, or RCVS) and decreased perfusion [12]. An alternate theory is that extensive vasogenic oedema leads to increased tissue perfusion pressure with subsequent impairment of the microcirculation leading to ischaemia [11]. This is supported by the time course and localisation of cytotoxic oedema, which often occurs following and adjacent to the development of significant vasogenic oedema [13].

The management of PRES is supportive and is often focused on blood pressure reduction, in cases where it is raised above baseline. The aim is to reduce diastolic blood pressure to around 100–110 mmHg, not exceeding a reduction greater than 20% within the first hour [12]. A more dramatic decrease in blood pressure risks cerebral, as well as coronary and renal, ischaemia. Seizures should be treated with antiseizure medication, electrolyte abnormalities should be corrected, and any precipitating medications withdrawn. Most patients improve over days to weeks but a minority are left with more persistent deficits, often as a result of cerebral infarction or haemorrhage. Recurrence is rare, occurring in less than 10% of patients [14].

Clinical Learning Points

- PRES typically presents with a rapid onset of headaches, seizures, altered consciousness and visual disturbance.
- HIV, even when viral load is suppressed, appears to be a predisposing factor, likely contributing to the development of PRES through endothelial dysfunction.
- Hypertension is commonly seen but is absent in around 20% of cases, or may occur after symptom onset as an autoregulatory consequence of end organ hypoperfusion.
- Ischaemic infarction is rare but when it occurs clinical deficits may be long lasting.
- Management of PRES and ischaemic infarction is supportive and often focused on blood pressure control. Overly rapid correction of blood pressure should be avoided to decrease the risk of hypoperfusion and further ischaemia.

Radiological Learning Points

- Vasogenic oedema leads to high T2 signal in predominantly the white matter, but cortical involvement can sometimes be seen.
- Usually the parieto-occipital lobes are affected in PRES, but changes can also occur in frontal and temporal lobes, basal ganglia, brainstem, and cerebellum.
- High DWI signal is common and can indicate 'T2 shine through' from vasogenic oedema. This is usually reversible, but when there are corresponding low ADC values this is suggestive of cytotoxic oedema and ischaemic infarction.
- MRI should be repeated in 1–2 weeks to ensure changes are resolving, as would be expected in PRES.
- CT venogram and intracranial angiogram are usually indicated to exclude differential diagnoses such as venous sinus thrombosis, RCVS and CNS vasculitis, however keep in mind that areas of arterial narrowing can sometimes be seen in PRES.

References

1. Hinchey J, Pao L, Mas J-L. A reversible posterior leukoencephalopathy syndrome. N Engl J Med. 1996;334(8):7.
2. Fugate JE, Claassen DO, Cloft HJ, Kallmes DF, Kozak OS, Rabinstein AA. Posterior reversible encephalopathy syndrome: associated clinical and radiologic findings. Mayo Clin Proc. 2010;85(5):427–32.

3. Granata G, Greco A, Iannella G, Granata M, Manno A, Savastano E, et al. Posterior reversible encephalopathy syndrome—insight into pathogenesis, clinical variants and treatment approaches. Autoimmun Rev. 2015;14(9):830–6.
4. Bartynski WS. Posterior reversible encephalopathy syndrome, part 2: controversies surrounding pathophysiology of vasogenic edema. AJNR Am J Neuroradiol. 2008;29(6):1043–9.
5. Nightingale S, Wood C, Ainsworth J. The posterior reversible encephalopathy syndrome in HIV infection. Case Rep. 2012;2012:bcr0120125647.
6. Birner B, Hirzel C, Wagner F, Waldegg G. Posterior reversible encephalopathy syndrome in an HIV-infected patient on antiretroviral treatment: what is the risk factor? Case Rep. 2018;2018:bcr2017221998.
7. Weiss ZF, Rich J, Wing EJ. Posterior reversible encephalopathy syndrome in a patient with HIV/AIDS and immune reconstitution syndrome: a case study and literature review. Oxf Med Case Rep. 2018;8:46.
8. Choudhary M, Rose F. Posterior reversible encephalopathic syndrome due to severe hypercalcemia in AIDS. Scand J Infect Dis. 2005;37(6–7):524–6.
9. Viehman JA, Khalil D, Barhoma C, Hanna RM. Mycobacterium avium-intracellulare otomastoiditis in a young AIDS patient: case report and review of the literature. HIV AIDS. 2013;5:61–6.
10. Singhal AB. Postpartum angiopathy with reversible posterior leukoencephalopathy. Arch Neurol. 2004;61(3):411–6.
11. Ay H, Buonanno FS, Schaefer PW, Le DA, Wang B, Gonzalez RG, et al. Posterior leukoencephalopathy without severe hypertension: utility of diffusion-weighted MRI. Neurology. 1998;51(5):1369–76.
12. Lamy C, Oppenheim C, Mas JL. Posterior reversible encephalopathy syndrome. In: Handbook of clinical neurology. Amsterdam: Elsevier; 2014. p. 1687–701. Available from: https://linkinghub.elsevier.com/retrieve/pii/B9780702040887001097.
13. Covarrubias DJ, Luetmer PH, Campeau NG. Posterior reversible encephalopathy syndrome: prognostic utility of quantitative diffusion-weighted MR images. AJNR Am J Neuroradiol. 2002;23:1038–48.
14. Roth C, Ferbert A. Posterior reversible encephalopathy syndrome: long-term follow-up. J Neurol Neurosurg Psychiatry. 2010;81(7):773–7.

Chapter 32
A Case of Mechanical Thrombectomy for Acute Ischaemic Stroke

Sumanjit K. Gill, David Doig, and Robert Simister

An 87 year old right handed male presented to the acute service at 05:46 am with left sided face arm and leg weakness with aphasia. There was a clear wake up time of 02:00 am, he was well when he went to sleep at 9pm the night prior. He had pre morbid Modified Rankin Score (mRS) of 0 and on presentation his NIHSS was 19. His medical history was of atrial fibrillation for which he took edoxaban (with the last dose taken >24 h prior) and prostate cancer. He reached the CT scanner at 06:10. The CT head showed a dense right MCA sign (Fig. 32.1) and no established infarction. The ASPECTS score was 8. Concurrent CT angiogram (Fig. 32.2) confirmed a completely occluded right middle cerebral artery and CT perfusion imaging showed mismatch with a relatively large penumbra volume of 91 ml and core volume of 6 ml (Fig. 32.3). His blood pressure was 121/56 mmHg. He was in atrial fibrillation with a controlled heart rate. His INR was 1.1, anti Xa level was 10ng/ml (well below the trough range for the lab). He was consented for treatment and given intravenous thrombolysis at 06:52 and transferred to the interventional radiology suite. The groin puncture time was at 08:31 which was 2.75 h after presentation to hospital. The procedure was technically successful with clot aspiration and post procedure Thrombolysis in Cerebral Infarction (TICI) score of 3 which represents complete restoration of flow. Later that day he had a CT head (Fig. 32.4) as he was persistently

S. K. Gill (✉)
Institute of Neurology, UCL, National Hospital for Neurology and Neurosurgery, London, UK

D. Doig
University College London Hospitals NHS Foundation Trust, London, UK
e-mail: david.doig@nhs.net

R. Simister
Comprehensive Stroke Service, The National Hospital for Neurology and Neurosurgery, UCLH Foundation Trust, Stroke Research Centre, London, UK
e-mail: robert.simister@nhs.net

S. K. Gill et al. (eds.), *Stroke Medicine*,
https://doi.org/10.1007/978-3-031-58188-5_32

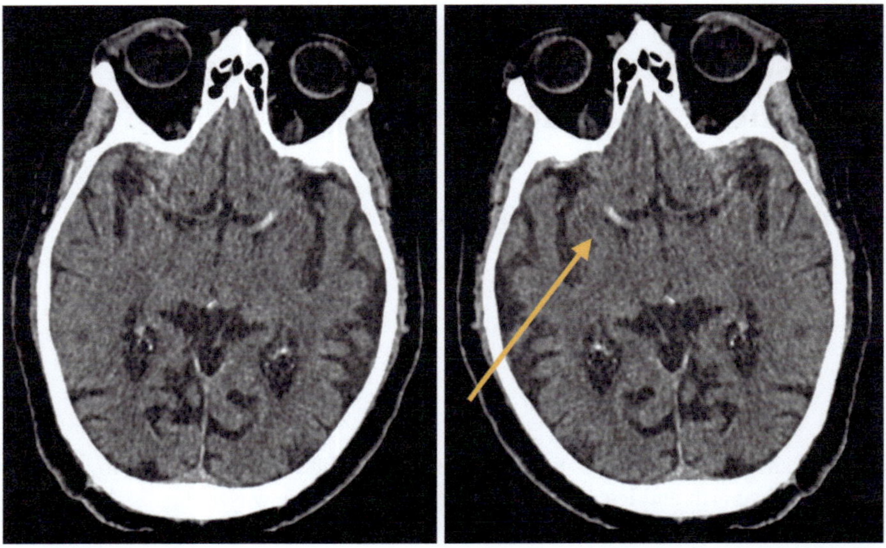

Fig. 32.1 Plain CT head with visible right thrombosed middle cerebral artery (arrow)

Fig. 32.2 CT angiogram confirmed occluded right middle cerebral artery with no flow (arrow)

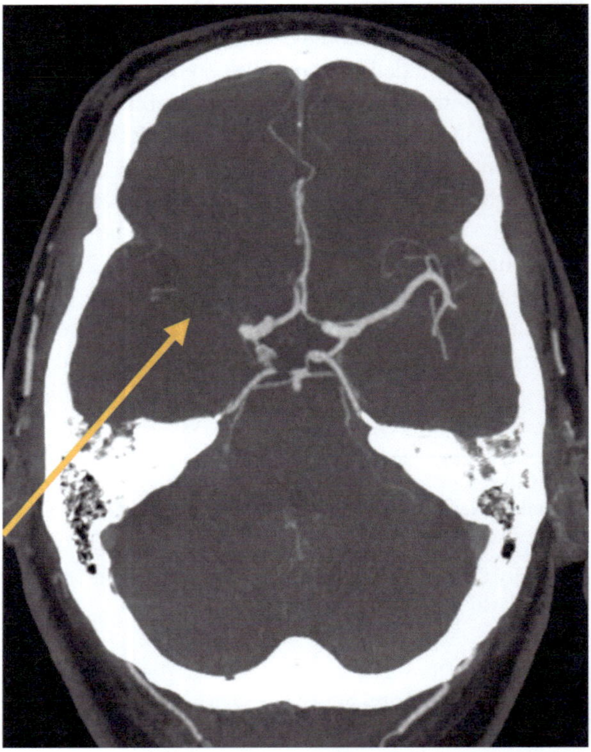

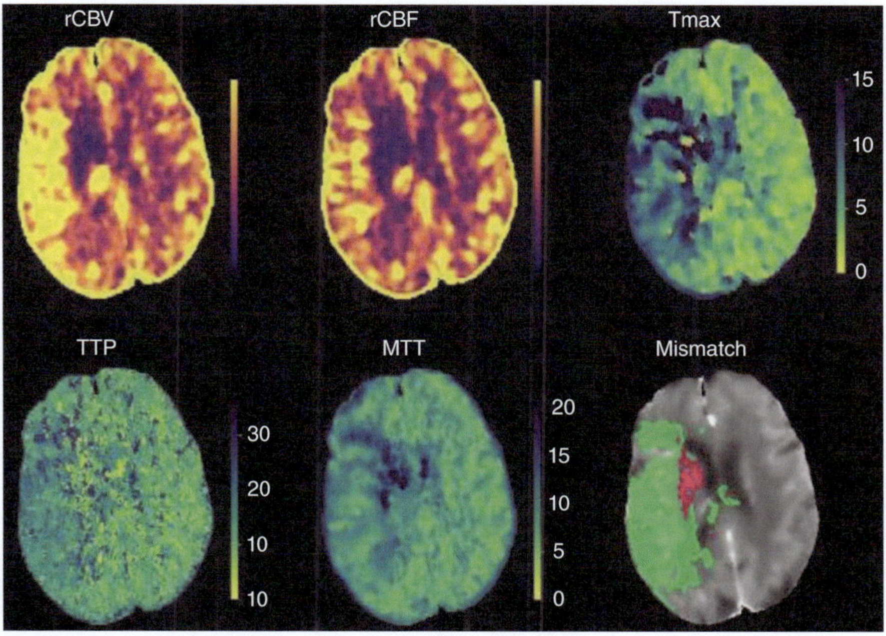

Fig. 32.3 CT perfusion imaging with penumbra (green) and ischaemic core (red) in the right middle cerebral artery territory in the bottom right image. The other images top row show: rCBV cerebral blood volume, rCBV cerebral blood flow, T_{max}. The remaining images on the bottom row left to right are: TTP time to peak, MTT mean transit time

drowsy. This showed an area of haemorrhagic transformation and contrast staining, this was more clearly seen as a basal ganglia haematoma the next day and had resolved on imaging after an interval (Fig. 32.5). His neurological assessment demonstrated a left sided hemianopia and inattention. He had 5/5 power throughout except for his left upper and lower limb which was graded at 1–2/5 throughout.

Mechanical thrombectomy is now established as an important treatment for acute ischaemic stroke in the context of large intracranial vessel occlusion. It involves aspiration or retrieval of the occluding clot and restoration of flow to blood starved brain tissue distal to the occlusion. Meta-analysis of the first positive studies exploring the impact of mechanical thrombectomy has identified that the number needed to treat significantly reduce the level of disability is 2.3 and that 46% of patients treated within 6 hours recover to full independence [1]. More recently, national guidance has widened criteria for treatment [2] up to 24 h since onset and with higher volumes of established new infarction at presentation but there are ongoing areas of uncertainty with respect to patient selection. In particular, further evidence is required to help clarify whether there is an upper age cut off, to determine the minimum ASPECTS score on the CT head at presentation. There is also a need to establish the role of CT perfusion imaging in patient selection in the context of longer times since onset and higher ischaemic burden with core infarction at presentation of more than 50 ml.

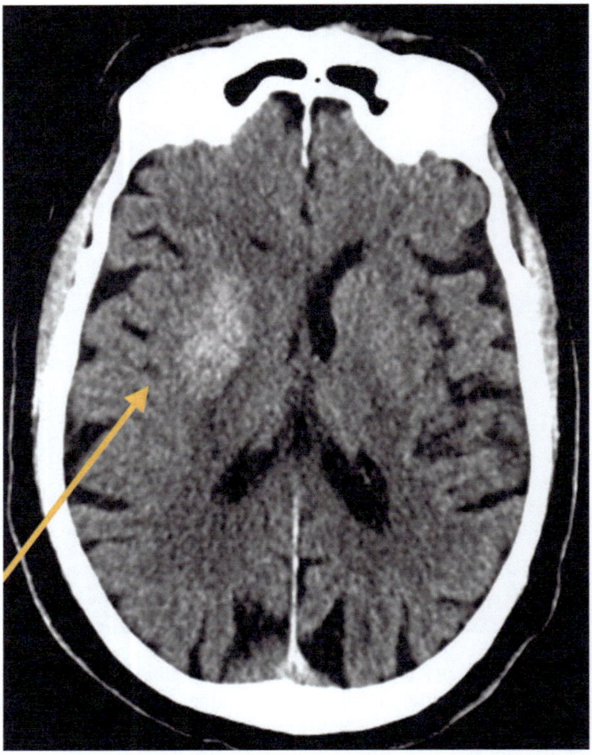

Fig. 32.4 Post thrombectomy plain CT showing a right sided area of contrast extravasation and haemorrhagic transformation

Our patient had a smaller core volume but still had a complication of contrast extravasation and haemorrhagic transformation—why? The first most obvious reason is his use of edoxaban although he had not taken a dose within 24 h and his anti Xa levels were low at 10 ng/ml. Other immediate potential factors are linked to blood pressure control during and after the thrombectomy procedure and the impact of restoration of blood flow on areas of recent completed infarct. Bleeding risk linked to thrombolysis treatment is also higher in very elderly patients. In our patient blood pressure was well managed and there were no cerebral microbleeds on subsequent MRI imaging, both factors influence the risk of haemorrhage.

The impact of thrombectomy with increasing patient age has not been formally studied. We do know that patients over 80 years are in general more likely to have moderate severe disability or be dead at one year follow up [3, 4]. This doesn't appear to be linked to their rate of symptomatic intracerebral haemorrhage or other procedural complication (arterial dissection, bleed or infection at the puncture site) [4] and the guidance remains to assess patients on a case by case basis. In an older person this would include evaluation of their pre existing disability, level of frailty, co morbidities and health beliefs about living life with disability.

The Alberta Stroke Programme (ASPECTS) is a topographic score which quantifies the amount of ischaemic injury in the middle cerebral artery brain territory

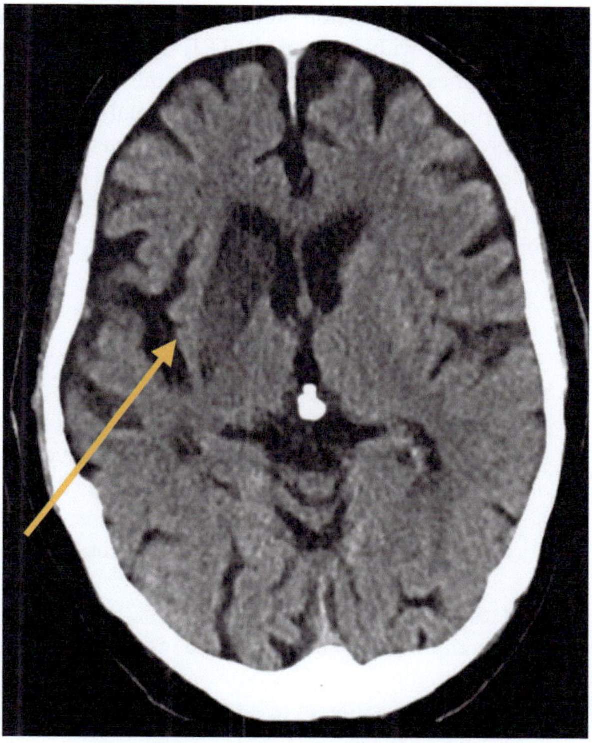

Fig. 32.5 Plain CT some months later showing resolution of oedema and midline shift and resorption of blood in the area of haemorrhagic transformation

seen on plain CT imaging and has become useful in aiding clinical decision making in selecting patients with middle cerebral artery infarction for the stroke physician. The ASPECTS score is a score out of a possible 10 points. A normal brain has a score of 10 and 1 point is subtracted from this number for each sub-region of the middle cerebral artery territory affected with visible acute stroke injury. The ASPECTS score can be calculated by trained clinicians but is increasingly measured by dedicated medical artificial intelligence systems. Until 2023, typical inclusion criteria for patient selection for treatment with thrombectomy included demonstration of a smaller middle cerebral artery territory infarction at presentation (recorded as an ASPECTS score on presenting CT > 5) [5] but recent studies have indicated that thrombectomy can still offer clinical value with lower ASPECTS scores i.e. >2 [2].

CT Perfusion imaging potentially adds further value to patient selection protocols which routinely consists of CT head and CT angiogram of carotids and intracranial vessels. The perfusion sequences can help to indicate the volume of brain tissue that has already infarcted (known as the infarct core) and, separately, the volume of any tissues that is not yet infarcted but which has reduced blood flow (known as the ischaemic penumbra). Perfusion is of particular utility with patient selection at longer times since onset and with larger infarct volumes on patient arrival.

A positive CT perfusion produces a picture seen in the imaging above with a core ischaemic area with prolonged MTT, T_{max} and reduced CBV and CBF. The mismatch signifies acute ischaemic tissue and a large potentially recoverable penumbral area [6]. This gives the physician a visual of the tissue at risk and also a measure of the core volume. The degree of progression of penumbral tissue to infarction will dependent on time from onset, the presence of collaterals and any spontaneous recanalization. The benefit to patients who are identified as having a large ischaemic core volume of reperfusion therapy is uncertain, it may be of some benefit to reduce oedema [7].

Key Clinical Learning Points

- Patients aged over 80 should be considered as candidates for mechanical thrombectomy after a careful evaluation of co-morbidities, frailty, medications and patient wishes
- Mechanical Thrombectomy is an effective, safe treatment for acute ischaemic stroke due to large vessel occlusion with a number needed to treat of 2.3 to reduce disability.
- Mechanical thrombectomy is a time dependent intervention and patients with large vessel occlusion who may be eligible should be transferred to a thrombectomy enabled hyperacute stroke unit as rapidly as possible with treatment possible up to 24 h after time of onset of acute ischaemic stroke for selected cases

Key Radiological Learning Points

- CT head imaging can demonstrate occlusion of intracranial arteries but this sign is not reliable without use of concurrent CT arteriography
- CT perfusion imaging is increasingly used to estimate infarct core and ischaemic penumbra i.e. the area of irreversibly infarcted tissue vs. potentially salvageable tissue
- Striatocapsular infarction is common after stroke associated with middle cerebral artery occlusion even with rapid treatment. This is because the clot occludes flow into the lenticulostriate end arteries feeding the capsular territory.
- Core ischaemic tissue has a reduced mean transit time with severely reduced cerebral blood flow and blood volume
- ASPECTS score is a useful tool to aid clinical decision making with low (<7) scores being strongly associated with death and disability

References

1. Goyal M, Menon B, et al. Endovascular thrombectomy after large vessel ischaemic stroke: a meta- analysis of individual patient data from five randomised trials. Lancet. 2016;387(10029):1723–31.
2. Stroke Association National Clinical Guidelines for Stroke. https://www.stroke.org.uk/professionals/resources-professionals/national-clinical-guideline-stroke. Accessed 7 October 2023.
3. Beuker C, Koppe J, et al. Association of age with 1 year outcome in patients with acute ischaemic stroke treated with thrombectomy: real world analysis in 18506 patients. J Neurol Neurosurg Psychiatry. 2023;94:631–7.
4. Meyer L, Alexandrou M, et al. Endovascular treatment of very elderly patients aged ≥90 with acute ischemic stroke. J Am Heart Assoc. 2020;9:e014447.
5. Warwick Pexman JH, Baber PA, et al. Use of the Alberta stroke program early CT score (ASPECTS) for assessing CT scans in patients with acute stroke. Am J Neuroradiol. 2001;22(8):1534–42.
6. Demeestere J, Wouters A, et al. Review of perfusion imaging in acute ischaemic stroke. Stroke. 2020;51:1017–24.
7. Broocks G, Hanning U, Flottmann F, Schönfeld M, Faizy TD, Sporns P, et al. Clinical benefit of thrombectomy in stroke patients with low ASPECTS is mediated by oedema reduction. Brain. 2019;142:1399–407.

Chapter 33
A Case of Moya Moya

Sumanjit K. Gill, David Doig, and Robert Simister

A 38 year old man presented to hospital with a left sided face, arm and leg weakness with marked inattention to the left hand side. His NIHSS was scored at 13. His blood pressure was 112/78 mmHg. He had a history of Moya Moya disease and coeliac disease. His Moya Moya had been diagnosed 2 years prior when he presented with transient ischaemic attack and was found to have imaging appearances in keeping with Moya Moya. The attacks were recurrent and began with paraesthesia on the left side with limb jerking and lasted a few minutes. He was a that time started on an anti epileptic medication and aspirin. His CT imaging on this occasion confirmed a right intraparenchymal haematoma in the region supplied by lenticulostriate collaterals (Fig. 33.1) with CTA (Fig. 33.2) showing an obliterative arteriopathy involving the right terminal carotid, right M1 segment of the middle cerebral artery and right A1 segment of the anterior cerebral artery. When reviewed in clinic several months later he noted to be able to walk without aides and was able to communicate normally. There was a discussion with the patient and he was informed of the possible need for surgery to stabilise his intracranial circulation. His case was discussed in a multidisciplinary meeting between stroke physicians, neurosurgeons and neuroradiology and it was decided he should have a formal angiogram to delineate cerebral vasculature and to have an EC-IC bypass procedure. The angiogram

S. K. Gill (✉)
Institute of Neurology, UCL, National Hospital for Neurology and Neurosurgery, London, UK

D. Doig
University College London Hospitals NHS Foundation Trust, London, UK
e-mail: david.doig@nhs.net

R. Simister
Comprehensive Stroke Service, The National Hospital for Neurology and Neurosurgery, UCLH Foundation Trust, Stroke Research Centre, London, UK
e-mail: robert.simister@nhs.net

S. K. Gill et al. (eds.), *Stroke Medicine*,
https://doi.org/10.1007/978-3-031-58188-5_33

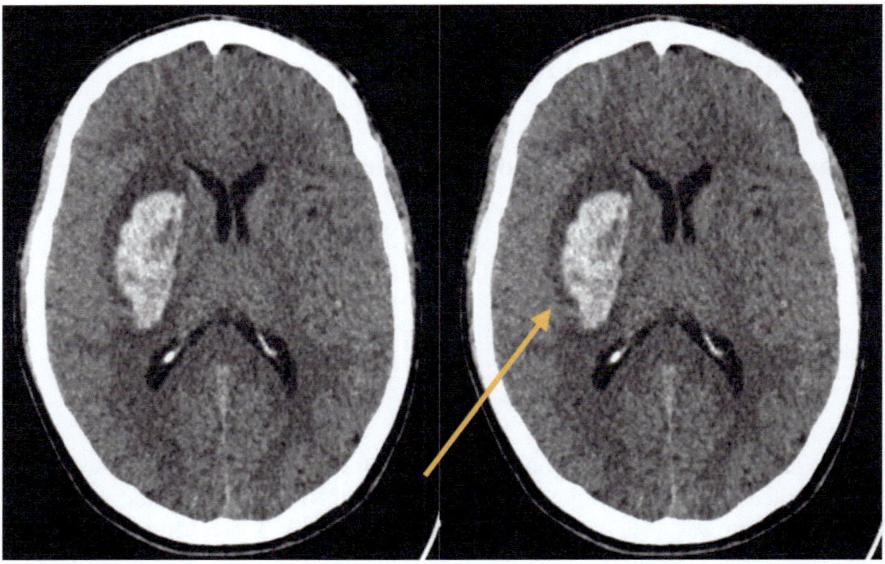

Fig. 33.1 An acute intraparenchymal haematoma measuring 5 × 2 × 4 cm with centre being on the right lentiform nucleus. There is partial effacement of the right lateral ventricle and midline shift indicating raised intracranial pressure in the right hemisphere

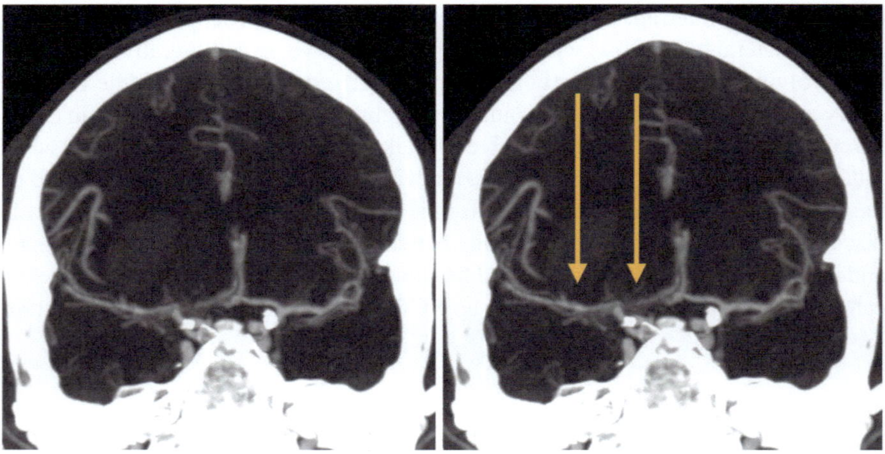

Fig. 33.2 A cerebral CT angiogram of the intracranial vessels showing an obliterative arteriopathy of the right M1, M2, A1 segment

confirmed occlusion of the right middle cerebral artery and a collateral vascularisation (Fig. 33.3). The superior temporal artery was of sufficient calibre to be able to use for a STA/MCA bypass. CT perfusion imaging confirmed reduced cerebral blood flow and blood volume in the right hemisphere.

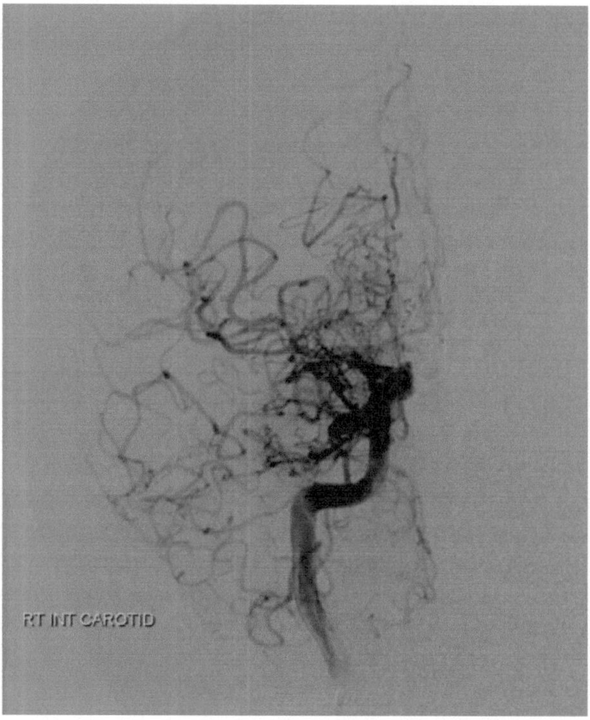

Fig. 33.3 Right internal carotid injection demonstrating proximal middle cerebral artery occlusion with 'puff of smoke' appearance of circle of willis collaterals

Three ways to proceed were considered and discussed with the patient:

1. Conservative management–this avoids taking risk with procedure but means there is an ongoing risk of both intracerebral haemorrhage and ischaemic stroke.
2. Direct bypass–this consists of connecting the superficial temporal artery, which normally supplies scalp, to the middle cerebral artery in an attempt to restore the blood flow in this artery and the brain supplied by it. It can be technically challenging and does carry significant risks, namely of stroke, failure, bypass occlusion, skin necrosis, epilepsy, bleeding, infection, medical complications, risk of general anaesthesia, permanent disability and death. However if all goes well this does reduce the risk of further strokes immediately.
3. Indirect revascularisation–this consists of applying muscle and the superficial temporal artery directly on the surface of the brain with the aim of stimulating the development of neovascularisation from these tissues to the brain. This is technically less challenging but has much more delayed effect, and until the full effect is observed, the risk of stroke remains virtually unaltered, which may take many months. This can be combined with a direct bypass, or carried out if direct bypass fails or is felt to be too high risk.

The patient decided to go ahead with the second option and four years after his initial TIA like episode he had his superior temporal artery anastomosed to the M4 segment of the middle cerebral artery. The surgery was uneventful and he was discharged 3 day later. Follow up at one year with repeat imaging confirmed good graft flow and the patient confirmed he had no further events.

Moya Moya disease is a rare cerebrovascular condition causing an obliterative vasculopathy which affects the large arteries causing both ischaemic stroke and also haemorrhage. It is characterised by obliterative disease of the terminal portion of the carotid artery with accompanying collateralisation of vessels giving a 'puff of smoke' appearance on imaging [1]. It is relentlessly progressive and significantly increases risk of both disability and death. It is most prevalent in East Asian countries and can be familial or sporadic raising a question about a possible gene locus—so far RNF213 which encodes for E3 ubiquitin ligase has been identified as a susceptibility gene [2]. Knockout zebrafish have abnormal growth of blood vessels indicating this gene is necessary for normal angiogenesis. This correlates with an earlier onset and severity and may be useful in prognosticating. Moya Moya can be staged using Suzukis angiographic staging process given in Table 33.1 [3] which helps understand how the process of prolonged hypoperfusion induces angiogenesis and compensates for reduced flow through affected vessels.

Treatment options are limited and are given in the case above—either conservative approach which confers an increasing risk of stroke or surgical procedures which also carry risk. The most common surgical procedure is of external carotid—internal carotid bypass [4]. One possible surgical complication not given in the case above is of post operative cerebral hyperperfusion—a sudden marked increase in cerebral blood flow causing reperfusion injury. One study of revascularisation surgery of the type our patient underwent had favourable long term outcome but a high incidence of cerebral hyperperfusion—18% which was associated with transient neurological events [5]. These did not appear to be of any long term significance in this instance but there is the potential for haemorrhagic stroke physicians should be aware of this possibility.

Table 33.1 Suzuki's staging process—a study detailing progression in 20 paediatric cases of Moyamoya disease

Stage 1: 'Narrowing of carotid fork'. On the angiographic exam, only the terminal portion of the internal carotid artery is stenosed
Stage 2: 'Initiation and appearance of basal moyamoya'. On the angiographic exam, stenosis of all the terminal branches of ICA (ACA and/or MCA) and deep moyamoya vessels are seen
Stage 3: 'Intensification of basal moyamoya'. On the angiographic exam, deep moyamoya vessels are intensified. MRA taken during this stage shows a "puff of smoke" appearance. The deflection of the anterior cerebral artery (ACA) and middle cerebral arteries (MCA) is noted
Stage 4: 'Minimization of basal moyamoya'. On the angiographic exam, deep moyamoya vessels begin to regress while transdural collaterals begin to appear. The deflection of the posterior cerebral artery (PCA) is noted
Stage 5: 'Reduction of moyamoya'. On the angiographic exam, continued regression of deep moyamoya vessels and progression of transdural collateral vessels are noted
Stage 6: 'Disappearance of moyamoya'. On the angiographic exam, deep moyamoya vessels have vanished and there is complete occlusion of the ICA. Blood supply to ACA and MCA areas is derived mainly from the external carotid artery

Medical treatment is also focussed on reducing the risk of recurrent ischaemic and haemorrhagic stroke. There are no randomised control trials and data is limited to retrospective studies so practice does vary. Antiplatelets in the form of aspirin and clopidogrel can be prescribed after a consideration of the balance of risk. Cilostazol is also sometimes used as it is unique for its vasodilatory properties. One prospective study of cilostazol was positive with ischemic stroke recurrence of 6% at 5 years with improved blood flow [6]. This is not strong enough evidence for a strong recommendation but may be considered as an alternative to surgery or in those with early disease.

Key Clinical Learning Points

- Moya Moya disease is a cause of recurrent intracerebral haemorrhage and ischaemic stroke and has a poor long term prognosis
- It can be familial or sporadic, paediatric or adult onset and is more prevalent in the East Asian population
- Multidisciplinary management of the condition is necessary with stroke physician working with neurosurgeon, neuroradiologist, neurovascular specialist nurse for proper case management—treatment options come with risk and should be carefully communicated with patients with additional time given for 'options talk'

Key Radiological Learning Points

- Moyamoya disease most often starts with obliterative disease of the terminal portion of the internal carotid artery
- Collateralisation of the arteries becomes prominent as the disease progresses and can give a 'puff of smoke appearance'
- Multiple imaging methods are required for clinical decision making and including MR angiogram, CT/MR perfusion imaging, digital subtraction angiogram, transcranial doppler

References

1. Ihara M, Yamamoto Y. Moyamoya disease: diagnosis and interventions. Lancet Neurol. 2022;21(8):747–58.
2. Kamada F, Aoki Y, et al. A genome wide association study identifies RNF213 as the first moyamoya disease gene. J Hum Genet. 2011;56:34–40.
3. Suzuki J, Takaku A, Sendai MD. Cerebrovascular 'moya moya disease'. Arch Neurol. 1969;20:288–99.

4. Hu J, Luo J, Chen Q. The susceptibility pathogenesis of moya moya disease. World Neurosurg. 2017;101:731–41.
5. Fujimura M, Tominaga T. Lessons learned from moyamoya disease: outcome of direct/indirect revascularisation surgery for 150 affected hemispheres. Neurol Med Chir. 2012;52(5):327–32.
6. Gonzalez N, Amin-Hanjani S, et al. Adult moyamoya and syndrome: current perspectives and future directions: a scientific statement from the AHA/ASA. Stroke. 2023;54:e465–79.

Chapter 34
A Case of Giant Cell Arteritis and Stroke

Sumanjit K. Gill, David Doig, and Robert Simister

A 76 year old was diagnosed with giant cell arteritis (GCA) and started on high dose steroids after left eye visual loss with optic nerve inflammation. His USS temporal arteries showed bilateral halo sign supporting a diagnosis of GCA. Six days later whilst out walking with a friend he had a sudden onset of confusion and when assessed by video triage with the ambulance service he was found to have full strength in his limbs despite being non compliant with a neurological examination. He was directed to accident and emergency and a few hours later when assessed he was found to have anew left lower limb weakness. He was then transferred to his local stroke service for assessment. He was complaining of a bilateral visual loss but it was impossible to clarify further due to his confusion. There was a lack of a pupillary reflex in the left eye. He had a plain CT (Fig. 34.1) which showed an area of hypodensity in the left occipital lobe and CT perfusion which conformed prolonged mean transit time in the same area. When reviewed by a neuroradiologist it was felt that despite the lack of mismatch on CT perfusion there was probable bilateral posterior circulation infarction. The CT angiogram showed a complete occlusion of the left vertebral artery (Fig. 34.2). He was now clearly outside of the thrombolysis time window and he was given high dose aspirin and admitted to the stroke unit.

S. K. Gill (✉)
Institute of Neurology, UCL, National Hospital for Neurology and Neurosurgery, London, UK

D. Doig
University College London Hospitals NHS Foundation Trust, London, UK
e-mail: david.doig@nhs.net

R. Simister
Comprehensive Stroke Service, The National Hospital for Neurology and Neurosurgery, UCLH Foundation Trust, Stroke Research Centre, London, UK
e-mail: robert.simister@nhs.net

S. K. Gill et al. (eds.), *Stroke Medicine*,
https://doi.org/10.1007/978-3-031-58188-5_34

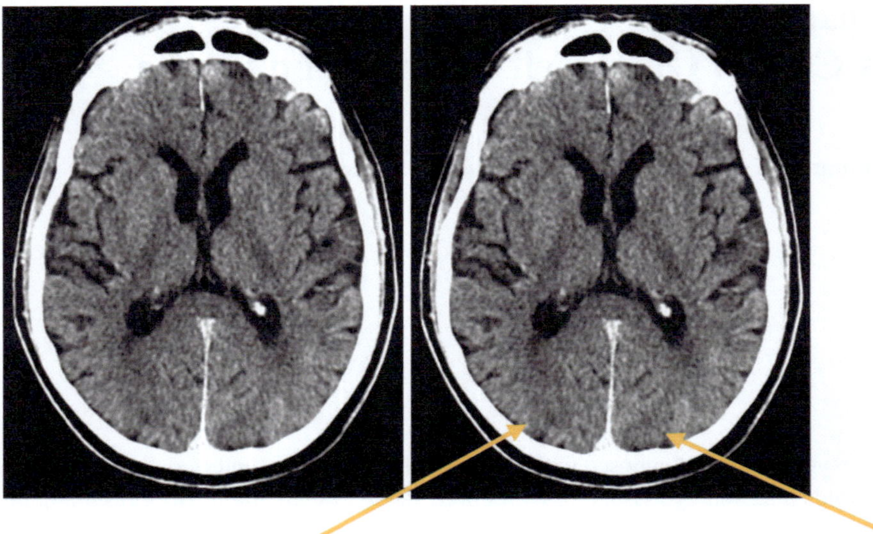

Fig. 34.1 Plain CT showing subtle occipital cortical hypoattenuation and parenchymal swelling

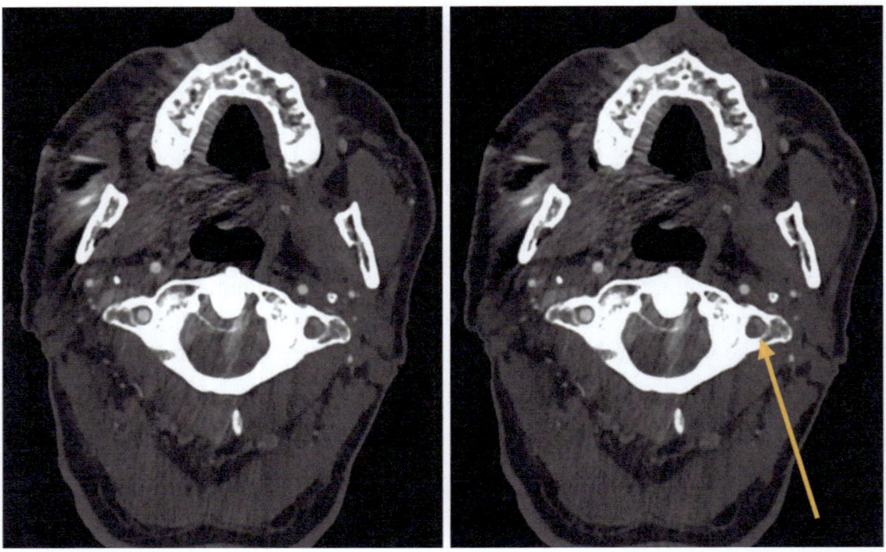

Fig. 34.2 CT angiogram showing lack of contrast opacification of the left vertebral artery

His MRI showed haemorrhagic transformation of bilateral occipital lobe infarcts with possible new thrombus in the right internal carotid artery and bilateral infarcts in multiple territories (Fig. 34.3). The vessel wall imaging was planned after a one week interval. He was reviewed by neuro ophthalmology and was found to have a bilateral ischaemic optic neuropathy. A CT of his chest, abdomen and pelvis was

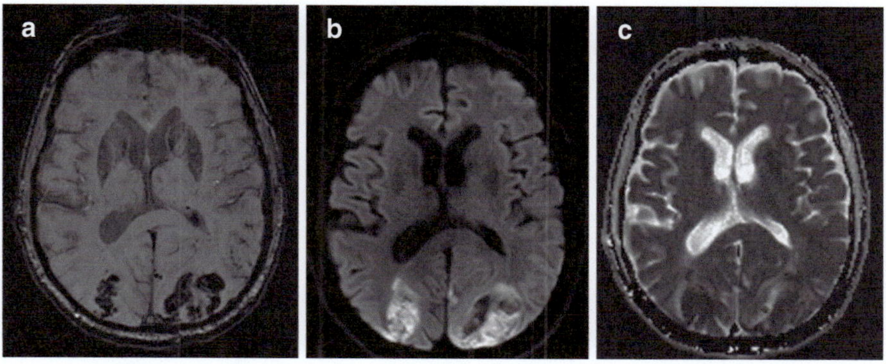

Fig. 34.3 Left to Right: (**a**) Susceptibility weighted sequences showing blood in bilateral posterior circulation territories. (**b**) B1000 image showing bilateral posterior circulation hyperintensity and bilateral multiple territory hyperintensities which are matched by areas of signal drop out shown in (**c**). ADC map

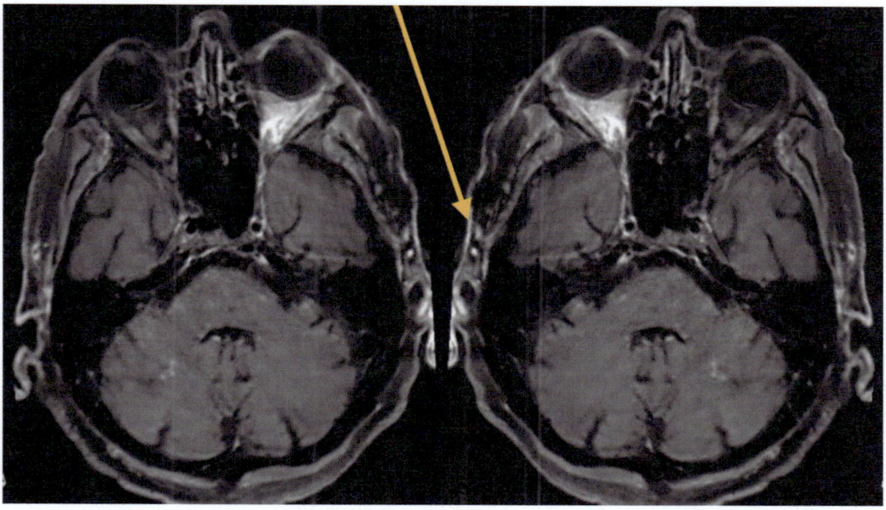

Fig. 34.4 Vessel wall MRI (fat-saturated black-blood T1-weighted post-contrast) showing pathological enhancement round the right superficial temporal artery

normal except for a right renal pole soft tissue mass. A decision was made to start a half treatment dose once a day low molecular weight heparin injection in view of the cardioembolic stroke appearances on imaging with new thrombus in the internal carotid artery. The cautious dosing was due to the bilateral transformation in the two larger infarcts which did worsen over the first two sets of CT imaging. Lupus anticoagulant was positive with anti cardiolipin antibodies negative. A temporal artery biopsy showed a transmural non-necrotising inflammation with mainly lymphocytes and histiocytes. Occasional giant cells are noted. Vessel wall imaging (Fig. 34.4) was initially reported as normal with no evidence of arterial inflammation.

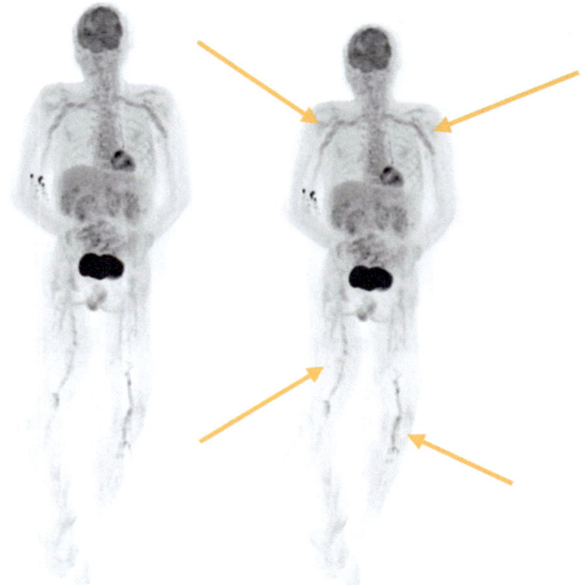

Fig. 34.5 Diffusely increased FDG uptake of the thoracic aorta, subclavian, axillary, internal mammary and femoral arteries (arrow)

Rheumatology made a decision to treat the vasculitis and start tocilizumab with infusion and weekly injection in conjunction with high dose steroids. PET scan showed diffusely increased FDG uptake of the thoracic aorta, subclavian, axillary, internal mammary and femoral arteries (Fig. 34.5). There was additional diffusely increased uptake of the vertebral arteries. To find such avid enhancement after 2 weeks of high dose steroids was recognised as unusual and the decision was made to repeat PET imaging after a week and consider adding further immunosuppression in the form of cyclophosphamide. It was concluded that the progressive accrual of ischaemic lesions with new thrombus seen in the carotid was more probably a consequence of the aggressive nature of his inflammatory disease rather than cardioembolism and there was no increase in his dose of low molecular weight heparin. The repeat PET confirmed on going active vasculitis and he was transferred to a stroke rehab unit after the addition of cyclophosphamide.

Giant cell arteritis has a known association with ischaemic stroke although remains relatively rare for it to present in this way [1]. A more common way to present is with manifestations of external carotid inflammation with headache, scalp tenderness or as in our case jaw claudication which was an element of history elicited from the patient later during his hospital stay. The literature contains small case series from which we have built our knowledge of the natural history and response to treatment. A case review of 47 cases [2] shows at that the mortality is relatively high at 53% (varying lengths of follow up) with 22% achieving full neurological recovery. A higher mortality was seen in those with extradural involvement and did not appear to be associated with prednisolone use at time of stroke onset. There was a tendency to affect the vertebrobasilar circulation as opposed to the anterior circulation. An attempt to correlate clinical and pathological findings was made earlier in 1972 [3] in an autopsy study which confirmed that vertebral arteries were more frequently affected and more severely with all three layers of the arterial wall inflamed. This corresponded to a higher number of brainstem or occipital lobe strokes. This was also the conclusion of a larger series in Dijon [4].

One atypical feature of our case was the absence of vessel wall enhancement on vessel wall imaging. Vessel Imaging has a high sensitivity of 88.4% and in a patient with such aggressive disease this initial negative report. It has been shown that after 5 days of corticosteroids imaging is less sensitive so this was thought to be the reason [5]. However review of imaging after discharge revealed some subtle change which was in keeping with pathological enhancement of the temporal artery. This was consistent with the aggressive disease seen on PET imaging. Another unexpected negative finding was the initially normal CT perfusion but this may be as CT perfusion varies in performance in differing anatomical locations [6]. The tendency is for it to be less sensitive for posterior circulation ischaemia.

Key Clinical Learning Points

- Giant cell arteritis is a cause of stroke which is relatively high mortality
- Giant cell arteritis is associated with strokes which happen more often in the posterior circulation as it causes inflammation with a predilection for the vertebral arteries
- Bilateral multi territory strokes can happen in strokes caused by systemic disease and are not always due to cardioembolism

Key Radiological Learning Points

- The sensitivity of CT perfusion imaging varies by anatomical location and is lower in the posterior circulation
- Halo sign on US temporal arteries is pathognomonic of giant cell arteritis
- Vessel wall imaging is highly sensitive and specific for visualising the inflammatory changes caused by giant cell arteritis. If imaging is initially normal—get the images reviewed again! Interpretation requires time and expertise and in the pressure of the moment the neuroradiologist may not be able to identify subtle change.

References

1. Kuganesan T, Huang AR. Stroke as an atypical initial presentation of giant cell arteritis. BMC Geriatr. 2018;18:55.
2. Alsolaimani RS, Bhavsar SV. Severe intracranial involvement in giant cell arteritis: 5 cases and a literature review. J Rheumatol. 2016;43:3.
3. Wilkinson I, Russell RW. Arteries of the head and neck in giant cell arteritis: a pathological study to show the pattern of arterial involvement. Arch Neurol. 1972;27:378–91.
4. Samson M, Jacquin A, Audia S, et al. Stroke associated with giant cell arteritis: a population-based study. J Neurol Neurosurg Psychiatry. 2015;86:216–21.
5. Klink T, Geiger J, et al. Giant cell arteritis: diagnostic accuracy of mr imaging of superficial cranial arteries in initial diagnosis – results from a multicentre trial. Radiology. 2014;273(3):844–52.
6. Edwards LS, Cappelen-Smith C, et al. Optimal CT perfusion thresholds for core and penumbra in acute posterior circulation infarction. Front Neurol. 2023;14:1092505.

Chapter 35
Treat the Child, Not the Number

Anoushka Alwis and Vijeya Ganesan

Clinical History

An 8-year-old boy with type 1 diabetes (T1D) had a raised systolic blood pressure (SBP) of 120 mmHg and frequent headache. MRI brain scan showed mature right frontal and left parietotemporal junction infarcts (Fig. 35.1). There was no concordant ictus, however parents recounted recent cognitive decline, less clear speech and reports of blurred vision. Daily amlodipine for ambulatory SBPs of 120–151 mmHg (>99th centile) was commenced after discussion with nephrologists. Subsequent brain MRA demonstrated bilateral arteriopathy and cerebral catheter angiography (CA) confirmed severe moyamoya (Fig. 35.2). Following neurovascular review, bilateral revascularisation surgery was offered, and amlodipine discontinued to promote brain perfusion. Within days he developed severe headache and visual disturbance responsive to intravenous fluids and high dose aspirin (5 mg/kg), with acute right temporoparietal infarction on brain MRI. Five weeks later he re-presented with left lower limb weakness.

A. Alwis (✉)
Great Ormond Street Hospital for Children NHS Foundation Trust, London, UK
e-mail: anouskha.alwis@gosh.nhs.uk

V. Ganesan
UCL Great Ormond Street Institute of Child Health, London, UK
e-mail: v.ganesan@ucl.ac.uk

S. K. Gill et al. (eds.), *Stroke Medicine*,
https://doi.org/10.1007/978-3-031-58188-5_35

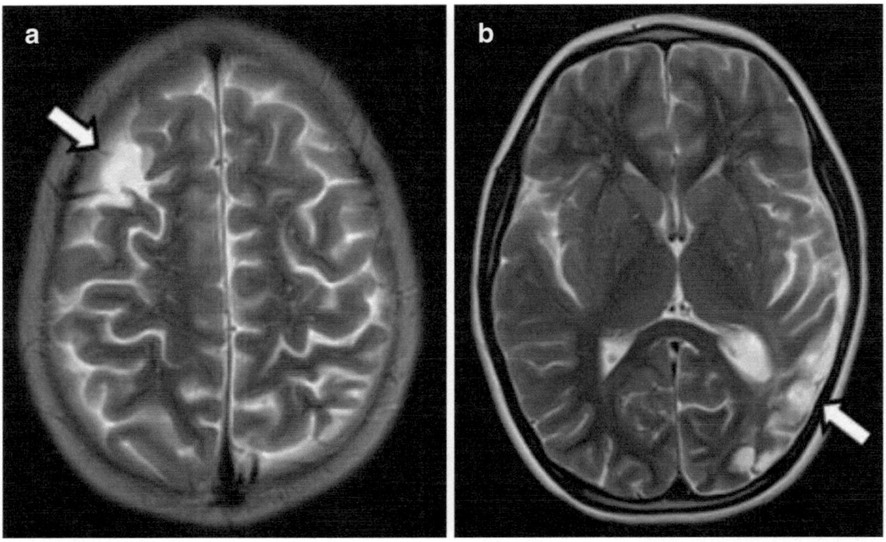

Fig. 35.1 Presenting MRI brain axial T2—weighted images showing mature infarction of (**a**) right frontal lobe (*arrow*) and (**b**) left parietooccipital region (*arrow*)

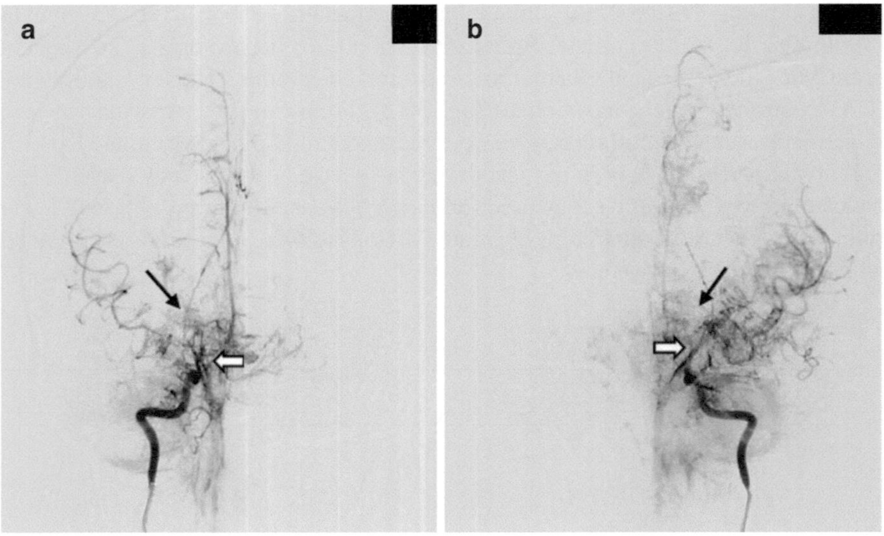

Fig. 35.2 Cerebral catheter angiogram right (**a**) and left (**b**) internal carotid artery injections in coronal projection. These show significant bilateral terminal ICA plus proximal MCA and ACA steno-occlusive disease (*white arrows*) with lenticulostriate collateral vessels (*black arrows*) consistent with severe moyamoya

Examination

His GCS was 15. Temperature, oxygen saturations, heart and respiratory rate were normal. SBP was 151 mmHg and blood glucose 9.6 mmol/L. Systemic examination was otherwise unremarkable. The left visual field was reduced as was acuity bilaterally to counting fingers. He was unable to identify objects unless through touch or sound, name the colour of a pen or write his name correctly. There was left lower limb weakness maximum at the ankle with foot drop and spasticity. Evolved left upper limb weakness largely resolved by 12 h with residual dysmetria. He had reduced proprioception of the left hallux and ankle. There was left gait ataxia with scissoring in assisted walking. Paediatric National Institutes of Health Stroke Scale (PedNIHSS) was 7.

Investigations

An urgent CT brain scan showed acute right anterior cerebral artery (ACA) territory infarction. Intravenous hydration was initiated, aspirin continued, and he was transferred for continuous monitoring and expert re-evaluation. After 48 h he developed recurrence of left upper limb weakness and MRI/A brain scan showed acute right precentral gyrus and parietooccipital infarction with no progression of arteriopathy (Fig. 35.3). An arterial line was sited and a target SBP of 110–140 mmHg (>90th centile) agreed with nephrologists. Fluid boluses and/or inotropes were to be administered for lesser BPs. Four days later he developed headache, transient SBP < 110

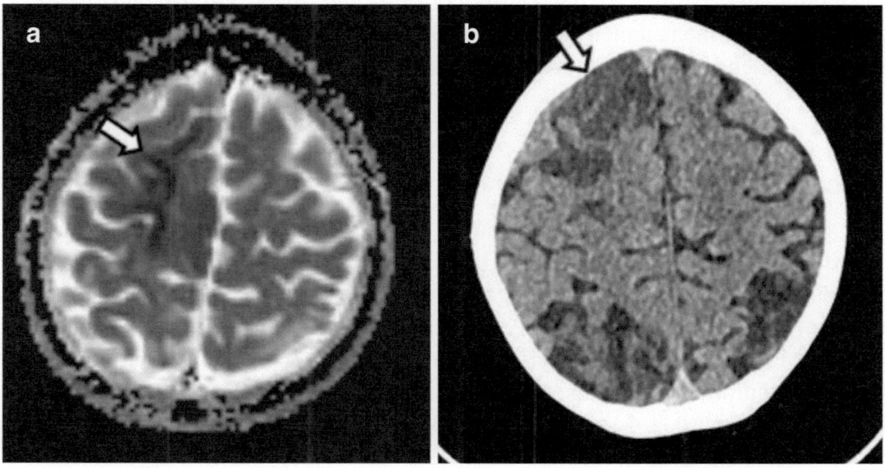

Fig. 35.3 (**a**) Re-presentation MRI brain axial apparent diffusion coefficient map showing right precentral gyrus diffusion restriction consistent with acute infarction (*arrow*) and (**b**) CT brain axial image showing extension of right frontal infarction after 4 days (*arrow*)

mmHg and extreme agitation. A repeat CT brain scan showed extension of right frontal infarction (Fig. 35.3).

In view of rapidly recurring arterial ischaemic strokes (AIS) he underwent bilateral pial synangiosis accepting a higher risk of perioperative stroke. For this reason, aspirin as not discontinued preoperatively. He was discharged home after a 3-week inpatient stay including neurorehabilitation. He had on-going difficulties with visual function, recall and following three-part instructions. Although independently mobile, residual left-lower limb weakness impacted balance and co-ordination. He subsequently developed a wound infection and dehiscence, likely predisposed by T1D. This responded well to surgical debridement, closure and prolonged antibiotics.

Cerebral CA at 15 months on aspirin showed no progression of arteriopathy and patent bilateral anastomoses supplying middle cerebral artery (MCA) territories. Right bypass perfusion was slower, and perfusion of anterior and posterior cerebral artery territories reduced, confirming a critical role for systemic BP in maintaining brain perfusion. He has on-going episodic headache, blurred vision and left-hand clawing with differentials of transient ischaemic attack (TIA) and symptomatic hypoglycaemia. An interictal EEG did not support seizure liability and most recent MRI brain shows no new infarcts. Glycaemic control is satisfactory and last ambulatory SBP monitoring confirmed measurements within target range (128–132 mmHg) with 67% systolic load. He remains off anti-hypertensive medication with no evidence of end organ damage. No cause for renovascular hypertension was found following renal ultrasound, dopplers and renal CA.

Electrodiagnostics confirmed marked bilateral macular pathway dysfunction and hemispheric dysfunction affecting the central left half field. Registration for visual impairment (VI) is in progress. He continues mainstream education with VI teacher support. Adaptations include sitting at the front of class, magnified learning materials and extra time for processing. He has lots of friends, but difficulties remembering their names. He uses a left ankle-foot orthosis and wheelchair for long distances. Joint medical management continues between neurovascular, ophthalmology, nephrology, endocrinology, community paediatric and therapy teams.

Discussion

Moyamoya is an angiographic descriptor of the ‘puff of smoke’ basal collaterals visualised in typically bilateral, progressive and steno-occlusive arteriopathy of the terminal internal carotid artery (ICA), ACA or MCA. Aetiology is not fully determined. Moyamoya disease describes idiopathic East Asia cases, a proportion of which are familial with linkage to several susceptibility loci e.g. 17q25.3 containing the RNF213 gene [1]. Moyamoya syndrome refers to association with other co-morbidity, typically neurofibromatosis, sickle cell disease or Down syndrome. TIAs and/or AIS are usual presentations in childhood with intracranial haemorrhage more prominent in adults. Additional sequalae include headache, epilepsy, neurodisability and increased mortality risk. Poor outcome factors include AIS presentation and posterior circulation involvement [2]. Treatment is supportive and includes increasing hydration, antithrombotic agents and surgery in select cases. Surgical revascularisation has been found safe and effective in children with progressive ischaemic symptoms. This family were counselling for increased perioperative AIS risk given previous report of high frequency preoperative TIA as a predictor [3].

The role of autoimmunity in moyamoya aetiology continues to be studied. Described higher prevalence of Graves' disease and T1D in some adult moyamoya cohorts would lend support to a link [4, 5]. In reported cases TD1 onset predates moyamoya with speculation that arteriopathy development is primed [6]. Although data on causation and natural history is scant this association presents real-life challenges to diagnosis and management. A delay in diagnosis and recognition of clinical recurrences may be anticipated given the overlap between neurologic symptoms of hypo- or hyperglycaemia and brain ischaemia. There is also the effect of serious TD1 related complications to consider. Habib reported a 9-year-old female with diabetic ketoacidosis, right-sided hemiplegia, periventricular white matter changes and left anterior circulation angiographic moyamoya. Fluid loss, blood hyperviscosity and hyperglycaemia-induced vasoconstriction were theorised to predispose cerebral ischaemia [7]. For surgical candidates, added to already scrupulous perioperative management of AIS risk, is the task of optimising glycaemia and vigilance around post-operative wound healing and infection. It is unknown whether moyamoya is accelerated by TD1 association and if good control has any bearing on this. Krebs et al. reported reduced adult-type common carotid intimal thickening in a 12-year-old poorly controlled TD1 following intensive diabetes treatment [8]. Concerning for this child is concurrent TD1, moyamoya and associated hypertension, all independent risk factors for AIS but also haemorrhagic stroke. Further modification of this by the addition of a statin is being considered but lacks specific evidence.

Headache in the presentation of moyamoya is reported in 47% of children [9], however its significance outside of acute stroke is poorly understood. Reported features include those of some primary headache disorders, most commonly migraine-like, but also tension and rarely cluster types [10, 11]. As a result, clinically differentiating moyamoya-related headache from more common aetiologies is made difficult. The International Classification of Headache Disorders 3rd Edition (ICHD-3) categorises headache attributable to moyamoya as secondary to genetic vasculopathy. Diagnostic criteria include recurrent headache in temporal relation to other features or diagnosis of moyamoya, which has significantly worsened with progressive disease or improved after revascularisation surgery [12]. This seems best applied to those with confirmed moyamoya in evaluating whether symptoms are likely related to disease or another cause. Deciding which children with new headache warrant brain imaging for moyamoya is challenging and needs to be balanced against potential procedural hazards of sedation or anaesthesia for scan. Recognising moyamoya risk factors may elude even the most astute clinician given the high prevalence of primary headache, rarity of moyamoya disease outside East Asia and syndrome association with numerous co-morbid conditions. As with other causes of secondary headache, the presence of focal or symptomatic neurology should contribute. Chiang et al. reviewed 8 adult and 3 paediatric cases of moyamoya-related headache and reported all to have other neurological signs or symptoms (e.g. paresis, seizures, dysarthria, ptosis) [11]. In our case, although the original question was likely one of a space occupying intracranial lesion, several headache 'red flags' (e.g. recent onset, persistence, early waking) and hypertension were present, prompting imaging and diagnosis. Postulated headache mechanisms include stimulation of intracranial nociceptors, cerebral hypoperfusion and hypertension [10, 11]. Yet targeting some of these for treatment may trigger further brain ischaemia (e.g. vasoconstrictor effects of triptans or calcitonin gene-related peptide antagonists) or interact with existing therapy (e.g. NSAIDs and aspirin). The prognostic significance of moyamoya associated headache also remains undefined. As Ganesan, it is unclear whether this indicates adequate collateral response (e.g. in the subset who have new onset headache post-revascularisation) or a still 'hungry', hypoxic brain [10].

Paediatric hypertension (BP $\geq$ 95th centile) is uncommon and usually a secondary phenomenon with renal (parenchymal or renovascular), cardiac and endocrine causes being prominent. Other than seizures and raised intracranial pressure, clinical approaches tend to consider the brain as target rather than cause. Treatment indications include marked hypertension with potential for clinical deterioration or impact on end organs (e.g. hypertensive encephalopathy, retinopathy or left ventricular hypertrophy). In such instances treatment at presentation has been recommended with a target BP of <90th centile in all hypertensive children [13]. This poses a significant management predicament. BP elevation is common in moyamoya but underappreciated. Whilst approximately 10% have coexisting renal artery stenosis, it is also a critical, central response to maintain brain perfusion in a dysregulated, 'pressure passive' circulation [10]. Reflex antihypertensive use in such scenarios may provoke AIS, as was likely in this case where amlodipine was commenced prior to knowledge of concurrent moyamoya. Yet left untreated severe hypertension creates significant cerebro- and cardiovascular risk, end organ damage and even mortality. It is therefore not possible to be prescriptive regarding BP treatment thresholds in moyamoya. This is a fine balance struck between neurologist and nephrologist who generally negotiate a target above which the child develops symptomatic cerebral hypoperfusion. Interestingly raised BP has been observed to reduce after surgical revascularisation, speculated the effect of offloaded cerebral circulation reliance [10]. Given this it may be reasonable to review antihypertensive requirement post-operatively in surgical patients.

Key Clinical Learning Points

- The full significance of headache in moyamoya is undetermined but has importance as a presenting symptom.
- T1D and moyamoya are associated. Neurologic manifestations of hypo- or hyperglycaemia may mask those of brain ischaemia, challenging management. Post-operative wound complications may be more predisposed.
- Where moyamoya-associated AIS is rapidly recurrent expedited revascularisation surgery to within the acute/subacute phase may be necessary. In such instances a higher than expected perioperative AIS risk should be discussed.
- T1D, moyamoya and related hypertension are independent cerebrovascular disease risks. Managing each individually is pragmatic but may result in their combined effect being overlooked.
- Elevated BP in moyamoya is often physiological to drive brain perfusion. Antihypertensive agents can precipitate AIS hence reflex use is discouraged. A target BP range providing thresholds for treatment should be agreed between neurology and nephrology teams.

Key Radiological Learning Points

- Consider brain imaging in a child with persistent headache and elevated blood pressure. Although rare underlying moyamoya is possible, particularly in the presence of risk factors.
- Moyamoya is an angiographic definition. Further correlation with clinical history and examination is required to determine aetiological factors and guide management.
- CCA flow rates are an indicator of cerebral perfusion. Slow flow emphasises the importance of systemic BP in maintaining brain perfusion.

References

1. Sigdel TK, Shoemaker LD, Chen R, Li L, Butte AJ, Sarwal MM, Steinberg GK. Immune response profiling identifies autoantibodies specific to Moyamoya patients. Orphanet J Rare Dis. 2013;8:45. https://doi.org/10.1186/1750-1172-8-45. PMID: 23518061; PMCID: PMC3648437.
2. Tho-Calvi SC, Thompson D, Saunders D, Agrawal S, Basu A, Chitre M, Chow G, Gibbon F, Hart A, Tallur KK, Kirkham F, Kneen R, McCullagh H, Mewasingh L, Vassallo G, Vijayakumar K, Wraige E, Yeo TH, Ganesan V, British Paediatric Neurology Association Moyamoya Study Group. Clinical features, course, and outcomes of a UK cohort of pediatric moyamoya. Neurology. 2018;90(9):e763–70. https://doi.org/10.1212/WNL.0000000000005026. PMID: 29483323.

3. Ng J, Thompson D, Lumley JP, Saunders DE, Ganesan V. Surgical revascularisation for childhood moyamoya. Childs Nerv Syst. 2012;28(7):1041–8. https://doi.org/10.1007/s00381-012-1743-7. Epub 2012 May 9. PMID: 22570164.
4. Bower RS, Mallory GW, Nwojo M, Kudva YC, Flemming KD, Meyer FB. Moyamoya disease in a primarily white, midwestern US population: increased prevalence of autoimmune disease. Stroke. 2013;44(7):1997–9. https://doi.org/10.1161/STROKEAHA.111.000307. Epub 2013 May 7. PMID: 23652271.
5. Chen JB, Liu Y, Zhou LX, Sun H, He M, You C. Prevalence of autoimmune disease in moyamoya disease patients in Western Chinese population. J Neurol Sci. 2015;351(1-2):184–6. https://doi.org/10.1016/j.jns.2015.02.037. Epub 2015 Feb 26. PMID: 25743224.
6. Hughes JW, Wyckoff JA, Hollander AS, Derdeyn CP, McGill JB. Moyamoya syndrome causing stroke in young women with type 1 diabetes. J Diabetes Complicat. 2016;30(8):1640–2. https://doi.org/10.1016/j.jdiacomp.2016.08.004. Epub 2016 Aug 12. PMID: 27592246; PMCID: PMC5050134.
7. Habib HS. Moyamoya disease presenting with ischemic stroke in association with diabetic ketoacidosis. J Pediatr Neurol. 2013;11:39–42.
8. Krebs A, Schmidt-Trucksäss A, Wagner J, Krebs K, Doerfer J, Schwab KO. Adult-like but regressive increase of intima-media thickness and roughness in a child with type 1 diabetes. Pediatr Diabetes. 2005;6(3):161–4. https://doi.org/10.1111/j.1399-543X.2005.00121.x. PMID: 16109073.
9. Lee S, Rivkin MJ, Kirton A, de Veber G, Elbers J, International Pediatric Stroke Study. Moyamoya disease in children: results from the international pediatric stroke study. J Child Neurol. 2017;32(11):924–9. https://doi.org/10.1177/0883073817718730. Epub 2017 Jul 17. PMID: 28715924.
10. Ganesan V. Moyamoya disease: to cut or not to cut is not the only question. A paediatric neurologist's perspective. Dev Med Child Neurol. 2010;52:10–3. https://doi.org/10.1111/j.1469-8749.2009.03527.x.
11. Chiang CC, Shahid AH, Harriott AM, Tietjen GE, Savastano LE, Klaas JP, Lanzino G. Evaluation and treatment of headache associated with moyamoya disease - a narrative review. Cephalalgia. 2022;42(6):542–52. https://doi.org/10.1177/03331024211056250.
12. International Headache Society. The international classification of headache disorders. 3rd ed. (ICHD-3). Available from: https://ichd-3.org/6-headache-attributed-to-cranial-or-cervical-vascular-disorder/6-8-headache-attributed-to-genetic-vasculopathy/6-8-3-headache-attributed-to-another-genetic-vasculopathy/. Accessed 11 January 2022.
13. Singh C, Jones H, Copeman H, Sinha MD. Fifteen-minute consultation: the child with systemic arterial hypertension. Arch Dis Child Educ Pract Ed. 2017;102(1):2–7. https://doi.org/10.1136/archdischild-2014-306487. Epub 2016 Jul 29. PMID: 27473151.

Chapter 36
A Child Misspelling Post-Craniotomy

Anoushka Alwis and Vijeya Ganesan

Clinical History

A 9-year-old boy with known hereditary haemorrhagic telangiectasia (HHT) had an unruptured right frontal lobe arteriovenous malformation (AVM) detected on MRI brain screening. Cerebral catheter angiography (CCA) (Fig. 36.1) demonstrated a large nidal venous varix. There was no headache, seizures or neurological deficit. He had epistaxis but no respiratory symptoms. His mother had a pulmonary AVM (PAVM). His brother had a ruptured cerebral AVM (CAVM) resected and symptomatic PAVM embolised. Expert multidisciplinary team (MDT) opinion was for elective microsurgery with pre-operative embolisation to reduce lifelong bleeding risk. Post-embolisation intracranial haemorrhage required emergency clot evacuation, CAVM resection and external ventricular drain (EVD) placement. Four days later, during physical therapy and coincident with EVD challenge, left-body weakness was noted. In retrospect there had been transient memory impairment and misspelling of text messages. His mother thought he had had a stroke.

A. Alwis (✉)
Great Ormond Street Hospital for Children NHS Foundation Trust, London, UK
e-mail: anouskha.alwis@gosh.nhs.uk

V. Ganesan
UCL Great Ormond Street Institute of Child Health, London, UK
e-mail: v.ganesan@ucl.ac.uk

S. K. Gill et al. (eds.), *Stroke Medicine*,
https://doi.org/10.1007/978-3-031-58188-5_36

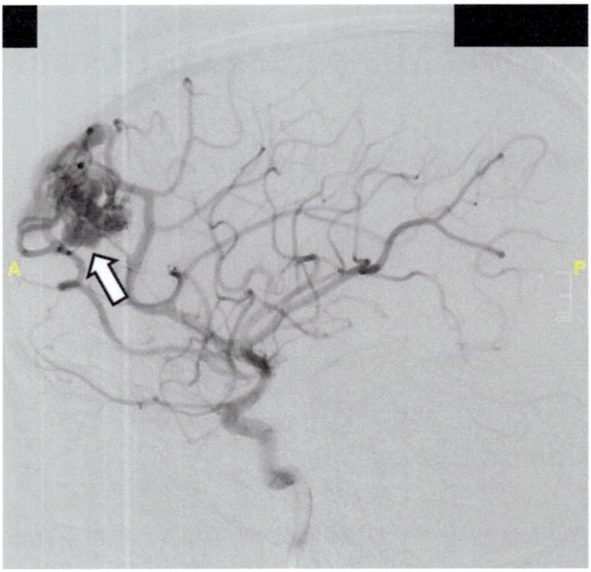

Fig. 36.1 Cerebral catheter angiogram (right internal carotid artery injection, lateral projection) showing right medial frontal lobe AVM involving the superior frontal gyrus. Arterial feeders are from the ipsilateral anterior cerebral artery. Venous drainage is predominantly antegrade through the superior sagittal sinus. A large venous varix (*arrow*) can be seen within the inferior portion of the 2 cm nidus

Examination

His GCS was 15. Temperature, blood pressure, heart and respiratory rate were normal. Oxygen saturations were 100% in air, other than for one episode of desaturation (90–92%) in the prior 48 h. There was mild lower left facial weakness. He leant left in sitting, was ataxic and had difficulty stepping with his left leg. There was transient left upper limb hypertonia and left-hand fisting. Cranial nerve examination, deep tendon reflexes and sensation were normal. Cardiorespiratory examination was unremarkable. Paediatric National Institutes of Health Stroke Scale (PedNIHSS) was 4.

Investigations

A CT brain scan for worsening headache at 48 h confirmed no EVD catheter displacement, hydrocephalous or acute intracranial haemorrhage (ICH). There were however new right middle cerebral artery (MCA) territory infarcts with mass effect and a hyperdense right MCA. MRI brain scan demonstrated acute infarction in right frontotemporal and parietal regions as well as corpus striatum. There were also bi-hemispheric white matter deep watershed infarcts. Head and neck MR angiography confirmed focal proximal right MCA narrowing; other craniocervical vessels were unremarkable with no dissection (Fig. 36.2). Given background HHT, paradoxical embolism via an asymptomatic PAVM was suspected.

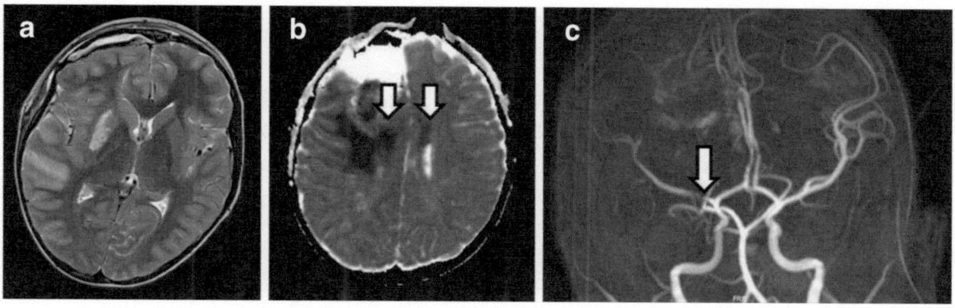

Fig. 36.2 MRI brain (**a**) axial T2—weighted, (**b**) apparent diffusion coefficient map, and (**c**) coronal intracranial angiogram images 72 h post-ictus. Post-craniotomy right frontal changes are evident with midline shift to the left in all three images. Acute infarction is seen in right basal ganglia, frontotemporal and parietal regions as high signal (**a**) plus bilaterally in (**b**) as white matter diffusion restriction in a deep watershed distribution (*arrows*). (**c**) shows significant focal right proximal M1 MCA narrowing (*arrow*) with non-visualisation of flow-related signal distally

Fig. 36.3 Pulmonary angiogram (main pulmonary artery injection) showing an AVM in the posterior medial segment of the right lung (*arrow*)

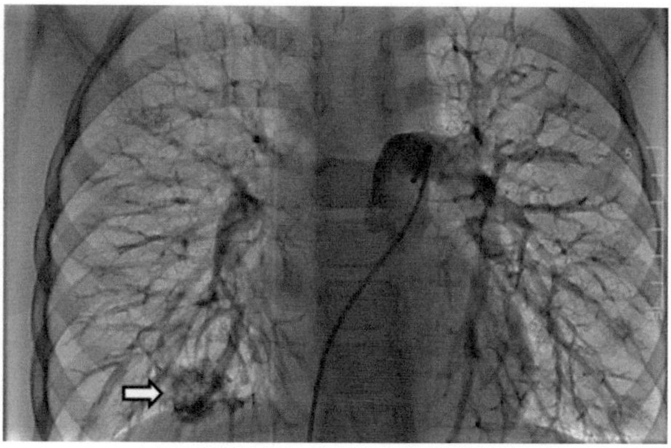

Aspirin was commenced in accordance with the Royal College of Paediatrics and Child Health (RCPCH) 2017 *Stroke in childhood* guidelines. Contrast CT chest confirmed a right lower lobe PAVM with concordant transthoracic contrast echocardiogram (TTCE) findings (early pulmonary venous return predominantly via right-sided veins). Following EVD removal and on recommendation by haematologists he was switched to low molecular weight heparin. Pulmonary angiography demonstrated a 5.6 mm main feeding artery to a saccular network of arterioles (Fig. 36.3). A week post-ictus he underwent PAVM embolisation by interventional cardiologists to prevent stroke recurrence. A thromboembolic source was not found following venous Doppler ultrasound of the inferior vena cava, iliac and lower limb deep veins. Anticoagulation maintenance with warfarin was opted for as most acceptable to him and his parents.

He made a good recovery with discharge home after 18-days, including inpatient neurorehabilitation. With prompting he could catch a ball and shoot a football. Graded school return was arranged with breaks for fatigue and poor concentration.

The family accessed psychological support, in particular for prognostic uncertainty and procedure-related anxiety.

A 4-month MRI brain scan showed no new infarcts or haemorrhage and contrast CT chest showed no reperfusion of the embolised PAVM or new arteriovenous communications. Warfarin was stepped down to aspirin with no clinical recurrence. Planned surveillance includes post-surgical CCA, lung function testing and ongoing review within a specialist HHT service.

Discussion

Hereditary Haemorrhagic Telangiectasia (HHT) is an autosomal dominant disorder of vascular malformations with an approximate prevalence of 1 in 5000 worldwide [1]. Iron deficiency anaemia (IDA) from chronic bleeding and major organ impairment, haemorrhage or other complications from shunting visceral AVMs cause significant morbidity and mortality. Diagnosis is by presence of three or more Curaçao criteria: spontaneous and recurrent epistaxis; multiple telangiectases (lips, oral cavity, fingers or nose); visceral lesions (gastrointestinal telangiectasia, pulmonary, hepatic, cerebral or spinal AVMs); and family history of a first degree relative with HHT [1]. 97% of those with definite clinical HHT have causative gene mutations in the transforming growth factor beta signalling pathway [1, 2]. Whilst not absolute, PAVMs and CAVMs; hepatic AVMs; and juvenile polyposis are reported prominent in endoglin (ENG), activin receptor-like kinase-1 (ACVRL1) and Mothers against decapentaplegic homolog 4 (SMAD4) mutations respectively [1, 3, 4]. Treatment is symptomatic and includes iron supplementation, systemic antiangiogenic agents (e.g. bevacizumab [1]) and AVM endovascular or surgical intervention where indicated.

Central to HHT management is securing the diagnosis with consciousness of often clinically silent visceral features [5]. This case demonstrates that despite diagnosis management may remain a challenge. Multi-organ involvement presents to numerous medical and surgical specialties and the implications of systemic aspects may be under appreciated. The age-dependent expression of manifest clinical sequelae (typically epistaxis in childhood; cutaneous telangiectases and gastrointestinal bleeding in adulthood) adds further complexity hence diagnostic criteria are not fully sensitive in children [1]. Yet visceral involvement may present at any age in view of likely congenital CAVMs [2] and PAVMs described in newborns [3].

CAVMs underlie 40–50% of haemorrhagic stroke (HS) in children [6]. The exact prevalence of HHT-associated CAVM in children is unknown; around 10% is documented in adults [1, 7]. Pre-diagnosis and screening presentations have been reported, including with neonatal ICH [8]. Secondary prevention by endovascular, radiosurgical, surgical or combined treatment modalities in appropriately selected patients can be effective with a favourable safety profile. Management aims to balance bleeding against treatment risk, including ICH, stroke, and death. Estimating natural history bleeding risk is challenging given heterogeneity of studies and lack of statistical data [6]. Higher risk in ruptured CAVMs is well described and treatment usually recommended. Treatment of unruptured, asymptomatic CAVMs is complex and requires specialist MDT evaluation including lesion subtype, size, location and angioarchitecture. Arteriovenous fistulas (AVFs) and nidal AVMs with arterial phase aneurysms, varicosities and venous stenoses carry increased HS risk [6]. RCPCH stroke guidelines recommend considering unruptured AVM treatment in children based on a higher cumulative rupture risk due to greater expected longevity.

Abnormally connected pulmonary arteries and veins in PAVMs cause right-to-left shunting and paradoxical embolic arterial ischaemic stroke (AIS). They are hence a target for stroke prevention. The majority of PAVMs are HHT-related and approximately 50% of adults with HHT have CT-detectable PAVMs [3]. Lack of paediatric PAVM data has led to non-inclusion in previous good practice guidance. Recommendations in the first *International Guidelines for the Diagnosis and Management of Hereditary Haemorrhagic Telangiectasia* (2009) were limited, suggesting PAVM screening in children on a case-by-case basis due to lack of evidence regarding best modality. Screening strategies vary and current practice includes only screening symptomatic children (e.g. dyspnoea, exercise intolerance, faltering growth, cyanosis, clubbing or previous complication) as these indicate treatment and there is risk of reperfusion and/or new PAVM development despite intervention. Requirement for intravenous access and sedation for more invasive screening (i.e. TTCE, contrast chest CT) especially in the young, presents further challenges. Endovascular treatment is reported safe in children, but not without complications. These include pleuritic chest pain, paradoxical device embolisation and device misplacement [9].

Recent larger paediatric case series document PAVM prevalence akin to adults: 22% (by clinical evaluation, oximetry for orthodeoxia, and CXR) [4], and 59% (by TTCE and/or contrast chest CT) [10]. Serious complications in untreated children have been reported. Faughnan et al. reported pre-treatment cyanosis in 25 (60%), stroke or cerebral abscess in 8 (19%) and haemoptysis in 3 (7%) of 42 children who underwent transcatheter embolotherapy [9]. Symptoms as an indicator of PAVM may also be problematic. Gefen at al. retrospectively reviewed 61 children with HHT and known PAVMs and found 34 (56%) asymptomatic. Of 27 with symptoms, exercise intolerance was reported in 16 (59%), but not consistently recognised or ascribed to alternate causes [11]. PAVMs may develop or small ones may enlarge throughout childhood, presenting further challenges to screening and intervention times. Mowers et al. retrospectively reviewed 129 children with HHT over 14 years. 76 (59%) had PAVMs; 67 detected on initial screening and a further 9 within a year of negative screening. 38 (50%) had or developed lesions large enough to embolized, of these 23 (60%) were asymptomatic and 8 (21%) had repeat intervention [10].

The September 2020 iteration of the international guidelines prioritised paediatric care. Updated recommendations included PAVM screening (CXR and oximetry or TTCE) in asymptomatic children at diagnosis and 5-year intervals. Chest CT was reserved as confirmatory when screening tests were positive. Treatment was advised for large PAVMs and those causing hypoxia to avoid serious complications. These would require follow-up per centre protocol for PAVM reperfusion and growth or development of new lesions. Treatment of asymptomatic PAVMs was recommended on a case-by-case basis. Extra vigilance to avoid intravenous (IV) air was advised during anaesthesia and IV access.

Hyperacute AIS therapy in HHT is undefined, indeed the British Thoracic Society have stated the safety of thrombolysis in PAVM-related AIS not established [3]. However, adult data suggest that with the majority of HHT patients with PAVMs diagnosed following associated AIS, likely a number have already received thrombolysis [12]. Topiwala et al. retrospectively reviewed >4 million USA-wide AIS admissions from 2005 to 2014 and reported equal rates of IV thrombolytics in non-PAVM and PAVM groups where PAVM and HHT prevalence were 822 (0.02%) and 106 (12.9%) respectively [13]. Whilst HHT is not an absolute preclusion, a number of thrombolysis contraindications may have relevance, including previous ICH, history of AVM and recent gastrointestinal bleeding [6]. Epistaxis and HHT family history are not documented contraindications but may be useful screening particularly in children where these may be the only diagnostic features. Mechanical thrombectomy may be a consideration in proven large vessel obstruction but would require rapid MDT discussion and careful counselling. Secondary prevention with anti-platelets and anticoagulation can be well tolerated, having considered individualised bleeding risk. Anticoagulants are higher risk and direct agents (e.g. rivaroxaban) are generally not advised. Combination or dual anti-antiplatelet therapy is also not recommended, but if unavoidable should be stepped down as soon as possible [1].

Adult data reports increased thrombotic risk in HHT, particularly in relation to IDA and factor VIII elevation. IDA is common in adults secondary to chronic epistaxis and/or gastrointestinal bleeding [14]. It is also a common childhood nutritional problem and an independent risk factor for paediatric AIS, hence worth considering as modifiable. A source of embolism was not found in this case, however combined procedural complications, major surgery, impaired mobility, IV access and transient mild anaemia may have favoured venous air or thromboembolism. Post-operative thromboprophylaxis is generally not indicated pre-adolescence however this patient had Thrombo-Embolus Deterrent (TED) stockings post-embolotherapy.

Key Clinical Learning Points

- Peri-operative stroke in children is rare, but important to appreciate given potential sequels of prolonged hospitalisation, neurorehabilitation, new neurodisability or death. Targeting co-morbid risk factors in high-risk groups is key to prevention.
- Childhood stroke recognition is challenging. Co-morbid risk factors in this case were HHT and an asymptomatic PAVM. This child's post-operative presentation, including new focal neurological deficit attributable to the operated hemisphere, likely confounded diagnosis. Parents can be a useful indicator, as sole witnesses to the event they often suspect stroke.
- HHT is a multi-system vascular disorder with clinically silent CAVMs predisposing to HS through rupture and PAVMS associated with paradoxical embolic AIS.
- Secondary prevention of PAVM-associated AIS is challenged by screening only symptomatic children as a proportion of clinically significant PAVMs are asymptomatic.
- Use of recently updated, best consensus guidelines alongside expert MDT and close, cross-speciality working is key to minimising serious disease and treatment risks.

Key Radiological Learning Points

- Neuroradiological findings in HHT include cerebral nidus-type AVM, AVF and capillary vascular malformations [1] or embolic infarction.
- In undifferentiated, new onset focal neurological deficit it is important to keep an open mind when interpreting imaging, particularly if anticipated findings are not confirmed e.g. new ICH or EVD catheter displacement in this case.
- A hyperdense MCA on CT brain represents intraluminal thrombus and is an early radiological feature of AIS.
- Bi-hemispheric infarcts of multiple arterial territories should raise suspicion of embolic AIS. In a child with known or possible HHT, PAVM is the primary diagnosis to exclude.

References

1. Faughnan ME, Mager JJ, Hetts SW, Palda VA, Lang-Robertson K, Buscarini E, Deslandres E, Kasthuri RS, Lausman A, Poetker D, Ratjen F, Chesnutt MS, Clancy M, Whitehead KJ, Al-Samkari H, Chakinala M, Conrad M, Cortes D, Crocione C, Darling J, de Gussem E, Derksen C, Dupuis-Girod S, Foy P, Geisthoff U, Gossage JR, Hammill A, Heimdal K, Henderson K, Iyer VN, Kjeldsen AD, Komiyama M, Korenblatt K, McDonald J, McMahon J, McWilliams J, Meek ME, Mei-Zahav M, Olitsky S, Palmer S, Pantalone R, Piccirillo JF, Plahn B, Porteous MEM, Post MC, Radovanovic I, Rochon PJ, Rodriguez-Lopez J, Sabba C, Serra M, Shovlin C, Sprecher D, White AJ, Winship I, Zarrabeitia R. Second international guidelines for the diagnosis and management of hereditary hemorrhagic telangiectasia. Ann Intern Med. 2020;173(12):989–1001. https://doi.org/10.7326/M20-1443. Epub 2020 Sep 8. PMID: 32894695.
2. McDonald J, Bayrak-Toydemir P, DeMille D, Wooderchak-Donahue W, Whitehead K. Curaçao diagnostic criteria for hereditary hemorrhagic telangiectasia is highly predictive of a pathogenic variant in ENG or ACVRL1 (HHT1 and HHT2). Genet Med. 2020;22(7):1201–5. https://doi.org/10.1038/s41436-020-0775-8. Epub 2020 Apr 17. PMID: 32300199.
3. Shovlin CL, Condliffe R, Donaldson JW, Kiely DG, Wort SJ, British Thoracic Society. British Thoracic Society clinical statement on pulmonary arteriovenous malformations. Thorax. 2017;72(12):1154–63. https://doi.org/10.1136/thoraxjnl-2017-210764. PMID: 29141890.
4. Hosman AE, de Gussem EM, Balemans WAF, et al. Screening children for pulmonary arteriovenous malformations: evaluation of 18 years of experience. Pediatr Pulmonol. 2017;52:1206–11. https://doi.org/10.1002/ppul.23704.
5. Shovlin CL, Letarte M. Hereditary haemorrhagic telangiectasia and pulmonary arteriovenous malformations: issues in clinical management and review of pathogenic mechanisms. Thorax. 1999;54(8):714–29. https://doi.org/10.1136/thx.54.8.714. PMID: 10413726; PMCID: PMC1745557.
6. www.rcpch.ac.uk/stroke-guideline.
7. Eker OF, Boccardi E, Sure U, Patel MC, Alicante S, Alsafi A, Coote N, Droege F, Dupuis O, Fialla AD, Jones B, Kariholu U, Kjeldsen AD, Lefroy D, Lenato GM, Mager HJ, Manfredi G, Nielsen TH, Pagella F, Post MC, Rennie C, Sabbà C, Suppressa P, Toerring PM, Ugolini S, Buscarini E, Dupuis-Girod S, Shovlin CL. European Reference Network for Rare Vascular Diseases (VASCERN) position statement on cerebral screening in adults and children with hereditary haemorrhagic telangiectasia (HHT). Orphanet J Rare Dis. 2020;15(1):165. https://doi.org/10.1186/s13023-020-01386-9. PMID: 32600364; PMCID: PMC7322871.
8. Delaney HM, Rooks VJ, Wolfe SQ, Sawyer TL. Term neonate with intracranial hemorrhage and hereditary hemorrhagic telangiectasia: a case report and review of the literature. J Perinatol. 2012;32(8):642–4. https://doi.org/10.1038/jp.2011.146. PMID: 22842803.
9. Faughnan ME, Thabet A, Mei-Zahav M, Colombo M, Maclusky I, Hyland RH, Pugash RA, Chait P, Henderson KJ, White RI Jr. Pulmonary arteriovenous malformations in children: outcomes of transcatheter embolotherapy. J Pediatr. 2004;145(6):826–31. https://doi.org/10.1016/j.jpeds.2004.08.046. PMID: 15580209.
10. Mowers KL, Sekarski L, White AJ, Grady RM. Pulmonary arteriovenous malformations in children with hereditary hemorrhagic telangiectasia: a longitudinal study. Pulm Circ. 2018;8(3):2045894018786696. https://doi.org/10.1177/2045894018786696. Epub 2018 Jun 19. PMID: 29916764; PMCID: PMC6055266.
11. Gefen AM, White AJ. Asymptomatic pulmonary arteriovenous malformations in children with hereditary hemorrhagic telangiectasia. Pediatr Pulmonol. 2017;52(9):1194–7. https://doi.org/10.1002/ppul.23686. Epub 2017 Jun 13. PMID: 28608633.
12. Brinjikji W, Iyer VN, Sorenson T, Lanzino G. Cerebrovascular manifestations of hereditary hemorrhagic telangiectasia. Stroke. 2015;46(11):3329–37. https://doi.org/10.1161/STROKEAHA.115.010984. Epub 2015 Sep 24. Erratum in: Stroke. 2015 Nov;46(11):e247. PMID: 26405205.

13. Topiwala KK, Patel SD, Pervez M, Shovlin CL, Alberts MJ. Ischemic stroke in patients with pulmonary arteriovenous fistulas. Stroke. 2021;52(7):e311–5. https://doi.org/10.1161/STROKEAHA.120.032073. Epub 2021 Jun 4. PMID: 34082575.
14. Faughnan ME, Palda VA, Garcia-Tsao G, Geisthoff UW, McDonald J, Proctor DD, Spears J, Brown DH, Buscarini E, Chesnutt MS, Cottin V, Ganguly A, Gossage JR, Guttmacher AE, Hyland RH, Kennedy SJ, Korzenik J, Mager JJ, Ozanne AP, Piccirillo JF, Picus D, Plauchu H, Porteous ME, Pyeritz RE, Ross DA, Sabba C, Swanson K, Terry P, Wallace MC, Westermann CJ, White RI, Young LH, Zarrabeitia R, HHT Foundation International - Guidelines Working Group. International guidelines for the diagnosis and management of hereditary haemorrhagic telangiectasia. J Med Genet. 2011;48(2):73–87. https://doi.org/10.1136/jmg.2009.069013. Epub 2009 Jun 23. PMID: 19553198.

Chapter 37
A Child with Vesicles and Weakness

Anoushka Alwis and Vijeya Ganesan

Clinical History

A previously well 9-year-old boy presented to A&E with transient inability to use his left hand. Parents were reassured after a normal neurological examination. Three months later, whilst fasting during Ramadan, he developed frequent falls and persistent left-body weakness. MRI brain scan showed acute right motor cortex and parietal lobe infarction plus chronic ipsilateral frontotemporal, parietooccipital, lenticulostriate and pontine infarction (Figs. 37.1 and 37.2). MRA demonstrated severe stenosis of right terminal internal carotid (ICA), proximal middle cerebral (MCA) and basilar (BA) arteries plus bilateral posterior cerebral artery (PCA) narrowing. He was symptom free for a week on high-dose aspirin before re-presenting with progressive left-body weakness. A repeat MRI brain showed new right MCA territory frontal lobe infarcts (Fig. 37.2). Low molecular weight heparin (LMWH) was added and he was transferred for the assessment of moyamoya. There was history of chickenpox four months prior.

A. Alwis (✉)
Great Ormond Street Hospital for Children NHS Foundation Trust, London, UK
e-mail: anouskha.alwis@gosh.nhs.uk

V. Ganesan
UCL Great Ormond Street Institute of Child Health, London, UK
e-mail: v.ganesan@ucl.ac.uk

S. K. Gill et al. (eds.), *Stroke Medicine*,
https://doi.org/10.1007/978-3-031-58188-5_37

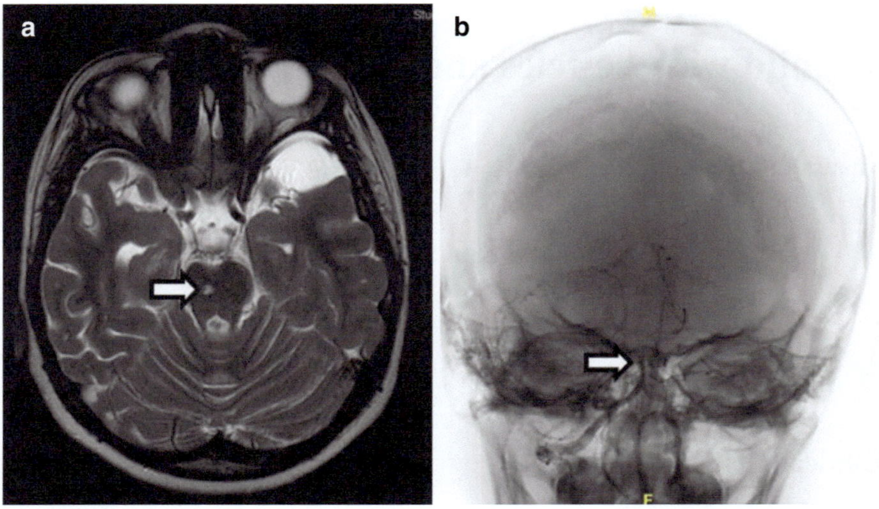

Fig. 37.1 (**a**) Presenting MRI brain axial T2—weighted image showing chronic pontine infarct (*arrow*). (**b**) Cerebral catheter angiogram (right vertebral artery injection, coronal projection) showing severe distal basilar artery stenosis with tip occlusion (*arrow*)

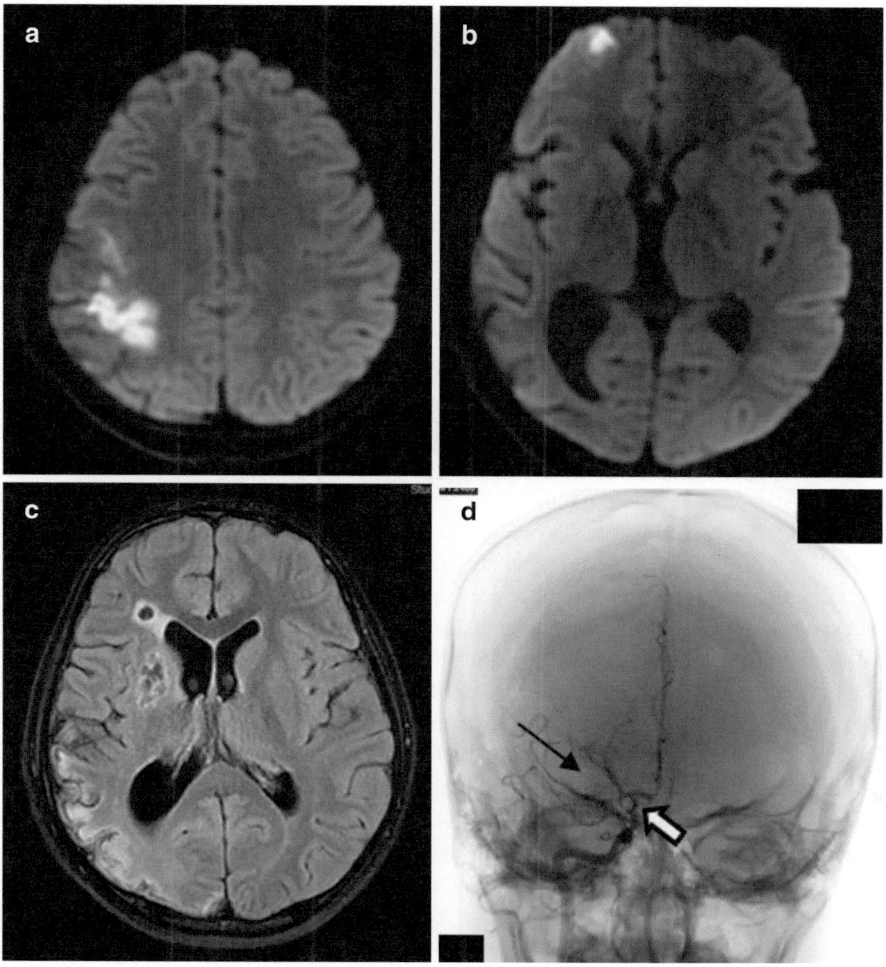

Fig. 37.2 MRI brain axial diffusion-weighted image showing acute right motor cortex and parietal lobe infarction at presentation (**a**) and new right middle frontal gyrus infarction a week later (**b**). Fluid attenuated inversion recovery image showing chronic right MCA territory infarction (**c**). Cerebral catheter angiogram (**d**) (right internal carotid artery injection, coronal projection) showing severe MCA M1 and M2 segment stenosis (*white arrow*) with ipsilateral lenticulostriate collateral vessels (*black arrow*)

Examination

His GCS was 15. Temperature, oxygen saturations, blood pressure, heart and respiratory rate were normal. There was left-sided weakness of the lower face, upper and lower limbs maximum in hand grip and foot eversion. There was associated left lower limb hyperreflexia, ankle clonus and an upgoing plantar. He had difficulties with left pincer grasp, rapid index finger tapping, left leg independent standing and foot taps. There was also left-sided disturbance of proprioception, light touch, pin-prick and temperature perception. Systemic examination was remarkable for a Body Mass Index (BMI) of 28.2 kg/m^2 (severe obesity). Paediatric National Institutes of Health Stroke Scale (PedNIHSS) was 4.

Investigations

In view of his progressive course securing a diagnosis became priority. Aspirin and LMWH were temporarily discontinued for cerebral catheter angiography (CA), lumbar puncture and peripheral central catheter insertion. Severe stenosis of right-sided supraclinoid ICA, anterior choroidal, posterior communicating artery origins and MCA M1 and proximal M2 segments was demonstrated. There were ipsilateral lenticulostriate and middle meningeal artery deep and superficial collaterals respectively (Fig. 37.2). There was also severe steno-occlusive disease of the distal BA and branches with MCA leptomeningeal collaterals (Fig. 37.1). The presence of collaterals suggested some chronicity. The left internal carotid circulation was normal. A working diagnosis of varicella zoster virus (VZV) vasculitis was made given temporal association with chickenpox. ESR was 50 mm/h. Following rheumatological evaluation including blood and urine markers, echocardiogram, ophthalmic assessment and renal CA, no evidence for an alternate vasculitic condition was found. Fabry disease screening and flexion/extension cervical spine X-rays for atlanto-axial instability were negative. CSF cell count and VZV PCR were also negative however VZV IgG index was positive, consistent with intrathecal VZV antibody synthesis.

He received neurorehabilitation and dietetic assessment during a 10-day admission and was treated with prolonged corticosteroids and aciclovir, rationalised by repeat CSF examination. Secondary stroke prevention with advice to remain well hydrated, daily aspirin and warfarin was continued. Aspirin was stopped after 2 months for mucosal bleeding. Three years later, on warfarin maintenance, there has been no clinical or radiological recurrence. Annual surveillance MRA shows persistent anterior and posterior circulation multi-segmental steno-occlusive arteriopathy with no progression. He has residual left-hand weakness and fatigue with self-care activities. An educational psychologist and school Special Educational Needs Coordinator have implemented extra time and memory aids to counter new difficulties with comprehension and recall. He is now morbidly obese (BMI 31.3 kg/m^2).

Discussion

There is increasing interest in the role of infection and related inflammation in paediatric arterial ischaemic stroke (AIS). It is an attractive hypothesis, potentially offering additional targets for stroke prevention and treatment. Well described mechanisms are septic emboli, cerebral vasculitis and cavernous sinus thrombosis caused by bacterial endocarditis, meningitis and orofacial infections respectively. There is also growing evidence for non-invasive childhood infections, including upper respiratory tract sources as triggers. The Vascular Effects of Infection in Paediatric Stroke Study (VIPS I) reported that infection in the week prior to ictus conferred a sixfold increase in AIS risk and serologic evidence of acute herpesviridae infections approximately doubled AIS probability. Most cases were asymptomatic, and findings were applicable across arteriopathic, cardioembolic and idiopathic subtypes [1–3]. Arteriopathy was prominent in previously well children and associated with a 21% one-year recurrence risk [4]. It has, however not been possible to establish a causal link through such epidemiological studies and current practice in screening for and treating infection in AIS varies.

Varicella ('chickenpox'), caused by herpesvirus VZV is a self-limiting illness of fever and cropping skin vesicles in most children. It is common, with three quarters of parents reporting a history in pre-school years [5]. Related AIS is rare, occurring in approximately 1 in 15,000 children but is an important association given antecedent infection in up to a third of cases [6, 7]. Affected children are usually under 10 years, otherwise well and have a history of varicella in the previous year. Following primary infection, the virus is hypothesised to access the trigeminal ganglion and spread transaxonally to the internal carotid circulation causing vessel wall infection and vascular remodelling [1, 6–9]. Presentation is generally within 4 months with hemiplegia secondary to proximal MCA stenosis and basal ganglia infarction [1, 6, 7]. This unilateral, unifocal entity is termed post-varicella arteriopathy (PVA), a subtype of focal cerebral arteriopathy which typically runs a monophasic course. Distinct to this is VZV vasculitis, a sequela of viral reactivation (herpes zoster) largely seen in adults causing diffuse symptoms, multifocal arteriopathy and recurrent multiple arterial territory brain infarction [1, 8, 9]. Overlap between these entities is possible given reports of PVA diagnosis revision to VZV vasculitis after clinical recurrence, progressive arteriopathy and CSF VZV marker positivity [9]. A degree of neurological impairment is seen in the majority with persistent hemiparesis and behavioural difficulties. Hemidystonia is reported in severe deficits and associated with poorer outcomes. Notable is a higher rate of recurrence than in non-varicella AIS, reflecting the underlying stenotic arteriopathy that persists in most. Less commonly this normalises or may progress [6, 7]. Given that there are no predictors for this, regular clinical and radiological surveillance with brain MRI and MRA is recommended.

This case reinforces the importance of interpreting radiological findings within a wider clinical context. Report of early 'moyamoya type vessels' raised suspicion of moyamoya, a typically bilateral, progressive and occlusive arteriopathy of terminal ICAs with 'puff of smoke' basal collaterals. Terminology such as 'moyamoya-like', 'moyamoya phenomenon' and 'quasi moyamoya disease' is often used to describe atypical, in particular unilateral cases with a similar vessel configuration and may confound the clinician. Moyamoya is an angiographic description and not specific for aetiology, hence careful clinical evaluation is required to delineate cause and treatment. This boy's unusual combination of severe, strictly unilateral ICA and distal BA stenotic disease with collaterals led to expanded investigation. Following diagnosis with VZV vasculitis his course stabilised with added anticoagulation, aciclovir, corticosteroids and intravenous hydration. Intravascular depletion and underperfusion of collateral circulation may have contributed to stroke recurrence given coincident fasting during Ramadan. Progression of major artery stenosis to angiographic moyamoya has been previously described after infection, including varicella. Ganesan et al. originally reported bilateral anterior and posterior circulation large vessel occlusion with collaterals in a 3-year-old boy with chronic right frontoparietal infarction within 6 months of varicella and subsequent transient ischaemic attacks [8]. In a further study of 24 children with VZV-related cerebral infarction, evolution of lenticulostriate collaterals were described in three, all of whom had clinical recurrence with major artery stenotic progression in two. The reason for a collateral response in some and not in the majority with similar proximal arterial disease was not clear [7, 8].

The management of VZV-associated AIS in childhood has a number of challenges. Delayed time to ictus (up to a year in some) and subclinical infection may impede recognition. A lack of confirmatory biomarkers is problematic for diagnosis and whilst positive serology may be supportive, inferring direct causality would be unreliable. It has been recommended that all children with AIS and recent varicella have infection screening to include CSF microscopy, VZV PCR and anti-VZV IgG [9]. This rarely occurs in practice and clinicians are frequently required to assess the risk-benefit of lumbar puncture and theoretical spinal haematoma versus further AIS with temporary anti-thrombotic cessation. CSF VZV detection by PCR is generally poor, particularly in PVA. In adult VZV vasculitis DNA is found in approximately a third but anti-VZV IgG positivity is in excess of 90% [9], thus offering increased sensitivity and hence a role for CSF examination in diagnosis.

Secondary prevention of VZV-related AIS is aspirin as first line with escalation to anticoagulation in recurrent disease. Those with recurrence, progressive arteriopathy, CSF VZV PCR or intrathecal antibody positivity usually receive additional aciclovir and corticosteroids for a prolonged period. There is no evidence to support a similar treatment paradigm in children with typical PVA [9]. Although chickenpox is a common childhood illness, primary prevention of related AIS is not straightforward. VIPS I reported routine childhood vaccination protective against AIS, speculated the effect of mitigating transient systemic inflammation by reducing infection exposure. The relative protection conferred by individual vaccines however was not determined [2, 9]. Whilst the USA and Australia routinely vaccinate children against varicella, this is not included in the UK schedule. The rate of severe varicella disease is low in children and an economic analysis by the Joint Committee on Vaccination and Immunisation deemed VZV vaccination not cost-effective in the short-to-medium term [5]. As highlighted by Askalan et al. recommending VZV vaccination to prevent AIS is likely to come under some scrutiny if the number needed to treat is 15,000 [6].

Finally, when thinking about long term risk factors for stroke and prevention in children, obesity (BMI >95th centile) is important to consider. That obesity increases stroke risk in adults is well documented and as obese children are more likely to become obese adults [10] it follows that this is carried forward. There is evidence that obese children have higher blood pressure, lipids and lipoproteins [11], increased risk of adult coronary artery disease [12] and young adult AIS [13]. Although normotensive with a normal blood glucose and lipid profile, this child was severely obese (BMI >99.6th centile) at presentation and remains so, despite attempted intervention, as he advances through adolescence. Childhood obesity is potentially modifiable, but challenged by under recognition, 'obesogenic' social environments and health inequalities [14]. Prevalence continues to rise in England with 40.9% of 10 to 11-year olds in England classified as overweight or obese in 2020/2021 [15]. Given it's 'modern-day epidemic' status, paediatric caregivers are likely to encounter children or young people with obesity and should use such opportunities to promote healthy weight.

Key Clinical Learning Points

- Considering urgent brain imaging in a child with a clear history of resolved acute neurological deficit is recommended to screen for stroke [16].
- Stuttering symptoms suggest underlying arteriopathy, a strong predictor of stroke recurrence. Inflammatory causes, including common infections are aetiologically prominent in children.
- History of varicella within a year of AIS should prompt assessment for VZV-arteriopathy and consideration of adjuvant aciclovir and corticosteroid treatment. Currently the most sensitive, available marker for diagnosis is a reduced serum/CSF anti-VZV IgG ratio [9].
- Maintaining intravascular volume is important in occlusive cerebral arteriopathy. This child's fasting state likely precipitated further strokes due to collateral circulation underperfusion.
- Childhood obesity is a modifiable stroke risk factor carried into adult life. Measures to promote healthy weight should be included in paediatric AIS care.

Key Radiological Learning Points

- VZV arteriopathy should be strongly suspected where there is MCA territory infarction and corresponding large vessel stenosis. Other or additional arterial and brain parenchymal involvement should prompt wider investigation, even with a history of recent varicella.
- Moyamoya is an angiographic description and has been reported post-varicella. The presence of collateral vessels indicates a compromised primary brain arterial circulation and suggests chronicity but does not specify cause.
- Factors determining progressive arteriopathy in VZV-related AIS are undetermined, hence periodic surveillance with brain MRI and MRA is an important aspect of management.

References

1. McCrea N, Fullerton HJ, Ganesan V. Genetic and environmental associations with pediatric cerebral arteriopathy. Stroke. 2019;50(2):257–65. https://doi.org/10.1161/STROKEAHA.118.020479. PMID: 30661495.
2. Fullerton HJ, Hills NK, Elkind MS, et al. Infection, vaccination, and childhood arterial ischemic stroke: results of the VIPS study. Neurology. 2015;85(17):1459–66. https://doi.org/10.1212/WNL.0000000000002065.
3. Elkind MS, Hills NK, Glaser CA, Lo WD, Amlie-Lefond C, Dlamini N, Kneen R, Hod EA, Wintermark M, de Veber GA, Fullerton HJ, VIPS Investigators. Herpesvirus infections and childhood arterial ischemic stroke: results of the VIPS study. Circulation. 2016;133(8):732–41. https://doi.org/10.1161/CIRCULATIONAHA.115.018595. Epub 2016 Jan 26. PMID: 26813104; PMCID: PMC4766042.
4. University of California San Francisco. Vascular effects of Infection in Pediatric Stroke (VIPS) Study II. Available from: https://pediatricstroke.ucsf.edu/vascular-effects-infection-pediatric-stroke-vips-study-ii. Accessed 29 December 2021.
5. Amirthalingam G, Ramsay M. Should the UK introduce a universal childhood varicella vaccination programme? Arch Dis Child. 2016;101:2–3.
6. Askalan R, Laughlin S, Mayank S, Chan A, MacGregor D, Andrew M, Curtis R, Meaney B, de Veber G. Chickenpox and stroke in childhood: a study of frequency and causation. Stroke. 2001;32(6):1257–62. https://doi.org/10.1161/01.str.32.6.1257. PMID: 11387484.
7. Miravet E, Danchaivijitr N, Basu H, Saunders DE, Ganesan V. Clinical and radiological features of childhood cerebral infarction following varicella zoster virus infection. Dev Med Child Neurol. 2007;49(6):417–22. https://doi.org/10.1111/j.1469-8749.2007.00417.x. PMID: 17518925.
8. Ganesan V, Kirkham FJ. Mechanisms of ischaemic stroke after chickenpox. Arch Dis Child. 1997;76(6):522–5. https://doi.org/10.1136/adc.76.6.522. PMID: 9245851; PMCID: PMC1717219.
9. Moraitis E, Ganesan V. Childhood infections and trauma as risk factors for stroke. Curr Cardiol Rep. 2014;16(9):527. https://doi.org/10.1007/s11886-014-0527-y.
10. Gov UK. Childhood obesity: applying all our health. 2020. Available from: https://www.gov.uk/government/publications/childhood-obesity-applying-all-our-health/childhood-obesity-applying-all-our-health. Accessed 29 December 2021.
11. Ilić M, Jerkan M. P56 obesity and accompanying risk factors important for the onset of aeroscellosis. Arch Dis Child. 2019;104:A178.
12. Nadeau KJ, Maahs DM, Daniels SR, Eckel RH. Childhood obesity and cardiovascular disease: links and prevention strategies. Nat Rev Cardiol. 2011;8(9):513–25. https://doi.org/10.1038/nrcardio.2011.86.
13. Gjaerde LK, Gamborg M, Ängquist L, et al. Association of childhood body mass index and change in body mass index with first adult ischemic stroke. JAMA Neurol. 2017;74(11):1312–8. https://doi.org/10.1001/jamaneurol.2017.1627. PMID: 28828465; PMCID: PMC5710582.
14. Gluckman P, Nishtar S, Armstrong T. Ending childhood obesity: a multidimensional challenge. Lancet. 2015;385(9973):1048–50. https://doi.org/10.1016/S0140-6736(15)60509-8. PMID: 25797547.
15. Population Health Team, NHS Digital. National child measurement programme, England 2020/21 School Year. Available from: https://digital.nhs.uk/data-and-information/publications/statistical/national-child-measurement-programme/2020-21-school-year. Accessed 29 December 2021.
16. The Royal College of Paediatrics and Child Health. Stroke in childhood - clinical guideline for diagnosis, management and rehabilitation. 2017. Available from: https://www.rcpch.ac.uk/resources/stroke-in-childhood-clinical-guideline. Accessed 29 December 2021.

Index

S. K. Gill et al. (eds.), *Stroke Medicine*,
https://doi.org/10.1007/978-3-031-58188-5

L

M

N

O

P

MIX
Papier aus verantwortungsvollen Quellen
Paper from responsible sources
FSC® C105338

If you have any concerns about our products,
you can contact us on
ProductSafety@springernature.com

In case Publisher is established outside the EU,
the EU authorized representative is:
Springer Nature Customer Service Center GmbH
Europaplatz 3, 69115 Heidelberg, Germany

Printed by Libri Plureos GmbH
in Hamburg, Germany